RECENT ADVANCES IN

Surgery

RECENT ADVANCES IN SURGERY

Contents of Number 17
Edited by: C. D. Johnson I. Taylor,

ISBN 0443 050163

You can place your order by contacting your local medical bookseller or the Sales Promotion Department, Churchill Livingstone, Robert Stevenson House, 1–3 Baxter's Place, Leith Walk, Edinburgh EH1 3AF, UK

Tel: (0131) 556 2424; Fax: (0131) 558 1278

Look out for *Recent Advances in Surgery* 19 in April 1996.
See page 252 for proposed list of contents.

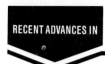
RECENT ADVANCES IN

Surgery

Edited by

I. Taylor MD ChM FRCS

Professor and Head, Department of Surgery,
University College London,
London, UK

C. D. Johnson MChir FRCS
Senior Lecturer in Surgery,
University of Southampton,
Southampton, UK

NUMBER EIGHTEEN

CHURCHILL LIVINGSTONE
EDINBURGH HONG KONG LONDON MADRID MELBOURNE NEW YORK
AND TOKYO 1995

CHURCHILL LIVINGSTONE
Medical Division of Pearson Professional Limited

Distributed in the United States of America by
Churchill Livingstone Inc., 650 Avenue of the Americas, New
York, N. Y. 10011, and by associated companies, branches and
representatives throughout the world.

First published 1995

ISBN 0 443 051321
ISSN 0143-8295

British Library Cataloguing in Publication Data
A catalogue record for this book is available from the British
Library

Library of Congress Cataloging in Publication Data
is available

The
publisher's
policy is to use
**paper manufactured
from sustainable forests**

Produced by Longman Singapore Publishers Pte Ltd
Printed in Singapore

Contents

Preface

In this volume we have continued with a similar format to that used in previous editions. We are conscious of the need to provide up-to-date reviews on topics of general interest as well as providing our readers with information on advances relating to modern surgical technology and to developments in the basic sciences which relate to surgical practice.

The specific topics of general interest which are covered include; modern hernia management (Kingsnorth), the critically ischaemic limb (Tennant and Ruckley), screening for colorectal cancer (Bennett and Hardcastle), parathyroid surgery (Goode), penetrating injuries to the chest (Ashraf and Grötte) and the management of advanced breast cancer (Fentiman). All surgeons are becoming increasingly aware of the sophisticated technology which is now available for therapy as well as diagnosis. We have included in this category important aspects on laser surgery (Evrard), non biliary aspects of laparoscopic surgery (Tate) and the non surgical management of oesophageal cancer (Robertson). Surgeons must also maintain a familiarity with the basic scientific principles involved in disease management; accordingly chapters relating to monoclonal antibodies in oncology (Yiu) and the pathophysiology underlying pancreatitis (Johnson) are extensively covered.

Finally broad overviews of recent advances in general surgery (Taylor) and paediatric surgery (Wheeler) are included to provide our readers with well referenced highlights from publications.

We hope that our readers, whether trainees or established consultants, will find this volume both enjoyable and educationally fulfilling. We are most grateful, once again, to our contributors for providing prompt and comprehensive reviews.

London   I. T.
Southampton 1995   C. D. J.

Contributors

Saeed Ashraf, MB BS, FRCS
Senior Registrar, Department of Cardiothoracic Surgery
Killingbeck Hospital, Leeds, UK

David H. Bennett, BSC, MB BS, FRCS
Research Fellow, Department of Surgery, University Hospital,
Nottingham, UK

Serge Evrard, MD, PhD
Professor of Surgery, Hopital Civil, Clinique Chirugicale A, Strasbourg,
France

Ian S. Fentiman, MD, FRCS
Consultant Surgeon, ICRF Clinical Oncology Unit, Guy's Hospital,
London, UK

Anthony W. Goode, MD, FRCS
Assistant Director, Professor of Endocrine and Metabolic Surgery, Royal
London Hospital, London, UK

Geir J. Grötte, MB BS, FRCS
Consultant Cardiothoracic Surgeon and Clinical Manager, Cardiothoracic
Unit, Manchester Royal Infirmary, Manchester, UK

J. D. Hardcastle, MChir, FRCS, FRCP
Professor of Surgery, Department of Surgery University Hosptial
Nottingham, UK

Andrew N. Kingsnorth, BSc (Hons), MB BS, MS, FRCS,
Senior Lecturer in Surgery, Department of Surgery, University of
Liverpool, Liverpool, UK

Jacques Marescaux,
Professor and Chairman of Digestive and Endocrine Surgery, Hospital
Civil, Strasbourg, France

Anthony R. Mundy, MS, FRCS, FRCP
Professor and Director of Urology, University College London Medical
School, Institute of Urology and Nephrology, London, UK

Charles S. Robertson, MB BS, DM, FRCS
Consultant in General Surgery and Surgical Gastroenterology, Worcester
Royal Infirmary, Worcester, UK

C. Vaughan Ruckley, MB, ChM, FRCS, FRCP
Consultant Surgeon and Professor of Vascular Surgery, Vascular Surgery
Unit, Edinburgh Royal Infirmary Edinburgh, UK

J. J. T. Tate, MS, FRCS,
Consultant Surgeon, Royal United Free Hospital, Bath, UK

William G. Tennant, BSc, MBChB, MD, FRCS
Senior Registrar in Vascular Surgery, Departement of Vascular Surgery,
Eastern General Hospital, Edinburgh, UK

Robert Wheeler, MS, FRCS,
Senior Registrar in Paediatric Urology, The Hospitals for Sick Children,
Great Ormond Street, London, UK

C. Y. Yiu, BSc, MS, FRCS,
Senior Lecturer and Consultant Surgeon, Department of Surgery,
Whittington Hospital, London, UK

1

Pathogenesis of pancreatitis

C. D. Johnson

Acute pancreatitis is a common surgical emergency, with presentation varying from a mild self-limiting attack of abdominal pain, to severe systemic upset and eventual death as a consequence of pancreatic necrosis There is a wide variety of causes of acute pancreatitis, which, once established, seems to follow the same pattern irrespective of the cause. Chronic pancreatitis presents with abdominal pain, either unremitting or episodic, and may be characterized by attacks of acute pancreatitis. Chronic pancreatitis is classified according to its various causes although, with the exception of obstructive pancreatitis, the clinical pattern, physiological disturbances and histological changes are very similar in different types. While potentially helpful in planning management, classification by causes does not help us to understand the mechanisms involved in the pathogenesis of pancreatic inflammation and does not explain how these two disease processes may develop.

This review will focus on experimental evidence and clinical information which illuminates our understanding of the pathogenesis of acute pancreatitis and chronic pancreatitis. It will be seen that there are common features which link the two diseases. While this analysis points to avenues for exploration to improve therapy, it has to be admitted that the mainstay of treatment and prevention at present is the identification and removal of the precipitating cause.

ACUTE PANCREATITIS

In most centres in the UK gallstones account for well over half the cases of acute pancreatitis and alcohol accounts for about one fifth to one quarter (Corfield et al 1985, Thomson et al 1987). A long list of drugs has been implicated in sporadic cases of acute pancreatitis, and a wide variety of infections may also precipitate an attack. Other causes are listed in Table 1.1. Hypercalcaemia is a doubtful cause of acute pancreatitis as in most recent series patients often have some other cause of acute pancreatitis (Sitges-Serra et al 1988), and the incidences of acute pancreatititis in patients with hypercalcaemia and of hypercalcaemia in acute pancreatitis do not exceed those seen in the general population.

Table 1.1   Causes of acute pancreatitis

Gallstones

Alcohol

Infection
  Mumps virus
  Coxsackie B virus
  ECHO virus
  Mycoplasma pneumoniae
  Q fever*

Postoperative
  ERCP (endoscopic retrograde cholangiopancreatography)
  Biliary surgery
  Cardiac bypass

Drugs
  Azathioprine
  Thiazides
  Oestrogens
  Frusemide
  Sulphonamides
  Valproate
  Corticosteroids
  L-Asparaginase
  Ethacrynic acid
  Phenformin
  (+ many other possibles)

Metabolic
  Hypertriglyceridaemia
  (Hypercalcaemia)[†]
  (Pregnancy)[†]
  Hereditary
  Duct obstruction
  Ischaemic
    Hypotension
    Hypothermia

Compiled from Clemens & Cameron (1989) and Lankisch (1988).
*Personal observation.
[†]The association of acute pancreatitis with hypercalcaemia and with pregnancy has not been supported by recent studies (Johnson 1991).

Mechanisms of acinar cell damage

The causes of acute pancreatitis can be categorized as either causing duct obstruction or producing cellular injury by a toxic effect. In some cases there may be both mechanisms at work; for example, gallstones obstruct the pancreatic duct at the ampulla, and may allow reflux of bile up the pancreatic duct. Although in earlier experiments injection pressures were used which have dubious physiological significance, Armstrong et al (1985) demonstrated that injection of infected bile at low pressures caused irreversible duct disruption, so it seems likely that, if bile reflux occurs, it will be harmful to duct and acinar cell membranes.

Steer et al (1984) investigated diet-induced pancreatitis and hyper-stimulation pancreatitis in experimental animals. They found a severe disturbance of the normal process of zymogen granule maturation and transport through the cell to the apical membrane (Fig. 1.1). In these experiments co-localization of digestive and lysosomal enzymes occurs within

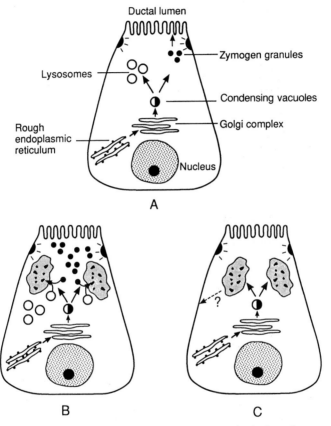

Fig. 1.1 **A** Pancreatic digestive and lysosomal enzymes are synthesized on ribosomes in the rough endoplasmic reticulum from where they are transported to the Golgi complex. Molecular sorting occurs in the Golgi complex and condensing vacuoles are formed which mature into zymogen granules that are ultimately discharged at the apical surface of the cell in response to secretagogue stimulation. Lysosomal enzymes are separated from digestive enzymes during condensing vacuole maturation, forming lysosomes. **B** In diet-induced pancreatitis, the discharge of zymogen granules is blocked, leading to their accumulation within the acinar cell. Subsequently they fuse with lysosomes, producing large vacuoles containing both pancreatic digestive enzymes and lysosomal enzymes, which are capable of activating trypsinogen. Digestive enzyme activation leads to acinar cell necrosis and pancreatitis. **C** In hyperstimulation pancreatitis there is interference with the process of condensing vacuole maturation leading to the formation of large vacuoles containing both digestive and lysosomal enzymes. Alternatively, zymogen granules and the large vacuoles may be discharged at the basolateral border of the cell, giving rise to interstitial oedema and pancreatitis. (Modified from Steer et al 1984 and reproduced with permission from Johnson & Imrie 1991.)

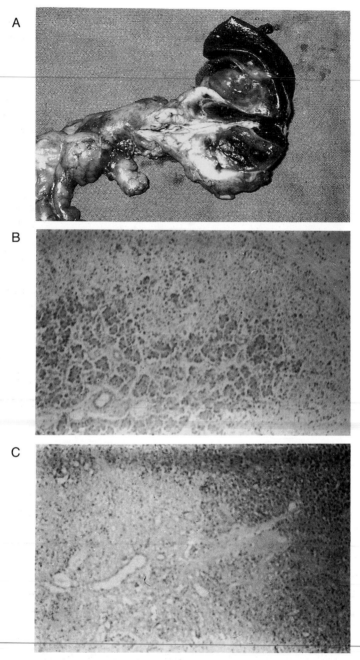

Fig. 1.2   Experimental pancreatitis produced by duct injection of bile throughout the whole pancreas, with subsequent devascularization of the pancreatic tail. **A** Macroscopic appearances at 48 h. There is oedema of the pancreatic head and necrosis of the pancreatic tail. **B** Oedematous pancreatitis in the pancreatic head. There is centrilobular necrosis and interstitial oedema. A lobular duct is seen at the bottom left. × 75. **C** Extensive perilobular necrosis and inflammatory infiltrate in the pancreatic tail with preservation of centrilobular acini. A lobular duct is seen on the left. × 75. In animals examined 1 week after induction of pancreatitis, the changes in the head resolved completely whereas the necrotic changes affecting the tail persisted.

the cells. This allows activation of digestive enzymes by cathepsin B. Steer's group has also demonstrated similar findings in obstructive pancreatitis. It seems that whatever causes injury to the cell, the mechanism by which damage occurs is the same.

Various models have demonstrated that acute pancreatitis can be made more severe, with haemorrhage and necrosis, by the addition of a period of ischaemia (Spormann et al 1989, Klar et al 1990). Our own studies in the pig have shown that retrograde bile injection alone causes transient oedematous pancreatitis with minimal centrilobular necrosis, which resolves after 1 week, but that the addition of devascularization with consequent ischaemia leads to extensive perilobular and panlobular necrosis (Fig 1.2). The changes seen in the ischaemic tissue resemble the changes seen in severe necrotizing pancreatitis (Foulis, 1980). A mechanism for the development of ischaemia in severe acute pancreatitis was proposed in the 1950s by Thal (1954). Papp et al (1966) confirmed an early reduction in capillary blood flow in experimental pancreatitis. This mechanism has been confirmed by elegant work from Dublin, using scanning electron microscopy and microvascular casting. Kelly et al (1989) showed damage to the microcirculation after retrograde bile injection, which affected not only the pancreas but other organs also. McEntee et al (1989) repeated these findings in caerulein infusion pancreatitis (Fig. 1.3).

Other mechanisms by which ischaemia added to oedematous experimental pancreatitis can convert it to haemorrhagic necrotic pancreatitis include haemorrhagic shock (Kyogoku et al 1992) and bradykinin infusion (Yatsumoto et al 1993). The common pathway by which these mechanisms produce cellular damage will be discussed below.

Consequences of acinar cell injury

Cells working under metabolic stress, or subjected to toxic damage, release powerful neutrophil activators, which seems to be the first consequence of acute pancreatitis. Following activation of neutrophils, cytokines are released and the immune response is rapidly activated. This has local and systemic effects which are beyond the scope of this chapter. Tumour necrosis factor is released early and transiently (Exley et al 1992, Paajanen et al 1994) and interleukin 6 (Viedma et al 1992, Heath et al 1993) leads to the subsequent elevation of serum C-reactive protein levels (Mayer et al 1984, Heath et al 1993). These changes may indicate severity, but offer nothing in terms of treatment.

Recently interest has focused on the role of platelet activating factor (PAF) in the acute inflammatory response. Increased release of PAF and increased activation of platelets have been detected in experimental and clinical pancreatitis. It is believed that activation of platelets may contribute to endothelial damage and to intravascular coagulation, which in turn may play a role in the development of pancreatic tissue ischaemia and in the failure of

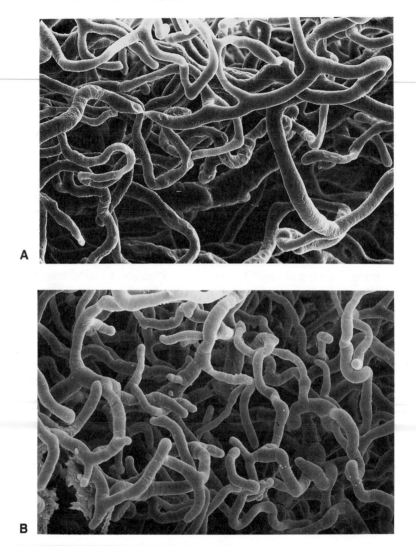

Fig. 1.3 **A** SEM (scanning electron-microscopic) view of pancreatic vascular cast in control animal. The microvascular bed is characterized by a dense network of interlacing vessels. × 650. **B** SEM view of a pancreatic vascular cast 4 h after induction of caerulein pancreatitis. Note the numerous blind-ending capillary buds and blebs of cast material on the surface of the cast. × 600. (Reproduced with permission from Johnson & Imrie 1991.)

distant organs. PAF antagonists have been developed, and preliminary studies of their use are encouraging, showing a reduction in inflammatory markers (Galloway et al 1994). Larger studies are in progress to confirm this effect and to demonstrate clinical benefit.

CHRONIC PANCREATITIS

Chronic obstructive pancreatitis causes diffuse fibrosis and destruction of acinar tissue as a result of long-standing obstruction of the main pancreatic duct. In contrast, chronic calcifying pancreatitis (which includes alcohol-related, tropical, hereditary, possibly hypercalcaemic, and idiopathic forms) produces a patchy destruction of acinar tissue (Sarles et al 1989). The pathogenesis of these patchy lesions is thought to be precipitation of secreted protein with plugging of ducts draining acini or lobules (Sarles et al 1990). In many cases, calcium crystal formation occurs on the basis of these protein precipitates and it seems likely that reduced secretion of lithostatin plays a significant part in the formation and growth of these crystals (Bernard et al 1994, Mariani et al 1994).

A direct toxic effect of alcohol on the pancreas appears to have been ruled out. The proposed mechanism — dehydrogenation of alcohol to acetaldehyde — produces concentrations much lower than those required to affect pancreatic secretion (Andersen et al 1980). However, Wilson et al (1992) demonstrated reduced lysosomal stability after exposure of rat lysosomes to cholesteryl oleate whereas ethanol and acetaldehyde had no effect. Cholesteryl oleate accumulates in the pancreas after alcohol consumption. The significance of this observation has not been fully elucidated, but it is conceivable that the reduced lysosomal stability could lead to increased co-localization of lysosomal enzymes and zymogens. Co-localization is known to be involved in cellular damage in acute pancreatitis, as discussed above.

The pathophysiological events of chronic pancreatitis have been best studied in relation to alcohol-related disease. However, the physiological and morphological changes in tropical and other forms of chronic pancreatitis appear to be identical. Chronic alcohol consumption increases protein concentration in pancreatic juice, particularly in basal secretion. Increased concentration of protein leads to protein precipitation and also favours calcium precipitation (Renner et al 1983, Clain et al 1981). The concentration of citrate in pancreatic juice is reduced in chronically alcoholic men (Boustière et al 1985) which will also favour calcium precipitation.

By analogy with the events that occur in acute pancreatitis, it is conceivable that obstruction to the flow of pancreatic juice as a result of protein and calcium precipitation could lead to cellular damage in focal areas of the pancreas secreting into an obstructed segment. The mechanism of cellular damage as a result of this metabolic stress appears to be related, in both acute and chronic pancreatitis, to the generation of free radicals.

OXYGEN FREE RADICALS

Oxygen free radicals are highly toxic, unstable reactive molecular species which contain an uneven number of electrons in the outer orbitals. Under normal conditions a small amount of oxygen undergoes a univalent reduction leading to the production of several toxic intermediates, including superoxide (O_2^-) hydrogen peroxide (H_2O_2) and hydroxyl radical ($OH^\bullet$). The xanthine oxidase system is the most common source of free radical generation. This system is activated in ischaemic conditions (Parks & Granger 1983). During reperfusion after ischaemia, oxygen reaches the tissues and is combined with hypoxanthine to generate free radicals. These free radicals can lead to tissue damage through degradation of hyaluronic acid and collagen (Halliwell 1978), and they damage cell membranes by a process of lipid peroxidation and fragmentation into malondialdehyde (Kellogg & Fridovitch 1975, Goldstein & Weissman 1977). This membrane damage affects not only the cellular membrane but also intracellular organelles such as lysosomes (Fong et al 1973).

Acute pancreatitis

Sanfey et al (1984) demonstrated the involvement of oxygen free radicals in the pathogenesis of acute pancreatitis using an isolated canine pancreas preparation. A variety of different aetiological agents led to pancreatic oedema. This process could be prevented by pretreatment with free radical scavengers such as superoxide dismutase and catalase. Pretreatment with allopurinol (a xanthine oxidase inhibitor) significantly modified the development of pancreatitis (Sanfey et al 1985) The role of the xanthine oxidase system in a variety of different experimental models has been confirmed by the protective effect of allopurinol (Sanfey 1991).

The role of oxygen free radicals is less well defined in the pathogenesis of haemorrhagic, necrotic pancreatitis. Lankisch et al (1989) found no benefit from allopurinol in pancreatitis caused by a choline-deficient diet or taurocholate injection. However, Gough et al (1990) demonstrated increased chemiluminescence in taurocholate-induced pancreatitis 15 min after injection. Superoxide dismutase injected immediately after the taurocholate significantly reduced chemiluminescence and serum amylase levels, and Schoenberg et al (1990) found reduced necrosis after injection of superoxide dismutase in caerulein-induced pancreatitis in the rat.

Free radicals are a potent source of neutrophil activation (Petrone et al 1980) and it is known that this is an early step in the development of haemorrhagic pancreatitis. Braganza & Rinderknecht (1988) proposed that the pathogenesis of haemorrhagic pancreatitis results from activation of leucocytes within the pancreas as a result of the generation of lipid oxidation products which are powerful chemoattractants. The damage to vessels demonstrated by microvascular casting techniques (Kelly et al 1989, McEntee et al 1989) could well result from free radical damage to vascular endothelium. The consequent impairment of blood flow would lead to tissue ischaemia and further free radical generation. Thus a vicious cycle develops with continuing cellular damage and further activation of neutrophils.

Clinical observations

There is growing evidence to implicate free radical generation in the pathogenesis of acute pancreatitis. Guyan et al (1990) found increased levels of lipid oxidation products in duodenal juice of patients who had had an attack of acute pancreatitis. Schoenberg et al (1988) showed increased lipid peroxidation products in pancreatic tissue from patients with acute pancreatitis. A variety of antioxidants such as selenium, glutathione, methionine and ascorbic acid have been shown to be present at reduced levels in the acute phase of pancreatitis (Braganza 1991). Ascorbic acid and its metabolites are reduced after recovery from pancreatitis, and the relative concentrations of these substances indicate a pre-existing deficiency (Scott et al 1993).

Attempts to modify the course of acute pancreatitis with antioxidant therapy have been limited, but remarkably successful. Braganza's group (Braganza 1991) treated 15 patients who had multiorgan failure, half of whom had severe pancreatitis. Median APACHE II scores were in excess of 30 in seven control patients and in seven patients treated with N-acetylcysteine (NAC) in addition to standard therapy. Seven of eight controls died, but only one of seven patients who received NAC died. Kuklinski et al (1991) found increased levels of malondialdehyde in subjects with acute pancreatitis. They randomized eight patients with acute necrotising pancreatitis to receive sodium selenite and nine control patients to standard therapy. Eight of the nine control patients died but there were no deaths in the therapy group. These impressive results require confirmation in larger studies, but they do suggest that such studies are worthwhile.

Chronic pancreatitis

Braganza's group has pointed out the deficiency of dietary antioxidants in patients with chronic pancreatitis (Rose et al 1986, Uden et al 1988). They subsequently composed a 'cocktail' of antioxidants which proved effective in pain relief and in reducing the number of acute attacks in a 20-week double-blind crossover trial (Uden et al 1990). Braganza has used these observations to suggest that free radical generation is an essential part of the pathogenesis of chronic pancreatitis. The observation that tobacco smoking is an independent risk factor for the development of chronic pancreatitis (Bourlière et al 1991) supports this theory, as smoking leads to inhalation of free radicals and depletion of antioxidant systems.

Role of free radicals

Oxygen free radicals appear to be at the focal point of the pathogenesis of both chronic and acute pancreatitis. However, the two conditions have different causes and different effects. Possible mechanisms are shown in Figs 1.4 and 1.5. In chronic pancreatitis, persistent low-grade release of oxygen free

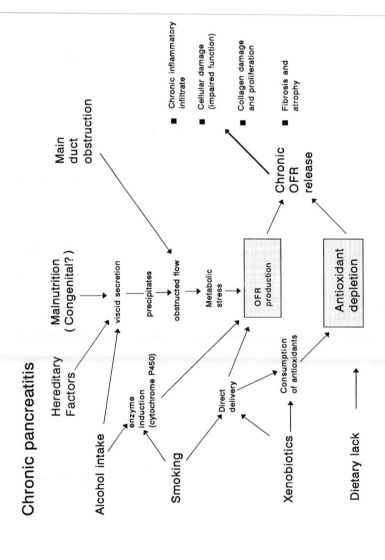

Fig. 1.4 Simplified schema for the pathogenesis of chronic pancreatitis. Oxygen free radical (OFR) release results from an imbalance between the supply of antioxidant and free radical production. Several known aetiological factors may have more than one mechanism of action. Chronic oxygen free radical release produces sublethal cellular damage and a chronic inflammatory response.

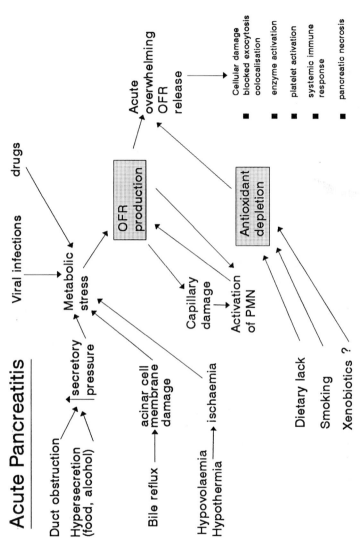

Fig. 1.5 A schematic presentation of the pathogenesis of acute pancreatitis. A variety of precipitating events leads to metabolic stress throughout the pancreas. The resulting oxygen free radical (OFR) production overwhelms defence mechanisms which may be depleted by prior dietary insufficiency or other factors. The distinguishing feature in acute pancreatitis is the presence of closed positive feedback loops involving capillary damage and ischaemia, and activation of neutrophils. The sudden surge of oxygen free radical release causes fatal cell damage, leading to enzyme activation in the pancreas and systemic platelet and immune response activation. Vascular injury causes pancreatic necrosis.

radicals leads to cellular damage with impaired function, changes in the nature of the pancreatic secretion, alterations in the connective tissue scaffolding of the pancreas (Slater 1984) and the eventual, usually patchy, destruction of glandular tissue. In contrast, in acute pancreatitis, there is a sudden and overwhelming generation of oxygen free radicals, which leads to capillary damage and neutrophil activation throughout the pancreas, with consequent pancreatic necrosis and a systemic immune response.

In reality, there will be overlap between these two processes, which can explain the clinical observation of acute exacerbations in chronic alcohol-related pancreatitis, for example. The interrelationship between these patho-genetic mechanisms is probably more complex than suggested by this simplified scheme.

IMPLICATIONS FOR THERAPY

These recent advances in our understanding of the pathogenesis of pancreatitis have not yet been translated into proven therapies. Both acute pancreatitis and chronic pancreatitis have been disappointing diseases to treat because, on the one hand, in acute pancreatitis the outcome seems to be determined early in the course of disease and the numerous therapies which seem promising when tested in the laboratory have failed to produce clinical benefits, presumably because of the obligatory delay between onset of disease and the start of therapy, and, on the other hand, in chronic pancreatitis the symptoms and disturbance of function seem to result from structural changes in the gland and so respond poorly to medical manipulation.

Chronic pancreatitis

Reduced citrate levels in the pancreatic juice of patients with chronic pancreatitis can be corrected by administration of oral citrate. While this may have a role in helping to clear stone fragments after extracorporeal lithotripsy, there is no evidence to support clinical benefit in terms of symptom relief from citrate therapy. Indeed, the focusing of treatment effort on pancreatic calculi seems misguided, as these are the final effect, rather than a cause, of the disease (Goggin & Johnson 1995).

The work of Braganza highlighting the effect of oxidative stress in the pathogenesis of chronic pancreatitis might lead to effective therapy in the shape of antioxidant supplements. However, the encouraging results reported for this approach (Uden et al 1990) have not been confirmed by others. This is perhaps because late-stage chronic pancreatitis is a reflection of significant structural alteration within the pancreas.

Acute pancreatitis

The conventional supportive management for patients with severe acute pancreatitis is well known. Advances in intensive care and general supportive therapy have reduced the mortality of this condition but further improvement in this area appears extremely difficult. The indications for surgical intervention have been reviewed in Taylor & Johnson (1993), and the timing of intervention has been discussed recently by Johnson (1993).

Gallstones

The most important advance in therapy of severe acute pancreatitis has been the recognition that early endoscopic sphincterotomy can reduce the complications and mortality of biliary pancreatitis (Neoptolemos et al 1988, Nowak et al 1990, Fan et al 1993). Each of these reports demonstrated a significant reduction in complications and deaths in patients with severe biliary pancreatitis who underwent endoscopic sphincterotomy within 24 or 48 h of admission. In total there were 28 complications and three deaths in 203 patients who underwent early endoscopic therapy, compared with 44 complications and 14 deaths in 173 patients managed expectantly. It is now clear that early endoscopic sphincterotomy should be offered to all patients with known or suspected gallstones, or other biliary pathology, who have acute pancreatitis that is predicted to be severe by the Glasgow, Ranson, or APACHE II scoring systems.

Free radicals

Despite the encouraging preliminary studies quoted above, confirmation of the beneficial effects of antioxidant therapy is awaited. At present, therefore, this form of therapy cannot be recommended, although it appears safe and is theoretically likely to be more effective than in chronic pancreatitis.

Systemic response

Attempts to modify the harmful consequences of acute pancreatitis have uniformly failed. However, a preliminary study of a PAF antagonist has given encouraging results (Galloway et al 1994). This novel approach to acute pancreatitis is currently under investigation in a multicentre study.

These cellular events and changes in the perfusion of the pancreas lead to activation of a systemic immune response. The earliest event seems to be activation of neutrophils, with release of elastase being the first detectable systemic consequence of severe pancreatitis (Dominiquez-Muñoz et al 1991). This phase of the disease is not yet amenable to treatment.

KEY POINTS FOR CLINICAL PRACTICE

- Relative pancreatic ischaemia is implicated in the pathogenesis of acute pancreatitis, and hypoxaemia is a common systemic manifestation of the disease. Attention to maintaining adequate arterial oxygen tension is essential.

- Hypovolaemia and hypotension often complicate acute pancreatitis. Full circulatory support is therefore essential to prevent pancreatic hypoperfusion.
- Only one convincing therapeutic measure has been established in the management of acute pancreatitis. Patients with a biliary aetiology and a predicted severe attack should undergo urgent endoscopic sphincterotomy, which reduces the risk of complication and death.
- Potential treatments under evaluation are antioxidant therapy and platelet activating factor antagonist therapy.
- Chronic pancreatitis has a multifactorial pathogenesis, although chronic oxygen free radical release may be the mechanism involved in tissue damage resulting from duct obstruction, juice precipitates and exposure to xenobiotics.
- Specific therapies in chronic pancreatitis are lacking. Attention should be directed to removal of any precipitating cause and establishment of a balanced diet.

REFERENCES

Armstrong CP, Taylor TV, Torrance HB 1985 Effects of bile, infection and pressure on pancreatic duct integrity. Br J Surg 72: 792–795
Bernard JP, Barthet M, Gharib B et al 1994 Quantification of human lithostathine by high performance liquid chromatography. Gut (in press)
Bourlière M, Barthet M, Berthezene P et al 1991 Is tobacco a risk factor for chronic pancreatitis and alcoholic cirrhosis? Gut 32: 1392–1395
Boustière C, Sarles H, Lohse J et al 1985 Citrate and calcium secretion in the pure human pancreatic juice of alcoholic and nonalcoholic men and of chronic pancreatitis patients. Digestion 32: 1–9
Braganza JM 1991 The pathogenesis of pancreatitis. Manchester University Press, Manchester, pp 178–197
Braganza JM, Rinderknecht H 1988 Free radicals and acute pancreatitis. Gastroenterology 94: 1111–1112
Clain JE, Barbezat GO, Marks IN 1981 Exocrine pancreatic enzyme and calcium secretion in health and pancreatitis. Gut 22: 355-358
Clemens JA, Cameron JL 1989 The pathogenesis of pancreatitis. In: Carter DC, Warshaw AL (eds) Pancreatitis. Churchill Livingstone, London, pp 1–30
Corfield AP, Cooper MJ, Williamson RCN et al 1985 Prediction of severity in acute pancreatitis: prospective comparison of three prognostic indices. Lancet 2: 403–407
Dominiquez-Muñoz et al 1991 Clinical usefulness of polymorphonuclear elastase in predicting the severity of acute pancreatitis: results of a multicentre study. Br J Surg 78: 1230–1234
Exley AR, Leese T, Holliday MP et al 1992 Endotoxaemia and serum tumour necrosis as prognostic markers in severe acute pancreatitis. Gut 33: 1126–1128
Fan ST, Lai ECS, Mok F et al 1993 Early treatment of acute biliary pancreatitis by endoscopic papillotomy. N Engl J Med 328: 228–232
Fong KL, McKay PB, Poyer JL et al 1973 Evidence that peroxidation of lysosomal membranes is initiated by hydroxyl free radicals produced during flavin enzyme activity. J Biol Chem 248: 7792–7797
Foulis AK 1980 Histological evidence of initiating factors in acute necrotising pancreatitis in man. J Clin Pathol 33: 1125–1131
Galloway SW, Formela L, Kingsnorth AN 1994 A double blind placebo controlled study of

BB-882 (a potent PAF antagonist) in human acute pancreatitis. Gut 35: Suppl 5: S35

Goggin PM, Johnson CD 1995 Pancreatic stones in chronic pancreatitis. In: Beger HG, Warshaw AL, Carr-Locke DEl et al (eds) The pancreas: a clinical textbook. Blackwell Scientific, Oxford (in press)

Goldstein IM, Weissman G 1977 Effects of the generation of superoxide anion on permeability of liposomes. Biochem Biophys Res Commun 75: 604–609

Gough D, Boyle B, Joyce WP et al 1990 Free radical inhibition and serial chemiluminescence in evolving experimental pancreatitis. Br J Surg 77: 1256–1259

Guyan PM, Oden S, Braganza JM 1990 Heightened free radical activity in chronic pancreatitis Free Radic Biol Med 8: 347–354

Halliwell B 1978 Biochemical mechanisms accounting for the toxic action of oxygen on living organisms, The key role of superoxide. Cell Biol Int Rep 2: 113–128

Heath DI, Cruickshank A, Gudgeon M et al 1993 Role of interleukin 6 in mediating the acute phase protein response and potential as an early means of severity assessment in acute pancreatitis. Gut 34: 41–45

Johnson CD 1991 Acute pancreatitis: do we need to know the cause? In: Johnson CD, Imrie CW (eds) Pancreatic disease: progress and prospects, Springer, London, pp 311–319

Johnson CD 1993 Timing of intervention in acute pancreatitis. Postgrad Med J 69: 509–515

Kellogg EW, Fridovich I 1975 Superoxide, hydrogen peroxide and singlet oxygen in lipid peroxidation by a xanthine oxidase system. J Biol Chem 250: 8812–8817

Kelly D, McEntee G, Cottell D et al 1989 Diffuse vascular injury is a critical factor in the extrapancreatic organ impairment of acute haemorrhagic pancreatitis. Digestion 34: 152

Klar E, Messmer K, Warshaw L et al 1990 Pancreatic ischaemia in experimental acute pancreatitis: mechanism, significance and therapy. Br J Surg 77: 1205–1210

Kuklinski B, Buchner M, Schweder R et al 1991 Akute Pankreatitis: eine 'Free Radical Disease'. Z Gesamte Inn Med 46: S145–S149

Kyogoku T, Manabe T, Tobe T 1992 Role of ischaemia in acute pancreatitis: haemorrhagic shock converts oedematous pancreatitis to haemorrhagic pancreatitis in rats. Dig Dis Sci 37: 1409–1417

Lankisch PG 1988 Aetiology of acute pancreatitis In: Glazer G, Ranson JHC (eds) Acute pancreatitis. Ballière Tindall, London, pp 167–181

Lankisch PG, Pohl U, Otto J et al 1989 Xanthine oxidase inhibitor in acute experimental pancreatitis in rats and mice. Pancreas 4: 436–440

McEntee GP, Leahy A, Cottell DC et al 1989 Three dimensional morphological study of the pancreatic microvasculature in caerulein induced experimental pancreatitis. Br J Surg 76: 853–855

Mariani A, Mezzi G, Malesci A 1994 Purification and assay of secretory lithostathine in human pancreatic juice by fast protein liquid chromatography. Gut (in press)

Mayer AD, McMahon MJ, Bowen M et al 1984 C-reactive protein: an aid to assessment and monitoring of acute pancreatitis. J Clin Pathol 37: 207–211

Neoptolemos JP, Carr-Locke DL, London NJM et al 1988 Controlled trial of urgent endoscopic sphincterotomy versus conservative treatment for acute pancreatitis due to gallstones. Lancet 2: 979–983

Nowak A, Nowakowaska-Dulawa, Rybicka J 1990 A prospective randomised trial of urgent endoscopic sphinterotomy vs conservative treatment for acute biliary pancreatitis. Hepatogastroenterology 37 (Suppl II A5)

Paajanen H, Laato M, Jaakala M et al 1994 Serum tumour necrosis factor compared to C-reactive protein in the early assessment of severity of acute pancreatitis. Br J Surg (in press)

Papp M, Makara GB, Hajtman B et al 1966 A quantitative study of pancreatic blood flow in experimental pancreatitis. Gastroenterology 51: 524–528

Parks DA, Granger DN 1983 Ischemia-induced microvascular changes. Role of xanthine oxidase and hydroxyl radical. Am J Physiol 245: G285–G289

Petrone WF, English DK, Wong K et al 1980 Free radicals and inflammation: superoxide-dependent activation of a neutrophil chemotactic factor in plasma. Proc Natl Acad Sci USA 77: 1159–1163

Renner IG, Rinderknecht H, Russell et al 1983 Pancreatic secretion after secretin and CCK stimulation in chronic alcoholics with and without cirrhosis. Dig Dis Sci 28: 1089–1093

Rose P, Fraine E, Hunt LP et al 1986 Dietary antioxidants and chronic pancreatitis. Hum

Nutr Appl Nutr 400: 151–164

Sanfey H 1991 Free radicals and antioxidants in pancreatic inflammation. In: Johnson CD, Imrie CW (eds) Pancreatic diseases: progress and prospects. Springer, London, pp 241–249

Sanfey H, Bulkley GH, Cameon JL 1984 The role of oxygen derived free radicals in the pathogenesis of acute pancreatitis. Ann Surg 200: 405–413

Sanfey H, Bulkley GB, Cameron JL 1985 The pathogenesis of acute pancreatitis: the source and role of oxygen derived free radicals in three different experimental models. Ann Surg 201: 633–639

Sarles H, Adler G, Dani R et al 1989 Classifications of pancreatitis and definition of pancreatic disease. Digestion 43: 234–236

Sarles H, Bernard JP, Gullo L 1990 Pathogenesis of chronic pancreatitis. Gut 31: 629–632

Schoenberg MH, Buchler M, Beger HG 1988 Lipid peroxidation products in the pancreatic tissue of patients with acute pancreatitis. Br J Surg 75: 1254

Schoenberg MH, Buchler M, Gasper M et al 1990 Oxygen free radicals in acute pancreatitis in the rat. Gut 31: 1138–1143

Scott P, Bruce C, Schofield D et al 1993 Vitamin C status in patients with acute pancreatitis. Br J Surg 80: 750–754

Sitges-Serra A, Alonso M, de Lecea C et al 1988 Pancreatitis and hyperparathyroidism. Br J Surg 75: 158–160

Slater TF 1984 Free radical mechanism in tissue injury. Biochem J 222: 1–15

Spormann H, Sokolowski A, Letko G 1989 Effect of temporary ischaemia upon development and histological patterns of acute pancreatitis in the rat. Pathol Res Pract 184: 507–513

Steer ML, Meldolesi J, Figarella C 1984 Pancreatitis. The role of lysosomes. Dig Dis Sci 29: 934–938

Thal A 1954 Studies on pancreatitis IV. The pathogenesis of bile pancreatitis. Surg Forum 5: 391–394

Taylor I, Johnson CD (eds) 1993 Recent advances in surgery. Churchill Livingstone, vol 16: pp 121–141

Thomson SR, Hendry WS, McFarlane GA et al 1987 Epidemiology and outcome of acute pancreatitis. Br J Surg 74: 398–401

Uden S, Acheson DWK, Reeves J et al 1988 Antioxidants, enzyme induction and chronic pancreatitis: a reappraisal following studies in patients on anticonvulsants. Eur J Clin Nutr 42: 561–569

Uden S, Bilton D, Nathan L et al 1990 Antioxidant therapy for recurrent pancreatitis: placebo controlled trial. Aliment Pharmacol Ther 4: 357–371

Viedma JA, Perez-Matea M, Dominguez JE et al 1992 Role of interleukin 6 in acute pancreatitis. Comparison with C-reactive protein and phospholipase A. Gut 33: 1264–1267

Wilson JS, Apte MV, Thomas MC et al 1992 Effects of ethanol, acetaldehyde and cholesteryl esters on pancreatic lysosomes. Gut 33: 1099–1104

Yatsumoto F, Manabe T, Ohshio G 1993 Bradykinin involvement in the aggravation of acute pancreatitis in rabbits. Digestion 54: 224–230

2

Non-biliary laparoscopic surgery

J. J. T. Tate

Laparoscopic cholecystectomy burst onto the surgical scene in 1989, 6 years ago, and rapidly became popular with both surgeons and patients. Immediately, a laparoscopic approach to other abdominal operations was considered and virtually every conceivable intraperitoneal operation has been described using endoscopic techniques. None has had the same impact as laparoscopic cholecystectomy but several now offer a realistic alternative to conventional operations. Whether and to what extent they will replace established procedures is unknown. The current position of non-biliary, intra-abdominal laparoscopic surgery is presented in this chapter.

INGUINAL HERNIA

Whilst not an intra-abdominal operation conventionally, it may become one with a laparoscopic approach and hence is included here. Laparoscopic hernia repair is controversial for several reasons including safety, cost and durability. Common to all laparoscopic hernia repairs is an approach from inside the abdominal wall, thus avoiding a painful groin incision. In the majority of descriptions this has been via the peritoneal cavity with a pneumoperitoneum (transperitoneal approach). The alternative is to open the potential space between the inside surface of the rectus muscles and the peritoneum (preperitoneal approach). This is achieved either by blunt dissection or by insertion of a balloon into the space which is expanded. The peritoneal cavity is not entered which should avoid the potential complications of laparoscopy. The disadvantage of the preperitoneal approach is that the anatomy is unfamiliar and the technique may be more difficult to learn.

Early operations

Various operative techniques have been described and several have been rapidly abandoned (MacFadyen et al 1993, Hanafy 1993). The 'plug and patch' repair is performed with no dissection and an intraperitoneal mesh. The 'plug' of rolled-up mesh is inserted into the hernial orifice with little regard to the size of the defect. Migration of the plug down a large hernia sac was not uncommon. The covering 'patch' was sometimes too small and the presence of mesh within the peritoneal cavity gave rise to concern that intestine might become adherent to it. The intraperitoneal 'on-lay' mesh technique is similar.

Laparoscopically guided sutured repair involves sutures placed percutaneously through the abdominal wall to close the hernial defect. This repair is under tension and the number of sutures employed is limited, often to a single stitch. These operations have no features to suggest they are physiologically advantageous and there is some evidence that they are associated with more technical failures (MacFadyen et al 1993).

The preperitoneal patch operation

Few surgeons used a preperitoneal repair until laparoscopic surgery was contemplated, but some results from an open approach are available (Stoppa et al 1986, Nyhus & Condon 1989). For laparoscopic surgery, a transperitoneal approach provides clear visualization of the hernial orifice and is the most popular (Fig. 2.1). The peritoneum is incised to create a preperitoneal pocket around the hernial defect. The sac is dissected off the cord and either reduced into the peritoneal cavity or circumcised. Injection of saline around the neck of the sac can aid dissection (Dunn 1993).

A non-absorbable mesh, usually polypropylene, is placed across the back of the inguinal canal to cover the hernial defect completely. It extends medially beyond the pubic tubercle and laterally beyond the deep ring. Most surgeons fix it in place with staples but there is a view that this is unnecessary. When staples are used, none should be placed beneath or lateral to the deep ring because of risk of injury to the iliac vessels and cutaneous nerves to the thigh respectively. The mesh elicits little inflammatory reaction and is rapidly covered in fibrin when it is lying flat against the muscles of the abdominal

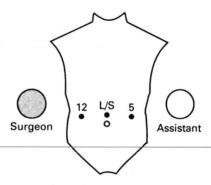

Fig. 2.1 Laparoscopic inguinal hernia repair — port positions. For left inguinal hernia, the staple gun is introduced through the right (contralateral) instrument port. Note that the laparoscope is placed supra-umbilically to allow a slightly wider field of view.

wall. Thus, it should be placed with no creases. Once the mesh is correctly placed, the peritoneal packet is closed.

The principles are the same for a preperitoneal approach but the excellent view of the hernial defect, which is useful to orientate the surgeon, is lost.

Results

There are many small series mostly presented as reports of technique or as abstracts. The largest series in the UK is a combined report from Hull and Stockport of 412 cases (Milkins et al 1993). Only three patients required conversion to open surgery and 93% were discharged home after an overnight stay. Return to work was 12 days (range 1–95) for unilateral hernia and 14 days (range 2–60) for bilateral. Median return to normal domestic activity was 3 and 5 days respectively. There were minor complications in 15%. Approximately half of these were fluid collections at the repair site, sometimes associated with a large indirect sac left within the inguinal canal, and all responded to needle aspiration, occasionally repeated. Major complications were 1.9% (urine retention, five; small bowel obstruction, two; mesh infection, one). Wound infection, at a port site, occurred in only three patients (0.8%) and the patient with a mesh infection had to have it removed.

Comparative studies are appearing but the open hernia technique varies and may not be a tension-free repair. Physical recovery is difficult to assess and established protocols are not always employed. Hospital stay may not be relevant as most hernia patients can be treated on a day case basis. In Adelaide, 80 day case patients were randomized into two groups, one having a tension-free open repair under local anaesthetic and the other laparoscopic preperitoneal repair with general anaesthesia (Maddern et al 1993). Mean operating time was the same for both operations, 35 min. One laparoscopic operation was converted to open for bleeding whilst three patients in the open group required conversion to general anaesthesia. There were no differences in pain, analgesia requirement and early postoperative mobilization at 3 days. Average time off work was 15.5 days for laparoscopic repair and 30 days for open. There was one early failure of the laparoscopic repair and two other complications (bleeding, one; small bowel obstruction, one).

Average operating time of 35–45 min for a unilateral hernia is likely although experience of 50–100 cases may be needed to reach this level. Initial cases will take 1.5–2 h (Winchester et al 1993).

Complications

The commonest complications are haematoma of the cord or subcutaneous tissues and emphysema or hydrocoele of the scrotum with a combined incidence of approximately 5% (MacFadyen et al 1993, Milkins et al 1993). The incidence may decrease with experience. Wound infections are not common, typically less than 2% but occasionally 10% in small series, and removal of the mesh because of sepsis is rare. Postoperative pain in the groin and upper thigh is reported in up to 2–5% of patients and is attributed to damage of the cutaneous nerve of the thigh or the genitofemoral nerve caused by staples placed lateral to the deep ring. Urinary retention can still occur with an incidence of 1–3%, probably less than with open surgery.

Anecdotal stories of life-threatening complications and major vascular injury have circulated but none have appeared in the literature. It is likely that they are genuinely rare. Several larger series include a few instances of bowel obstruction which has two aetiologies. First, if the mesh becomes exposed, the small intestine can become adherent and adhesion obstruction or ileus results. Second, if closure of peritoneal incision is inadequate, a loop of small bowel can enter, producing an internal hernia (Hendrickse & Evans 1993). Closure of the preperitoneal pocket with a continuous suture may avoid this. Incisional hernia through a cannula site can occur with any laparoscopic operation (Whiteley 1993).

Controversies — safety, cost, recurrence rates

The Royal College of Obstetrics and Gynaecology survey of laparoscopy in 11 000 patients found mortality of 0.1% and serious complications 0.7% (Chamberlain & Brown 1978). This is the level of morbidity added to any transperitoneal laparoscopic repair but may, perhaps, be reduced if the Hasson cannula and 'open' laparoscopy or a preperitoneal approach are widely adopted.

The requirement for general anaesthesia is a potential safety concern but probably not a major problem in practice. Any patient unfit for general anaesthesia cannot have a laparoscopic operation. When patients are fit, there are few differences in recovery between general, spinal or local anaesthesia once the patient has left hospital. Laparoscopic hernia repair is entirely suitable as a day case procedure once sufficient experience is gained. However, general anaesthesia does have cost implications for drugs and staff including the additional recovery time before discharge from the ward (Maddern et al 1993).

Use of prosthetic mesh for herniorrhaphy is more expensive than sutures but fixation of the mesh with titanium staples, generally only available in disposable applicators, is the major additional cost. Use of a disposable port to introduce the applicator and/or disposable instruments, such as scissors, adds further cost. If reduced time off work is the major benefit, laparoscopic hernia repair is financially unattractive unless the hospital is reimbursed for these additional costs. The question of whether the mesh needs to be fixed therefore assumes additional importance.

Long-term follow-up is non-existent and 6–18 months is typical. At this point only technical failures can be observed but these are gratifyingly few at 0.8–1.5%. Virtually all are thought to have been due to use of too small a mesh rather than displacement of the mesh. Five-year data are required and these will be of most value as part of a randomized trial. A very large study will be needed to generate sufficient power to show whether there is a statistically significant difference in recurrence rate for laparoscopic and conventional hernia repair and, for both types, technique will need to be standardized. Thus, reliable information about the recurrence rate of laparoscopic preperitoneal repair is many years away.

Lichtenstein repair

The gold standard against which laparoscopic hernia repair must be judged has changed over the last 5 years also. Of the newer conventional operations, first the Shouldice technique and now the Lichtenstein repair have usurped traditional operations. Lichtenstein's operation, which has been slightly revised (Lichtenstein et al 1989, Amid et al 1993), has the advantage of being simple to learn, suitable for all types of hernia, large or small, and offers rapid postoperative recovery. It is ideal as a day case procedure and suitable for local anaesthesia. In his own series of 3125 patients, Lichtenstein reports follow-up of 87% of patients with four recurrences at 1–8 years (Amid et al 1993). A multicentre study of the technique in 3019 patients showed recurrence rates of 0–0.8% and infection at 0–0.5% (Shulman et al 1992). This is the standard against which laparoscopic hernia repair should be measured in randomized trials.

Summary

Overall, it is likely that the differences between tension-free laparoscopic preperitoneal repair and tension-free Lichtenstein repair will be small and the need to develop laparoscopic hernia repair at all has been questioned (Condon 1993, Rutkow 1992). Avoiding the swelling and discomfort of a groin incision may be a significant advantage even though the requirement for general anaesthesia is a disadvantage. Reliable assessment of recovery at home and durability of the repair are key issues and are the most difficult aspects to research. For certain indications — bilateral hernia, complex recurrent hernia, obesity — laparoscopic repair has much to offer. In both laparoscopic and Lichtenstein operations, the size of the mesh and its correct placement over the defect are crucial and should be audited as part of any study.

DIAGNOSTIC LAPAROSCOPY AND APPENDICECTOMY

Diagnostic laparoscopy

Malignant disease

Diagnostic laparoscopy is valuable because percutaneous ultrasound, CT (computed tomography) and MRI (magnetic resonance imaging) all fail to detect the presence of some metastatic deposits of the liver or peritoneum that alter the stage of disease and may mean that planned surgery is not the best form of palliation (Cuesta et al 1992). For oesophageal and gastric cancer, laparoscopy was 50% better for the detection of metastases than CT or ultrasound and achieved a sensitivity of 88% (Watt et al 1989). In a series of 88 pancreatic cancer patients with a clear CT or MRI, one quarter had metastases visible on laparoscopy (Warshaw et al 1990). Of 16 patients thought to have operable liver tumours, laparoscopy showed previously unrecognized features in eight patients which rendered them inoperable and spared them an unnecessary laparotomy (Babineau et al 1994)

The emerging application of laparoscopic ultrasound will enhance diagnostic laparoscopy further. Originally a rigid instrument with a linear array was used; now probes are available with flexible tips and built-in colour Doppler. Laparoscopic ultrasound is especially valuable in the liver and pancreas (Mile set al 1992, Cuesta et al 1993). For colorectal cancer, ultrasound-detected lesions in the liver would not necessarily alter the primary treatment but would affect subsequent adjuvant therapy or the need for liver resection.

A practical problem with intraoperative ultrasound at open surgery is whether the surgeon or radiologist should do it. At laparoscopy, using a picture-in-picture video mixer, a simultaneous image of the position of the probe and the ultrasound image obtained can be displayed making interpretation much easier. This can be viewed simultaneously in the operating theatre and the radiology department so the radiologist does not have to interrupt his schedule to attend the operation.

The acute abdomen

Diagnostic laparoscopy for the acute abdomen, largely in patients suspected to have appendicitis, has been promoted for more than a decade but not widely adopted. Appendicectomy is usually done by trainees who do not have the experience or confidence in laparoscopy to use it routinely. Also, the value of diagnostic laparoscopy depends, largely, on the clinical skill in making the diagnosis of acute appendicitis; if a false positive diagnosis is infrequent (less than 20%) the benefits are small. One report showed a significant reduction in the number of normal appendices removed after laparoscopy compared with a control group (Olsen et al 1993). However, the clinical diagnosis was wrong in 60% of patients and hospital stay was not reduced by leaving the appendix in situ. Use of computer-aided diagnosis would probably be of more value than laparoscopy in this situation.

Up to 19% of normal-looking appendices show inflammation histologically, while 8% of inflamed-looking appendices are normal (Lau et al 1986). Hence, there is debate as to whether a normal appendix should be removed. There is an ethical objection to doing unnecessary surgery and complications can occur, especially wound infection. Removal of the appendix prevents a missed diagnosis and eliminates appendicitis as a diagnosis if the patient returns with similar symptoms in the future. Absence of a conventional appendix scar could, in itself, cause confusion in the future (Dawson et al 1992). Thus, diagnostic laparoscopy may be of most value in selected groups such as the elderly or females (Paterson-Brown 1993), or when acute appendicitis is a possibility and the surgeon is concerned as to the choice of incisions (midline or grid-iron). Alternatively, maximum yield is obtained if it is used in all cases (Manson et al 1993).

For trauma, laparoscopy is possibly of value in haemodynamically stable patients with a penetrating injury such as a stab wound. It can be determined immediately whether the peritoneal cavity has been breached; patients with superficial wounds alone do not require hospital admission (Fabian et al 1993). If the peritoneum has been perforated, a visceral injury can often be identified but it cannot be excluded; up to 20% of intestinal injuries were not seen in one series (Ivatury et al 1994). The relative merits, if any, of laparoscopy versus peritoneal lavage and clinical monitoring has yet to be established. Laparoscopy is of limited value in blunt trauma as it is difficult to see retroperitoneal structures and the spleen (Fabian et al 1993).

Laparoscopic appendicectomy

Operative technique

Most surgeons use a three-port technique but the position of the ports varies (Fig. 2.2). The choice depends on the surgeon's preferred orientation of instruments to the viewing axis and a one- or two-handed technique, but a port situated just above each pubic tubercle allows for 'invisible' scars (Tate et al 1993a). As the major advantage of laparoscopic appendicectomy is reduction in wound infections, it is important to remove the appendix through a cannula without it touching the wound edges, using a larger port if necessary (Tate et al 1993b). The appendix stump is commonly ligated with loop ligatures and it has been shown that invagination of the stump is not necessary (Engstrom & Fenyo 1985). However, pericaecal and pelvic collections are noted in some series (Tate et al 1993c), and it has been claimed that use of a stapling device to divide the appendix avoids this (Lujan et al 1994).

The technique of laparoscopic-assisted appendicectomy involves laparoscopic mobilization, after which the appendix is brought through a stab incision to the surface for division. Good results were reported from Australia (Browne 1990), but the wound is contaminated in many patients with risk of subsequent wound infection.

Results

Laparoscopic appendicectomy is almost unique among laparoscopic operations because data are available from several prospective randomized trials

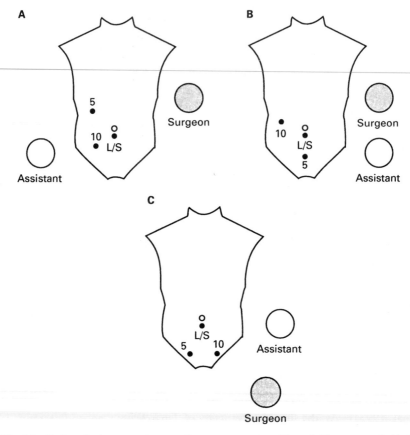

Fig. 2.2 Options for laparoscopic appendicectomy — port positions. **A** The surgeon holds the camera and one instrument. The assistant holds the appendix retracted through the right iliac fossa port; stands opposite surgeon. **B** Surgeon uses both hands; camera assistant stands next to surgeon. Appendix removed via umbilicus. **C** Two-handed method with 'invisible' scars.

(Attwood et al 1992, McAnena et al 1992, Tate et al 1993d, Kum et al 1993, Lujan et al 1994) which are summarized in Table 2.1. Overall, there is little advantage during the early postoperative course from laparoscopic appendicectomy. Once at home, recovery may be faster after laparoscopic surgery (Attwood et al 1992). The major difference is wound complication rates which are significantly reduced from around 20% for open surgery (Krukowski et al 1988) to less than 5% for laparoscopic surgery. In addition, the wounds of laparoscopic appendicectomy are more cosmetically acceptable overall.

Laparoscopic appendicectomy probably costs more than the open operation, but this may be more than balanced by savings from reduced wound infections which often accrue costs from nursing visits, dressings and antibiotics as well as increased time off work.

Table 2.1 Results of randomized comparison of laparoscopic and open appendicectomy

Author (Country)	n	% female	Age (years)	Hospital stay (days)	Analgesic (dozes i.m.)	Recovery time	Wound infection	Operation time (min)	Laparoscopic conversion
Attwood et al 1992 (Eire)	62	na	21 vs 27	2.5 vs 3.8*	na	Laparoscopy faster	0 vs 1	61 vs 51	2 of 30
McAnena et al 1992 (Eire)†	65	57	18 vs 24	2.2 vs 4.8*	1 vs 5*	na	1 vs 4*	52 vs 48	2 of 29
Kum et al 1993 (Singapore)	137	65	31 vs 33	3.2 vs 4.2	1.0 vs 1.3	19 vs 32 days	0 vs 5*	43 vs 40	na
Tate et al 1993d (Hong Kong)	140	39	31 vs 33	3.5 vs 3.6	1.7 vs 1.9	No difference	7 vs 10	70 vs 47*	14 of 70
Lujan et al 1994 (Spain)†	200	40	30 vs 26	4.8 vs 6.0*	na	na	1 vs 7*	51 vs 46	5 of 100

All results are listed as laparoscopic group first (laparoscopic vs open).
* Statistically significant difference.
† These studies not true randomization.
na, data not provided.

Operating time is generally longer than for open surgery but less than 1 h. Whilst the difference may be statistically significant it is probably of no practical or clinical significance. Conversion rates are between 10% and 20% typically but are very low in some of the largest series (Gotz et al 1990). Laparoscopic appendicectomy is applicable to virtually all patients, including pregnant women, although the conversion rate increases if presentation is delayed as dissection of the intensely inflamed appendix is difficult (Tate et al 1992).

Summary

Laparoscopic appendicectomy does not offer great advantages over the conventional operation in terms of patient recovery. However, it is certainly no worse and septic complications, which are common, can be reduced. Uniquely, the small morbidity of laparoscopy itself is balanced by the ability to more accurately diagnose the cause of symptoms in patients who do not have appendicitis. The impressive cosmetic results are an additional benefit that will be appreciated by many patients. It is undoubtedly a good training procedure. It appears that the logistics of out-of-hours surgery, theatre staff who remain unfamiliar with equipment and untrained surgeons are preventing the wider use of laparoscopic appendicectomy; these issues should be addressed.

COLORECTAL SURGERY

Development of technique

There is no doubt that it is technically possible to remove any or all of the large bowel through an insignificant incision after laparoscopic mobilization and ligation of the main vascular pedicle. From the randomized appendicectomy studies, it is apparent that there is little or no difference between laparoscopic wounds and a conventional grid-iron incision, so it is questionable whether it is necessary to remove resected colon any other way than via a small muscle-splitting incision. Most surgeons prefer to site the incision so that it allows access for a conventional anastomotic technique under direct vision and subsequent removal of the specimen (Monson et al 1992, Larach et al 1993, Scoggin et al 1993, Tate et al 1993e, Wexner et al 1993, Van Ye et al 1994) (Fig. 2.3). Intracorporeal anastomosis is possible after right colonic resection with a side-to-side stapled technique (but the problem of specimen removal remains) while, for left-sided resection, removal of tissue through the lumen of the distal bowel and subsequent trans-anal stapled anastomosis is possible. The technical difficulties of these methods suggest limited application.

Of the various procedures, right hemicolectomy and sigmoid colectomy are technically easiest and mobilization of the transverse colon the most difficult

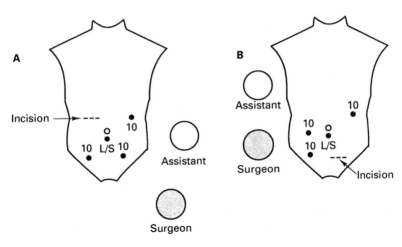

Fig. 2.3 Laparoscopic colon resection — port positions. **A** Right hemicolectomy. The surgeon stands on the patient's left side or between the legs. One of the lower abdominal ports is larger if the vascular pedicle is stapled rather than ligated. Left upper port is for bowel retraction by assistant. **B** Sigmoid colectomy. In females, an intrauterine sound is helpful to elevate the uterus.

(Geis et al 1994). The ureters can be identified in 90% of cases without difficulty but ureteric injury has been reported (Larach et al 1993), as have major vascular injury (Wexner et al 1993), visceral injury (Tate et al 1993e, Wexner et al 1993) and removal of the wrong bowel segment (Monson et al 1992), reflecting the high level of technical difficulty. The view into the pelvis during dissection for low rectal tumours is excellent but identification of the tissue plane laterally is a problem and bleeding is easily encountered which further hinders progress.

The advantages of laparoscopic-assisted bowel surgery are reduced postoperative pain and ileus (Tate et al 1993e, Van Ye et al 1994). These factors should shorten hospital stay and the time to full recovery. For benign disease, laparoscopic surgery should be advantageous. However, most benign neoplasias can be dealt with at colonoscopy. For diverticular disease the bowel is often surrounded by adhesions and difficult to dissect. For inflammatory bowel disease, the author's initial results with right hemicolectomy for Crohn's disease have been good with no increase in technical difficulty or complications, a hospital stay of less than 1 week and rapid return to normal activities, but patients with a mass on palpation or ultrasound were excluded. Total colectomy is limited by the technical difficulty of dissecting the transverse colon rather than the pathology, and operating time is 3–4 h. While laparoscopic surgery is potentially valuable for all these indications, it is for cancer surgery that it would have the greatest impact.

Colorectal cancer

The problem is whether laparoscopic surgery is an adequate cancer treatment (O'Rourke & Heald 1993, Kmiot & Wexner 1994). Ligation of the vascular pedicle does not seem to be a problem as the numbers of lymph nodes harvested at laparoscopic and open surgery are similar (Monson et al 1992, Tate et al 1993e, Van Ye et al 1994). However, en bloc excision of the specimen and lateral soft tissue margins is vital for rectal carcinoma and probably for other sites also (Heald 1988, Quirke et al 1986). Data are few; at St Mary's Hospital, London, seven patients having laparoscopic assisted abdominoperineal resection had tumour excision equal to 16 open patients (Lewis et al 1993). However, much of the dissection around the tumour could have been carried out by the perineal operator. Further randomized prospective studies with full involvement of the pathology department and three-dimensional sectioning of the specimens are needed. Many surgeons will not be convinced that laparoscopic cancer surgery is safe until 5-year follow-up data are available, but good pathological studies would provide a solid basis for continued use of laparoscopic techniques.

Implantation of viable malignant cells into the wound is a second area of concern and may occur more frequently than at open surgery (Fusco & Paluzzi 1993, O'Rourke et al 1993). On removal of a resected tumour through a small wound, contact with the wound edges must be avoided. Wound infection rates for laparoscopic colectomy of 5–18% confirm that contamination occurs. An alternative theory is that circulation of gas during laparoscopic surgery disseminates spilled malignant cells and the cannula wounds provide a fertile 'soil'. It is essential that the best methodology for preventing loss of viable cells into the peritoneal cavity is adopted.

Results

Most series are difficult to categorize because a wide range of operations and indications are mixed together. At St Mary's Hospital, London, 40 patients were treated (35 for cancer), with an equal split between right- and left-sided resections (Monson et al 1992). Operating time was 2.5 h (range 2–5) for right hemicolectomy and 4 h (range 2.5–5.5) for left hemicolectomy. This was the initial experience and seven cases were converted to open surgery; despite this median hospital stay was 8 days (range 5–14) compared with 14 days for previous, conventionally treated patients. There were six complications, none attributable to the laparoscopic technique, and one death from myocardial infarction. Fifty-one patients in an American study included 24 with carcinoma, one presenting with perforation and one with obstruction (Phillips et al 1992); the wisdom of attempting such cases is open to question. Overall operating time was 2.3 ± 0.9 h, stay 4.6 ± 4.1 days, and there were only four major complications including one death from pneumonia in a 95-year-old. Other American studies have also achieved an average stay 5–7 days or less.

A report from the Cleveland Clinic Florida of 74 patients included 32 total colectomy (ulcerative colitis and polyposis) and 32 segmental resection (12 for cancer) (Wexner et al 1993). For segmental resection, median operating time was 2.9 h (range 1.5–5.5), duration of ileus 3 days (range 2–7) and hospital stay 7 days (range 4–20). Corresponding figures for total colectomy were 3.9 h (2.5–6.5), 3.5 days (2–7) and 8.1 days (4–19). In all 74 operations, there were 10 (14%) intraoperative complications, including four bowel injuries and two major vascular injuries, and 15 (20%) postoperative complications.

A small prospective, but unrandomized, comparative study of 25 patients with sigmoid or proximal rectal cancer (laparoscopic-assisted 11, open 14) found postoperative pain was significantly reduced (2.6 ± 0.2 versus 7.4 ± 2.1 doses of pethidine) as was time to reintroduction of solid diet (2.5 ± 0.2 versus 3.6 ± 0.3 days) in laparoscopic patients (Tate et al 1993e). Hospital stay was reduced but the difference just failed to reach significance. Operating time was significantly longer (3.5 ± 0.5 versus 2.0 ± 0.5 h) and there was a relatively high rate of major complications in the laparoscopic group including one small injury requiring subsequent laparotomy.

Stoma formation

For palliative operations, laparoscopic surgery is particularly suitable. Resection of bulky tumours is often not possible but not all patients with liver metastases have a locally advanced primary. Where a stoma is all that is required, both end colostomy and loop colostomy and ileostomy can be created. The technique is to prepare the stoma and the tunnel in the abdominal wall before placing a trocar/cannula through the peritoneum at the site of the stoma because the pneumoperitoneum disappears once the peritoneum is opened (Lyerly & Mault 1994). Alternatively, a 3.5 cm disposable cannula can be used to create a sufficiently large tunnel through the abdominal wall (Lange et al 1991). Discharge is possible 48 h postoperatively, assuming the patient has learnt to manage the stoma!

Rectopexy

As a benign condition which often occurs in elderly patients, full thickness rectal prolapse appears an ideal subject for laparoscopic surgery (Lyerly & Mault 1994). Laparoscopic rectopexy has been discussed widely and cases presented at clinical meetings, but few published results are available. The excellent view into the pelvis should be beneficial, but some of the technical problems of a sutured or prosthetic mesh rectopexy have yet to be overcome.

Summary

Laparoscopic colectomy is an exciting challenge and much technical detail has been learned. If laparoscopic treatment is as good as open surgery it will be a worthwhile advance because patient recovery is likely to be significantly enhanced. Handling of tissue can be more of a problem than in any of the other areas covered in this chapter and instrumentation is still evolving. However, the key question of whether laparoscopic surgery is safe treatment for cancer has not yet been adequately addressed and considerable caution is required.

UPPER GASTROINTESTINAL TRACT SURGERY

Reflux and hiatus hernia

Hiatus hernia surgery is a more frequent indication than peptic ulceration for minimally invasive surgery in place of prolonged medical treatment. Initial reports and much data have come from Belgium (Dallemagne et al 1991, de Gheldere et al 1993, Cadiere et al 1994).

Laparoscopic cardiopexy, using the transplanted falciform ligament, has been described with adaptation of the original open procedure (Nathanson et al 1991). However, it has not become popular, probably because the technical difficulty of laparoscopic fundoplication is no greater and few surgeons are familiar with the technique. Surgeons who use the Angelchik prosthesis are now able to do so laparoscopically (MacPhee 1993). It is a simple operation and should allow a rapid recovery. The debate over its value is not significantly altered by the ability to place it through a very small incision.

Fundoplication has emerged as the most favoured laparoscopic option (Fig. 2.4). The indications remain the same as for open surgery and patients with oesophageal dysmotility should be avoided. Most surgeons use a five-port technique taking care in retracting the stomach to avoid serosal tearing. Creation of a retro-oesophageal window allows the gastric fundus to be brought around, creating a 360° wrap. Major complications include pneumo-

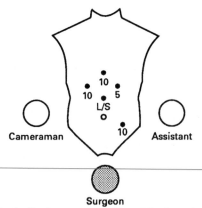

Fig. 2.4 Laparoscopic fundoplication — port positions. The lower left port is used to retract the stomach and the epigastric port to retract the left lobe of the liver. The surgeon uses the other two instrument ports. Note laparoscope placed well above umbillicus for improved view of hiatus.

thorax and perforation of the oesophagus which can occur as the window is being made, particularly if the oesophagus is dissected into the chest.

Several controversies still have to be addressed, including whether to divide the short gastrics, whether to include the vagii in the wrap and whether to suture the wrap to the oesophagus. Most surgeons close the oesophageal hiatus and use an intraoesophageal bougie to determine how tight to make the wrap. The bougie has to be inserted after oesophageal mobilization which is another cause of perforation. The length of the wrap varies considerably between surgeons.

For patients with abdominal adhesions a thoracoscopic approach can offer a solution and may be preferable in obese patients with a large hiatus also (Salo et al 1993). Additionally, a thoracic operation may reduce the incidence of a gastrogastric wrap. This is not mentioned in any report except one from Australia (Watson et al 1993) in which five of 54 patients required revisional surgery within 6 months, in two for gastric obstruction secondary to gastrogastric wrap. Subsequent barium meal studies on 28 patients showed the same situation in seven (25%) although they were asymptomatic. For a very large incarcerated hiatus hernia in an elderly patient causing respiratory embarrassment, laparoscopic reduction is a quick and valuable operation and the hiatus can be repaired if the patient is sufficiently fit (Cuschieri et al 1992).

Results

The following results are for fundoplication (Watson et al 1993, Bittner 1994, Cadiere et al 1994, McKernan & Laws 1994). Operating time is approximately 2 h and average postoperative stay as low as 3–4 days. Methods of scoring outcome vary but 'good/excellent results' have been reported in 80–87% of patients at up to 6 months. No longer-term follow-up data are available. Dysphagia has been a significant problem in 8–20% of cases but is usually transient. Inability to complete the operation laparoscopically is 14–15%, although several series claim no conversions and one records 50% (Cuschieri et al 1994), reflecting treatment of unselected patients. Complications have been few, but two large series (80 and 116 patients) (Cadiere et al 1994, Hunter 1994) show an incidence of pneumothorax of 2–3% and one detailed report (Bittner 1994) had three in 35 cases (including one tension pneumothorax) with two oesophageal perforations also. The surgical technique was subsequently altered.

Comparative data are limited, but a prospective randomized trial has been undertaken at the Royal Hallamshire Hospital, Sheffield. Initial results in 30 patients showed operating time was doubled for laparoscopic surgery whilst hospital stay was only slightly reduced at 3–4 days (median 3) for laparoscopic and 3–11 days (median 4) for open operation. Symptom outcome in both groups was not significantly different at 3 months but return to work was 1–6 weeks (median 2) after laparoscopic and 3–12 weeks (median 8) after open surgery. In a mixed group of patients, one Belgian study reported hospital stay of 6.7 days after laparoscopic surgery, 8.6 days after laparotomy and 13.6 days after thoracotomy (de Gheldere et al 1993).

Summary

Laparoscopic fundoplication is undoubtedly feasible and can probably provide similar results to open surgery with significant improvements in recovery. The exact technique appears to vary considerably and this may have important consequences. More physiological data would be helpful and longer follow-up is essential before the operation can be fully endorsed but it shows promise.

Peptic ulcer

Time cannot go backwards to suit laparoscopic surgery. Thus, truncal vagotomy with pyloroplasty/pyloromyotomy/balloon dilation or nothing at all is unlikely to be acceptable just because it is relatively easy to perform laparoscopically. Mouiel & Kathouda (1993) have been in the forefront of laparoscopic ulcer surgery and they have adopted posterior truncal vagotomy and anterior seromyotomy, espoused by Taylor for open surgery. In their 34 patients the mean operating time was 90 min (range 55–190 min) with hospital stay of 3–5 days. Ulcer healing was achieved in 33 patients and average basal acid output was reduced by 78% with maximum output reduced by 83% at 2–18 months follow-up. Major complications were few and two patients suffered delayed gastric emptying. Five ports are required. The position of the seromyotomy and its depth are important: too close to the lesser curve causes bleeding, and too far away an incomplete vagotomy. It must be deep enough to divide the nerve fibres but not to perforate the mucosa. This is a technique in which training in an animal model is valuable. Good results were claimed in an American study of 12 patients in which the seromyotomy was achieved by multiple firings of an endoscopic linear-cutting staple device along the lesser curve (Hannon et al 1992).

Laws & McKernan (1993) tried the Taylor operation but reverted to highly selective vagotomy (HSV) because they were familiar with it at open surgery. Their report, like others in the American literature, is long on technique but short on detailed results. Seven patients stayed 1–7 days postoperatively and most were at work after 1 week. Operating time was 2 h and several disposable clip applicators were used to divide the nerve fibres. Similar results were achieved by a Belgian group who claim a 70% reduction in hospital stay and 50% for overall recovery (despite a lack of comparative data) (Dallemagne et al 1994). In a German report of 15 patients, theatre time was 2.5–3.75 h and the authors found the operation 'difficult' (Helmo & Czarnetzki 1993). Neither of these papers included pH studies. Comment on the value of the Congo Red test was made.

For intractable recurrent ulcer after previous anti-ulcer surgery, thoraco-scopic vagotomy is a simple operation which may prove to be the treatment of choice (Chisholm et al 1992).

Summary

There is too little information to draw conclusions except that HSV is possible but more difficult than the Taylor operation. Similar improvements in recovery to those reported for anti-reflux surgery can be expected. Long-term follow-up data are needed; meanwhile inclusion of physiological studies would serve to increase confidence that the results of open surgery are being matched.

Perforated duodenal ulcer

Suturing of an omental patch to cover or plug a perforated duodenal ulcer can be achieved laparoscopically with relative ease (Sunderland et al 1992, Karanjia et al 1993). A synchronous acid-reducing procedure can be done if indicated (Laws & McKernan 1993). It can be difficult to locate the exact site of the perforation with an end-viewing laparoscope placed at the umbilicus in the presence of contamination and oedema; moving the laparoscope to an epigastric position for a 'birds-eye' view is helpful. Hospital stay may be determined by the disease rather than the type of surgery; ten patients aged 23–91 years (median 46) in a French study stayed 6–11 days, median 8 days, postoperatively (Benoit et al 1993), and in a similarly aged group of 15 patients in Hong Kong the average stay was 5.3 days. However, avoidance of a large incision is appealing.

Mortality from perforated peptic ulcer is age-related and if the patient is shocked as well as elderly it approaches 100% (Irvin 1989). In these patients, anaesthetic time may be very important and a laparoscopic operation usually takes longer than a conventional one. A quick laparotomy may be preferable to a small laparoscopic incision. Use of fibrin glue to seal the perforation is an alternative method that is quick, simple and ideal as a laparoscopic procedure. Use of a gelatin plug covered with fibrin (Tate et al 1993f) and an omental patch fixed in place with fibrin rather than sutures (Benoit et al 1993) have been reported. Results of a randomized study of fibrin sealant and suturing are awaited.

A compromise is to confirm the diagnosis by laparoscopy and perform only a peritoneal lavage if the perforation is seen to have been sealed spontaneously by omentum or adherence of the gallbladder or convert to a mini-laparotomy to suture the ulcer if there is an on-going leak (Walsh et al 1993). It is known that non-operative treatment is as effective as surgery (Crofts et al 1989), but it does not improve results in the elderly and requires close clinical monitoring to identify the small number of patients not responding. It could be concluded from these reports that peritoneal toilet is not of great importance, as long as leakage from the perforation has ceased. Use of a contrast meal to determine which patients require surgery is an obvious but little-used solution (Donovan et al 1979).

OTHER OPERATIONS

Hepatic cysts

Symptomatic liver cysts, especially solitary lesions, are ideal for laparoscopic treatment by transhepatic fenestration (Tate et al 1994). The more common polycystic liver disease will inevitably progress but, hopefully, laparoscopic surgery will cause few adhesions and the procedure can be repeated (Morino et al 1994). Minor wedge resections of the liver can be performed with endoscopic staplers. The creation of a cholecystojejunostomy for malignant jaundice can be achieved which, although a compromised treatment compared to Roux-en-Y hepaticojejunostomy, is appealing for a group of patients with short life expectancy.

Splenectomy

Life-threatening haemorrhage could occur during laparoscopic splenectomy but is unreported as yet. A Belgian group have treated seven patients with ITP (Cadiere et al 1993). Operation time was 4 h, postoperative stay 3 days and average blood loss 262 ml. The spleen was removed by placing it in a bag in the abdomen, bringing the neck of the bag onto the surface and then pulverizing it.

Adrenalectomy

The patient is usually placed in a lateral position on the operating table and the gland approached by dissection lateral to the colon. The approach to the right side may be easier than to the left. A Japanese series of 13 cases achieved success in 11 with two conversions for bleeding and adhesions (Matsuda et al 1993). Average operating time was 5 h. Laparoscopic removal of a phaeochromocytoma has been reported (Gagner et al 1992).

Oophorectomy

Laparoscopic oophorectomy has been widely reported in the gynaecological literature and textbooks. Application of this operation to palliative treatment of advanced breast cancer is likely to increase because 'medical' oophorectomy is unreliable. Many women may still favour non-operative treatment because of psychological resistance to loss of the ovaries.

KEY POINTS FOR CLINICAL PRACTICE

- All review articles become superseded by new developments; those on laparoscopic surgery have a particularly short sell-by date.
- Cholecystectomy is the ideal laparoscopic operation and no other has produced such a dramatic difference in such a large number of patients.
- There are some dangers unique to laparoscopic surgery and just because an operation can be done does not mean it should be done. 'Beware of zealots of the Society to Preserve the Linea Alba . . . more concerned with quick discharges than with lifetime cures' was one surgeon's comment on anti-ulcer operations but it is equally applicable to many others.
- However, although laparoscopic surgery is still under development, a positive view is justified and it appears to have an important future.
- Currently, there is a huge opportunity to establish good clinical trials which will become the reference points for abdominal surgery in the next century.

REFERENCES

Amid PK, Shulman AG, Lichtenstein IL 1993 Critical scrutiny of the open 'tension-free' hernioplasty. Am J Surg 165: 369–371
Attwood SEA, Hill ADK, Murphy PG et al 1992 A prospective randomised trial of laparoscopic versus open appendectomy. Surgery 112: 497–501
Babineau TJ et al 1994 Role of staging laparoscopy in the treatment of hepatic malignancy. Am J Surg 167: 151–154
Benoit J, Champault GG, Lebhar E et al 1993 Sutureless laparoscopic treatment of perforated duodenal ulcer. Br J Surg 80: 1212
Bittner HB 1994 Laparoscopic Nissen fundoplication. Am J Surg 167: 193–198
Browne DS 1990 Laparoscopic-guided appendicectomy. A study of 100 consecutive cases. Aust NZ J Obstet Gynaecol 30: 231–233
Cadiere GB, Bruyns J, Himpens J et al 1993 Laparoscopic splenectomy. Br J Surg 80 (Suppl): S 43
Cadiere GB, Houben JJ, Bruyus J et al 1994 Laparoscopic Nissen fundoplication: technique and preliminary results. Br J Surg 81: 400–403
Chamberlain G, Brown J 1978 Report of the Working Party of the Confidential Enquiry into Gynaecological Laparoscopy. Royal College of Obstetricians and Gynaecologists, London
Chisholm EM, Chung SCS, Sunderland GT et al 1992 Thoracoscopic vagotomy: a new use for the laparoscope. Br J Surg 79: 254
Condon RE 1993 Discussion. Arch Surg 128: 784–785
Crofts TJ, Park KGM, Steele RJC et al 1989 A randomized trial of non-operative treatment for perforated peptic ulcer. N Engl J Med 320: 970–973
Cuesta MA, Meijer S, Borgstein PJ 1992 Laparoscopy and assessment of digestive tract cancer. Br J Surg 79: 486–487
Cuesta MA, Meijer S, Borgstein PL et al 1993 Laparoscopic ultrasonography for hepatobiliary and pancreatic malignancy. Br J Surg 80: 1571–1574
Cuschieri A, Shimi S, Nathanson LK 1992 Laparoscopic reduction, crural repair and fundoplication of large hiatal hernia. Am J Surg 163: 425
Cuschieri A, Shimi SW, van der Veldin G et al 1994 Laparoscopic prosthesis fixation rectopexy for complete rectal prolapse. Br J Surg 81: 138–139
Dallemagne, Weets JM, Jehaes C et al 1991 Laparoscopic Nissen fundoplication. Surg Laparosc Endosc 1: 138
Dallemagne B, Weets JM, Jehaes C et al 1994 Laparoscopic highly selective vagotomy. Br J Surg 81: 554–556
Dawson JW, Tate JJT, Robertson CS 1992 The missing appendix. Br J Surg 79: 973

de Gheldere C, Collard JM, Otte JB et al 1993 Laparoscopic Nissen fundoplication: rationale for a new approach. Br J Surg 80 (Suppl): S 62–63

Donovan AJ, Vinson TL, Maulsby GO et al 1979 Selective treatment of duodenal ulcer with perforation. Ann Surg 189: 627–636

Dunn DC 1993 Method of separating the peritoneal sac from the spermatic vessels during laparoscopic repair of inguinal hernia. Br J Surg 80: 746

Engstrom L, Fenyo G 1985 Appendicectomy: assessment of stump in vagination versus simple ligation: a prospective randomised trial. Br J Surg 72: 971–972

Fabian TC, Croce MA, Stewart RM et al 1993 A prospective analysis of diagnostic laparoscopy in trauma. Am Surg 217: 557–565

Fusco MA, Paluzzi MW 1993 Abdominal wall recurrence after laparoscopic assisted colectomy for adenocarcinoma of the colon. Dis Colon Rectum 36: 858–861

Gagner M, Lecroix A, Bolte E 1992 Laparoscopic adrenalectomy in Cushing's syndrome and phaeochromocytoma. N Engl J Med 327: 1033

Geis WP, Coletta AV, Verdeja JC et al 1994 Sequential psychomotor skills development in laparoscopic colon surgery. Arch Surg 129: 206–212

Gotz F, Pier A, Bacher C 1990 Modified laparoscopic appendicectomy in surgery: a report on 388 operations. Surg Endosc 4: 100–102

Hanafy M 1993 Laparoscopic hernia repair: a review. Min Invasive Ther 2: 229–236

Hannon JK, Snow LL, Weinstein LS 1992 Linear gastrectomy: an endoscopic staple-assisted anterior highly selective vagotomy combined with posterior truncal vatogtomy for treatment of peptic ulcer disease. Surg Laparosc Endosc 2: 254–257

Heald RJ 1988 The 'holy plane' of rectal surgery. J R Soc Med 81: 503–508

Helmo B, Czarnetzki 1993 Laparoscopic highly selective vagotomy for duodenal ulcer disease. Br J Surg 80 (Suppl): S45

Hendrickse CW, Evans DS 1993 Intestinal obstruction following laparoscopic inguinal hernia repair. Br J Surg 80: 1432

Hunter JG 1994 Laparoscopic Nissen fundoplication. Am J Surg 167: 199

Irvin TT 1989 Mortality and perforated peptic ulcer: a case for risk stratification in elderly patients. Br J Surg 76: 215–218

Ivatury RR, Simon RJ, Stahl WM 1994 A critical evaluation of laparoscopy in penetrating abdominal trauma. J Trauma (in press)

Karanjia ND, Shanahan DJ, Knight MJ 1993 Omental patching of a large perforated duodenal ulcer: a new method. Br J Surg 80: 65

Kmiot WA, Wexner SD 1994 Laparoscopy in colorectal surgery: a call for careful appraisal. Br J Surg (in press).

Krukowski ZH, Irvin ST, Denholm S et al 1988 Preventing wound infection after appendicectomy: a review. Br J Surg 75: 1023–1033

Kum CK, Ngoi S, Goh PMY et al 1993 Randomized controlled trial comparing laparoscopic and open appendicectomy. Br J Surg 80: 1599–1600

Lange V, Meyer C, Shardey HM et al 1991 Laparoscopic creation of a loop colostomy. J Laparoendosc Surg 1: 307–312

Larach SW, Salomon MC, Williamson PR et al 1993 Laparoscopic assisted colectomy: experience during the learning curve. Coloproctology 1: 38–41

Lau WF, Fan ST, Yiu TF et al 1986 The clinical significance of routine histopathologic study of the resected appendix and safety of appendiceal inversion. Surg Gynecol Obstet 162: 256–258

Laws HL, McKernan BJ 1993 Endoscopic management of peptic ulcer disease. Ann Surg 217: 548–556

Lewis C, Darzi A, Goldin R et al 1993 Laparoscopic abdominoperineal resection of the rectum: assessment of adequacy of excision. Br J Surg 80 (Suppl): S46

Lichtenstein IL, Shulman AG, Amid PK et al 1989 The tension free hernioplasty. Am J Surg 157: 188–193

Lujan IA, Robles C, Parrilla P et al 1994 Laparoscopic versus open appendicectomy: a prospective assessment. Br J Surg 81: 133–135

Lujan JA, Parrilla P, Robles R et al 1994 Laparoscopic appendicectomy in acute appendicitis assessment in 200 patients, Br J Surg (in press)

Lyerly HK, Mault JR 1994 Laparoscopic ileostomy and colostomy. Ann Surg 219: 317–322

McAnena OJ, Austin O, O'Connell PR et al 1992 Laparoscopic versus open appendicectomy:

a prospective evaluation. Br J Surg 79: 818–820

MacFadyen BV, Arregui M, Corbitt J et al 1993 Complications of laparoscopic herniorrhaphy. Surg Endosc 7: 155–158

McKernan JB, Laws HL 1994 Laparoscopic Nissen fundoplication for the treatment of oesophageal reflux disease. Am Surg 60: 87–93

MacPhee WM 1993 The laparoscopic placement of the Angelchik anti-reflux prosthesis. Min Invasive Ther 2: 5–10

Maddern GJ, Devitt P, Malyeha P et al 1993 Laparoscopic versus open inguinal hernia repair. Br J Surg 80 (Suppl): 538–539

Manson WG, Reed MWR, Phillips WS 1993 Emergency laparoscopic surgery. Br J Surg 80: 1212

Matsuda T, Terachi T, Yoshida O 1993 Laparoscopic adrenalectomy: the surgical technique and initial results of 13 cases. Min Invasive Ther 3: 123–128

Miles WFA, Patterson-Brown S, Garden OJ 1992 Laparoscopic contact hepatic ultrasonography. Br J Surg 79: 419–420

Milkins RC, Lansdown MJR, Wedgewood KR et al 1993 Laparoscopic hernia repair: a prospective study of 409 cases. Min Invasive Ther 2: 237–242

Monson JRT, Darzi A, Carey PD et al 1992 Prospective evaluation of laparoscopic assisted colectomy in an unselected group of patients. Lancet 340: 831–833

Morino M, De Giuli M, Festa V et al 1994 Laparoscopic management of symptomatic non-parasitic cysts of the liver. Ann Surg 219: 157–164

Mouiel J, Kathouda N 1993 Laparoscopic vagotomy for chronic duodenal ulcer disease. World J Surg 17: 34–39

Nathanson LK, Shimi S, Cuschieri A 1991 Laparoscopic ligmentum teres (round ligament) cardiopexy. Br J Surg 78: 947–951

Nyhus LM, Condon RE 1989 Hernia. JB Lippincott, Philadelphia; pp 154–174

Olsen JB, Myren CJ, Haahr PE 1993 Randomised study of the value of laparoscopy before appendicectomy. Br J Surg 80: 922–923

O'Rourke NA, Heald RJ 1993 Laparoscopic surgery for colorectal cancer. Br J Surg 80: 1229–1230

O'Rourke N, Price PM, Kelly S et al 1993 Tumour inoculation during laparoscopy. Lancet 342: 368

Paterson-Brown S 1993 Emergency laparoscopic surgery. Br J Surg 80: 279–283

Phillips EH, Franklin M, Carroll BJ et al 1992 Laparoscopic colectomy. Ann Surg 216: 703–707

Quirke P, Durdey P, Dixon MF et al 1986 Local recurrence of rectal adenocarcinoma due to inadequate surgical resection. Lancet 2: 996–999

Rutkow IM 1992 Laparoscopic hernia repair the socioeconomic tyranny of surgical technology. Arch Surg 127: 1271

Salo JA et al 1993 Thoracoscopic fundoplication. Ann Chir Gynaecol 82: 199–201

Scoggin SD, Frazee RC, Snyder SK et al 1993 Laparoscopic assisted bowel surgery. Dis Colon Rectum 36: 747–750

Shulman AG, Amid PR, Lichtenstein IL 1992 The safety of mesh repair for primary inguinal hernias: results of 3019 operations from 5 diverse surgical sources. Am Surg 58: 225–257

Stoppa RE, Warlaumont CR, Verhaeghe PJ et al 1986 Prosthetic repair in the treatment of groin hernias. Int Surg 71: 154–158

Sunderland GT, Chisholm EM, Lau WY et al 1992 Laparoscopic repair of perforated peptic ulcer. Br J Surg 79: 785

Tate JJT, Dawson JW, Lau WY et al 1992 Which patients should undergo laparoscopic appendicectomy? Gut 33: 516 (Abstract)

Tate JJT, Chung SCS, Li AKC 1993a Laparoscopic appendicectomy: a two-handed technique. Br J Surg 80: 758

Tate JJT, Lau WY, Li AKC 1993b Removal of bulky tissue at laparoscopic surgery. Aust NZ J Surg 63: 221–223

Tate JJT, Dawson JW, Chung SCS et al 1993c Conventional versus laparoscopic surgery for acute appendicitis. Br J Surg 80: 761–764

Tate JJT, Dawson JW, Chung SCS et al 1993d Laparoscopic versus open appendicectomy: prospective randomized trial. Lancet 342: 633–637

Tate JJT, Kwok S, Dawson JW et al 1993e Prospective comparison of laparoscopic and conventional anterior resection. Br J Surg 80: 1396–1398

Tate JJT, Dawson JW, Lau WY et al 1993f Sutureless laparoscopic treatment of perforated duodenal ulcer. Br J Surg 80: 235

Tate JJT, Lau WY, Li AKC 1994 Transhepatic fenestration of liver cyst: a further application of laparoscopic surgery. Aust NZ J Surg 64: 264–265

Van Ye TM, Cattey PR, Henry LG 1994 Laparoscopic assisted colon resection compares favourably with open technique. Surg Laparosc Endosc 4: 25–31

Walsh CJ, Khoo DE, Motson RW 1993 Laparoscopic repair of perforated peptic ulcer (Letter). Br J Surg 80: 127

Warshaw AL, Gu W-Y, Wittenberg J et al 1990 Preoperative staging and assessment of resectability of pancreatic cancer. Arch Surg 125: 233–237

Watson DI, Jamieson GG, Britten-Jones R et al 1993 Pitfalls of laparoscopic Nissen fundoplication. Br J Surg 80 (Suppl): S64

Watt I, Stewart I, Anderson D et al 1989 Laparoscopy, ultrasound and computed tomography in cancer of the oesophagus and gastric cardia. Br J Surg 76: 1036–1039

Wexner SD, Cohen SM, Johansen OB et al 1993 Laparoscopic colorectal surgery: a prospective assessment and current perspective. Br J Surg 80: 1602–1605

Whiteley MS 1993 Herniation at the site of cannula insertion after laparoscopic cholecystectomy (Letter). Br J Surg 80: 1488

Winchester DJ, Dawes LG, Modelski DD et al 1993 Laparoscopic inguinal hernia repair — a preliminary experience. Arch Surg 128: 781–784

3

Non-surgical treatment of oesophageal cancer

C. S. Robertson

The treatment of patients with malignant dysphagia remains challenging. Surgical resection is still generally accepted as the best treatment for suitable patients providing good palliation and occasionally cure (Hennessey & O'Connell 1986, Watson 1988, Bancewicz 1990, Muller et al 1990). However, the majority of patients with oesophageal cancer are unsuitable for surgical treatment because of advanced disease at presentation, associated medical problems or age. The predominant symptom is difficulty in swallowing of a degree that varies but eventually progresses to complete dysphagia. Without some form of palliation these patients have a poor quality of life, rapid weight loss (mostly due to starvation) and an unpleasant death. The aim of palliation is the complete relief of dysphagia with minimum morbidity and maximum quality of life both during and after treatment. Although quality rather than quantity of life is more important, for many patients survival will be prolonged because of improved nutrition as a result of treatment (Fellows et al 1984). However, it must be remembered that this group of patients has a poor prognosis with any treatment having a mean survival of 4 months, although approximately 5% will survive 1 year.

Non-surgical treatments may be broadly divided into endoscopic techniques which relieve obstruction of the oesophageal lumen, and radiotherapy and chemotherapy which may, in addition, alter the natural history of the disease process (Table 3.1). As yet there is no consensus regarding the method or combination of methods best suited to treat an individual patient. Usually the technique chosen reflects the patient's circumstances, the geometry of the cancer and the local facilities and expertise. Fortunately, failure to palliate these patients is rare as it is unusual not to establish a passage through the growth, a prerequisite for success for most of these treatments.

PALLIATIVE ENDOSCOPIC TECHNIQUES

All of the endoscopic techniques may be performed using intravenous sedation and analgesia. Oesophageal dilatation alone is an inadequate treatment as dysphagia returns rapidly, but it is usually required prior to most of the endoscopic techniques.

Table 3.1 Non-surgical treatments of oesophageal cancer

Endoscopic techniques to palliate dysphagia	Potentially curative non-surgical therapies

• Intubation
   Silicone rubber
   Metal mesh
• Laser
   Contact
   Non-contact
• Photodynamic therapy
• Contact bipolar diathermy electrocoagulation
• Ethanol injection
• Intracavitary radiotherapy
	• Photodynamic therapy for early tumours
	• External beam radiotherapy alone
	• External beam radiotherapy and
	   intracavitary radiotherapy
	• Multimodal treatment
	   External beam radiotherapy and
	      combination chemotherapy
	   ± Palliative endoscopic techniques

Intubation

Oesophageal intubation was the first technique described to palliate malignant dysphagia (Symonds 1887) and probably remains the most commonly used method (Den Hartog-Jager et al 1979; Ogilvie et al 1982). Intubation should ideally be performed endoscopically and under X-ray screening. Most of the various systems currently available involve sliding a prosthetic tube, carried on a flexible introducer, along a guidewire through the stricture. Alternatively the tube is carried into position on the shaft of the endoscope itself. With experience, successful tube placement should be possible in approximately 95% of cases but there are certain limitations to use of a tube. Tube lie can be a problem. In particular, gross angulation of the lumen through the tumour or an inadequate gut lumen distal to the tube can both impair tube drainage. Tubes are also not well tolerated and there is a real risk of airway compression and pulmonary aspiration if placed close to the cricopharyngeal sphincter. When placed across the cardia, gastro-oesophageal reflux can be troublesome but this should not preclude an attempt at its use (Iftikhar et al 1989). About 25% of patients require tube servicing, usually for food blockage, occasionally for tube displacement and, in long-term survivors, for overgrowth of the tube ends by tumour. All these problems can usually be solved easily by further endoscopic manoeuvres. Although with good aftercare a soft and nutritious diet is possible, it is important to tell patients that the quality of swallowing after intubation is never normal. In cases of dysphagia due to external compression and cases complicated by tracheo-oesophageal fistula, intubation is the treatment of choice. However, for complete occlusion of a large malignant fistula a modified prosthesis may be necessary. The Wilson Cook fistula prosthesis (Fig. 3.1) is a modified tube with a sponge-filled balloon on its shaft which expands and blocks the fistula when positioned correctly (Lux et al 1987). Full expansion of the cuff can be confirmed fluoroscopically. An alternative solution is to wrap a standard tube with several layers of polyvinyl alcohol sponge which swells in situ to occlude the fistula (Robertson & Atkinson 1986).

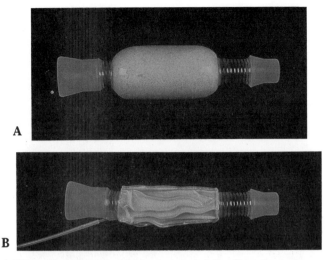

Fig. 3.1   A Wilson Cook fistula prosthesis: **A** expanded; **B** collapsed.

The major benefits of intubation are that it is inexpensive, is accomplished at one treatment session and provides immediate relief of dysphagia. Another merit of intubation is that, when other treatments have failed, intubation usually still remains an option. The major hazard is oesophageal perforation which occurs in about 10% of cases. However, mortality has fallen to under 10% due to prompt diagnosis and treatment with antibiotics, combined with early fine-bore enteral tube feeding until the leak has sealed (Hine & Atkinson 1986). The most recent development in intubation is the introduction of self-expanding metal stents (Fig. 3.2). These should make tube placement technically easier, more comfortable for the patient and safer to perform because of the smaller delivery system with the stent in its collapsed state (Knyrim et al 1991, Kozarek et al 1992). Problems have been reported with tumour ingrowth through the metal mesh but these have been addressed by wrapping the mesh with a silicone membrane (Schaer et al 1992). These stents are expensive but may prove cost effective if fewer admissions are required to maintain swallowing. More long-term data are required (Lightdale 1992).

Laser photocoagulation

Since Fleischer's first description in 1982 of laser therapy to palliate oesophageal cancer (Fleischer et al 1982) it has rapidly become an accepted modality (Bown et al 1987, Krasner et al 1987) (Fig. 3.3). However, the initial high capital cost of a laser has limited its use. Laser recanalization involves vaporizing tumour using the neodymium yttrium aluminium garnet (Nd:YAG laser) Exophytic tumours are more suitable for laser therapy. Sharply angulated tumours at the cardia or near cricopharyngeus are less suitable, as

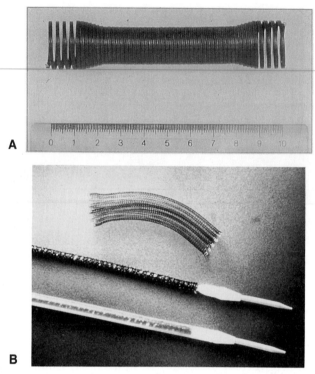

Fig. 3.2   Examples of the new self-expanding metal stents. **B** shows stent with its introducer.

are tumours longer than 6 cm in length (Fleischer & Sivak 1985). Laser therapy was initially described with the laser fibre held away from the tumour surface (non-contact method) but recently probes of sapphire and metal have been developed to concentrate the thermal energy on the tumour (contact method). Using contact probes a lower power of laser light can be used for treatment, thus reducing the risk of perforation.

High-power Nd:YAG laser therapy

A thin quartz fibre fixed in a Teflon catheter transmits the laser light. The catheter also contains a coaxial channel down which a constant jet of gas is passed to keep the tip of the fibre cool and clear by blowing away debris. When the laser is fired any tissues on the fibre tip are instantly coagulated leading to rapid heating which may damage the tip of the probe. Frequent cleansing of the tip is therefore essential and can make prolonged treatment tedious. Typical power settings range from 50 to 100 W and the energy is delivered in 1–2 second pulses from a distance of about 1 cm from the tumour surface. Ideally lasering starts from the distal tumour margin and progresses circumferentially up to the proximal margin. This technique means the

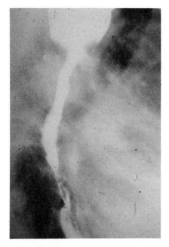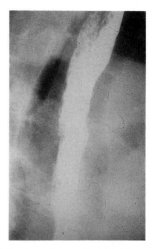

Fig. 3.3 Barium swallow before (left) and after (right) laser therapy for oesophageal cancer.

oesophageal lumen is always in view and should reduce the incidence of perforation.

Low-power contact Nd:YAG therapy

Low-power contact therapy is performed with power settings reduced to 10–20 W. Microendoprobes of varying shapes can be attached to the tip of the quartz fibre and used to burn and cut through tumour. This technique may be especially useful where there is total luminal obstruction when the risk of perforation with the non-contact method is highest. Contact probes produce less smoke and do not have to be carefully cleaned during treatment, but treatment is slower. As yet there is no clear advantage with respect to the number of treatment sessions, relief of dysphagia or complications between the contact and non-contact methods (Ell et al 1986, Radford et al 1989).

A delay of up to 1 week between initial treatment and relief of dysphagia is typical and regrowth of tumour always requires visits for further treatment. Treatment protocols vary between units but a typical regime would be two to three initial treatments in the first week. This rapidly recanalizes the lumen and is followed by monthly assessments with further laser treatment as necessary. Successful palliation is reported in approximately 85% of cases (Overholt 1992). Mild chest pain and a transient pyrexia are common but not usually serious. Perforation and creation of a tracheo-oesophageal fistula are the serious risks which occur in 5–10% of cases, but mortality is less than 5% (Tytgat 1990) which compares favourably with other palliative procedures.

In a prospective non-randomized comparison of laser versus intubation, the palliation of dysphagia was similar for both, but the perforation rate was significantly lower after laser treatment (2% versus 13%). However, laser-treated patients underwent more procedures and therefore had longer overall hospital stays (Loizou et al 1991). This lack of superiority of either technique has been confirmed in other studies (Alderson & Wright 1990, Hahl et al 1991).

In an assessment of quality of life between laser and intubation, both therapies resulted in a significant initial improvement in quality of life which deteriorated in the terminal phase of the disease. There was, however, no statistically significant difference between laser or intubation at any stage of treatment (Loizou et al 1992).

Photodynamic therapy

An area of current interest in laser treatment is photodynamic therapy (PDT). This involves sensitization of a tumour with a substance preferentially retained in malignant tissue — the photosensitizer. In PDT of oesophageal cancer the photosensitizer haematoporphyrin derivative is injected intravenously 48 h prior to endoscopy. At endoscopy the tumour is exposed to light of 630 nm wavelength (red light) from a tunable argon pumped dye laser or a gold metal vapour laser. Necrosis follows damage to the tumour vasculature by cytotoxic singlet oxygen liberated from the activated photosensitizer. The amount of damage produced in PDT is related to the light dose, its wavelength and penetration into the tissues as well as the concentration of the photosensitizer in the tissues. The laser energy is transmitted through a quartz fibre with an end diffuser to distribute the light circumferentially. The fibre is passed under direct vision into the lumen of the tumour and approximately 300 J/cm are delivered starting distally and moving proximally. The total laser light dose for each 2 cm of tumour takes approximately 25 min (Marcon 1993). Movement of the laser tip may occur over this prolonged treatment time so careful endoscopic monitoring is essential. The treatment causes only small elevations in tissue temperature of 2–4°C. At present PDT is of limited clinical use as it is only effective in the treatment of superficial cancers involving the mucosa and submucosa (Kato et al 1986). These early cancers are rare and their selection requires accurate staging, probably best achieved with endoscopic ultrasound. With advanced cancers, tumour necrosis following PDT is incomplete and may be delayed up to 1 week, thus providing poor palliation. There is also a risk of major haemorrhage. Chest pain may occur following the treatment but serious complications such as stricture or perforation rarely occur due to the superficial nature of the treatment. Future developments in PDT are expected when new photosensitizers (e.g. benzoporphyrins or phthalocyanines) are available (Lambert 1992). Their shorter half-life and enhanced concentration in tumours should improve efficacy and safety. All present, patients are instructed to avoid direct sunlight for 1 month to prevent serious sunburn due to the prolonged clearance of the drug.

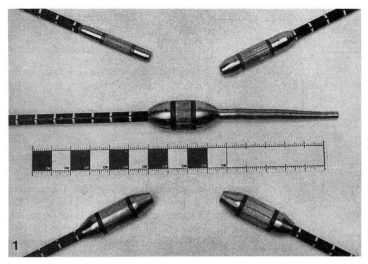

Fig. 3.4   Contact bipolar diathermy probes used for electrocoagulation.

Electrocoagulation with diathermy probes

Electrocoagulation using contact bipolar diathermy probes has been developed to recanalize oesophageal cancers (Johnston et al 1987) as a cheaper alternative to laser. The probes consist of an olive-shaped tip on a flexible insulated shaft (Fig. 3.4). They are passed over an endoscopically placed guidewire and are available with olive diameters from 6 to 15 mm. Pairs of electrodes are arranged longitudinally around the circumference of the olive tip between which current passes and generates heat. One probe in the set has electrodes on only one half of its circumference allowing treatment of non-circumferential tumours. Thermocoagulation can be performed under fluoroscopy but is best performed under direct vision by passing a paediatric endoscope alongside but kept proximal to the probe to avoid damage to the scope (Reilly & Fleisher 1991). This allows accurate positioning of the probe and avoids burning normal tissues. These probes are inexpensive to buy and simple to maintain and use. A recent comparative trial has shown it to be as efficacious and safe as laser treatment (Jensen et al 1988). Comparable results were also found in a comparison with endoscopic intubation (McIntyre et al 1989). This treatment is especially useful for tumours of the upper-third of the oesophagus and cardia sites which would otherwise be a problem to palliate with either tube (Robertson & Morris 1989) or laser (Jensen et al 1988). (Fig. 3.5).

Cytotoxic injection

Tumour necrosis following endoscopic injection of absolute ethanol is the most recently described technique for oesophageal recanalization (Payne-

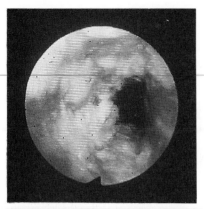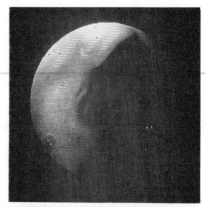

Fig. 3.5 Endoscopic views of an oesophageal cancer before (left) and after (right) bipolar diathermy.

James et al 1990) but to date there have been few publications on its use. Its attraction is that it is a cheap and simple technique only requiring a needle injection catheter. It is probably best suited to polypoid lesions. Endoscopic injection of 5-fluorouracil and the sclerosants 2.5% sodium morrhuate and polidocanol have proven ineffective (Wright & O'Conner 1990, Angelini et al 1991).

POTENTIALLY CURATIVE TECHNIQUES

Radiotherapy

In contrast to endoscopic methods, radiotherapy offers the possibility of inhibiting the local progression of the primary cancer. Traditionally radiation has been given by external beam from a linear accelerator or cobalt source. More recently intracavitary radiotherapy has become available.

The optimum dose for external beam radiotherapy is unknown but the minimum accepted for radical treatment is 5000 cGy and more than 6000 cGy often leads to unacceptable side-effects. Fractionation is safer than a single large treatment dose and gives better treatment tolerance and flexibility. With a daily dose of 200 cGy and five treatments per week, a full course of treatment lasts 5 weeks. It has been estimated that up to 20% of patients are unable to complete a full course of treatment because of poor tolerance (Wara et al 1976). In order to limit side-effects, various treatment techniques are available such as using two or three fields and a split course regimen. A postirradiation stricture and the creation of an oesophagorespiratory fistula are serious complications that may arise. The debilitating effects of radiotherapy may also detract from the quality of life remaining to the patient. To date, there have been no randomized trials of radiotherapy versus surgery in squamous cancer of the oesophagus. Radiotherapy series are biased as most patients have been deemed unfit for surgery making interpretation of the data difficult.

Pearson's survival rates of 44% at 1 year and 22% at 5 years with radiotherapy as the primary treatment of squamous cancers have never been reproduced (Pearson 1966). However, a more recent highly selected series from Manchester reported a 40% 1-year survival and an 8.3% 5-year survival (Slevin & Stour 1989). Unfortunately, there is no information available on the relationship between radiotherapy and the relief of dysphagia which can be quite variable and may take several weeks. For cancer of the cervical oesophagus, radiotherapy is the treatment of choice as pharyngolargyngectomy with its major morbidity can be avoided. Adenocarcinoma of the oesophagus has often been considered radioresistant but there are data showing little difference in survival rates between patients with adenocarcinoma and squamous carcinoma affecting the cardia treated by radiotherapy (Cederquist et al 1978, Earlam and Johnson 1990). This is particularly relevant as adenocarcinoma of the oesophagus and cardia is increasing in incidence (Lund et al 1989).

Intracavitary irradiation (brachytherapy)

Intracavitary irradiation is arousing interest as a result of the development of the Selectron (Nucleotron, Zeersum, The Netherlands), a remote-control afterloading machine which makes the procedure simple and safe (Rowland & Pagliero 1985, Hishikawa et al 1991). The Selectron applicator tube is passed over an endoscopically placed guidewire and positioned across the tumour using fluoroscopy. The applicator is fixed at the mouth and the patient is transferred to a protected treatment room and connected to the Selectron machine. A microprocessor controls the pneumatic transfer of caesium-137 pellets or iridium wire (Burt et al 1989) down a flexible tube inserted into the applicator. The treatment is timed so that 1500 cGy are given. In this situation the treatment is given as a single high-dose fraction to try to obtain rapid palliation. The great merit of brachytherapy is that the radiation dose is highest to the tumour while adjacent normal tissues are relatively spared, although some patients develop a troublesome oesophagitis.

The combination of a lower dose of external beam radiotherapy given with intracavitary treatment is an attractive new development (Montemaggi et al 1991, Agrawal et al 1992), but so far there are few published data on such combinations and no randomized trials. Intubation or intraluminal debulking by endoscopic methods in combination with external beam radiotherapy may also allow prolonged palliation and perhaps longer survival (Sargeant et al 1992) but few data are as yet available (Bown 1991). Oliver et al (1990) made a retrospective comparison of the effect of radiotherapy after the intubation of squamous cancers. There was no significant survival advantage in the group given radiotherapy and they had increased morbidity and a prolonged hospital stay.

The role of radiotherapy in relieving local discomfort from systemic metastases should also not be forgotten.

Chemotherapy and multimodality treatment

A systemic approach to treatment has been advocated as the results of locoregional treatment alone with either surgery or radiotherapy have been disappointing, and autopsy series report high incidences of systemic metastases (Anderson & Lad 1982, Kavanagh et al 1992).

This is the rationale for using chemotherapy, which alone has no place but as part of a multimodal approach combined with either radiotherapy (Coia et al 1988, Gill et al 1990, 1992) or surgery has given encouraging results. Response rates with single agent chemotherapy have been poor but a measurable response rate of 20–30% has been obtained when cyclical combination chemotherapy has been used, with the highest tumour response rates reported for combinations including cisplatin and 5-fluorouracil. Wayne State University in Detroit has recently reported combined chemotherapy (5-fluorouracil cisplatin × 4 cycles) and radiotherapy (5000 cGy) compared with radiotherapy (6400 cGy) alone in patients with either squamous or adenocarcinoma of the thoracic oesophagus (Herskovic et al 1992). One hundred and twenty-one patients were randomized and there was a modest but statistically significant improvement in survival in the combined chemotherapy/radiotherapy group (median survival at 24 months: 8.9 versus 12.5 months; $P < 0.001$), and they developed fewer local and distant metastases. However, this was at the expense of more severe and life- threatening side-effects including the only death in the study. The full treatment regimen was demanding, lasted 100 days and there was no demonstrable improvement in quality of life. The benefits of this form of treatment are therefore still debatable.

The optimal timing of radiotherapy with chemotherapy is not known but some investigators have suggested that induction chemotherapy may be more effective than concomittant treatment. This is because areas of radionecrosis may become sanctuary sites for chemotherapy-resistant tumour cells. In addition, the combined toxic effect of simultaneous treatment may limit the dose of chemotherapy that can be given. This issue has yet to be resolved by clinical trials. Combination chemotherapy is also being given preoperatively but it is not clear in this neoadjuvant setting if patient survival is improved. Results from current randomized trails are awaited.

SUMMARY

Clearly, there are a number of different therapeutic options for the treatment of the obstructed oesophageal lumen. There are also new methods of potentially altering the natural history of the disease. Although such treatment combinations may confer benefit, they must be subjected to the scrutiny of the controlled trial, with objective data being collected on both quality of life and palliation of dysphagia. These unfortunate patients should not be abandoned to therapeutic nihilism.

It must be appreciated that aftercare is also important as recurrent problems with swallowing after all palliative treatments are common. These are not always due simply to mechanical obstruction; they may also arise from recurrent laryngeal nerve palsy (Griffin et al 1992) resulting in aspiration on swallowing and the development of a tracheo-oesophageal fistula.

Treatment is probably best in specialized units with expertise in the full range of therapeutic endoscopy and oesophageal surgery and ready access to radiotherapy and oncology services. It may even be shown eventually that non-surgical treatment can provide a better result, in terms of quality and quantity of life, than attempted curative resection.

KEY POINTS FOR CLINICAL PRACTICE

- Oesophagectomy still offers the best palliation and chance of cure for oesophageal cancer.
- Therapeutic endoscopy to palliate dysphagia is indicated for patients unsuitable for surgery.
- A range of endoscopic techniques should be available as they are often complementary.
- The roles of radiotherapy including brachytherapy and multimodal treatments which include chemotherapy are still not clearly defined.
- Intubation remains the quickest and most versatile endoscopic method to relieve malignant dysphagia.
- In the future, self-expanding metal stents may have an important role.

REFERENCES

Agrawal RK, Dawes PJDK, Clague MB 1992 Combined external beam and intracavitary radiotherapy in oesophageal carcinoma. Clin Oncol (R Coll Radiol) 4: 222–227

Alderson D, Wright PD 1990 Laser recanalisation versus endoscopic intubation in the palliation of malignant dysphagia Br J Surg 77: 1151–1153

Anderson I, Lad T 1982 Autopsy findings in squamous cell carcinoma of the oesophagus. Cancer 50: 1587

Angelini G, Pasini AF, Ederle A et al 1991 Nd:YAG laser versus polidocanol injection for palliation of oesophageal malignancy: a prospective randomised study. Gatrointest Endosc 37: 607–610

Bancewicz J 1990 Cancer of the oesophagus. BMJ 300: 3–4

Bown, SG, Hawes R, Matthewson K et al 1987 Endoscopic laser palliation for advanced malignant dysphagia. Gut 28: 799–807

Bown SG 1991 Palliation of malignant dysphagia: surgery, radiotherapy, laser intubation alone or in combination? Gut 32: 841–844

Burt PA, Notley HM, Stout R 1989 A simple technique for intraluminal irradiation in oesophageal tumours using high dose rate microselectron. Br J Radiol 62: 748–750

Cederquist C, Nielsen J, Berthelsen A et al 1978 Cancer of the oesophagus: II, Therapy and outcome. Acta Chir Scand 144: 233–240

Coia LR, Paul AR, Engstrom PF 1988 Combined radiation and chemotherapy as primary management of adenocarcinoma of the oesophagus and gastro-oesophageal junction. Cancer 61: 643–649

Den Hartog-Jager FCA, Bartelsman JFWM, Tytgat GN 1979 Palliative treatment of oesophago-gastric malignancy by endoscopic positioning of a plastic prothesis. Gastroenterology 77: 1008–1014

Earlam RJ, Johnson L 1990 101 oesophageal cancers: a surgeon uses radiotherapy. Ann R Coll Surg Engl 72: 32–40

Ell B, Hochberger J, Lux G 1986 Clinical experience of non-contact and contact Nd:YAG laser therapy in operable tumour stenoses of the oesophagus and stomach. Lasers in Med Sci 1: 143–146

Fellows IW, Greensmith J, Atkinson M 1984 The nutritional effects of endoscopy intubation for carcinoma of the oesophagus of cardia. Clin Nutr 2: 167–168

Fleischer D, Sivak M Jr 1985 Endoscopic Nd:YAG laser therapy as palliation for oesophagogastric cancer. Gastroenterology 89: 827–831

Fleischer D, Keesler F, Haye O 1982 Endoscopic Nd:YAG laser therapy for carcinoma of the oesophagus: a new palliative approach. Am J Surg 143: 280–283

Gill PG, Jamieson GG, Denham J et al 1990 Treatment of adenocarcinoma of the cardia with synchronous chemotherapy and radiotherapy. Br J Surg 77: 1020–1023

Gill PG, Denham JW, Jamieson GG et al 1992 Patterns of treatment failure and prognostic factors associated with the treatment of oesophageal carcinoma with chemotherapy and radiotherapy either as sole treatment or followed by surgery. J Clin Oncol 10: 1037–1043

Griffin SM, Chung SCS, Van-Hasselt CA et al 1992 Late swallowing and aspiration problems after oesophagectomy for cancer. Malignant infiltration of the recurrent laryngeal nerves and its management. Surgery 112: 533–536

Hahl J, Salo J, Ovaska J et al 1991 Comparison of endoscopic Nd:YAG laser therapy and oesophageal tube in palliation of oesophagogastric malignancy. Scan J Gastroenterol 26: 103–108

Hennessey TPJ, O'Connell R 1986 Carcinoma of the hypopharynx, oesophagus and cardia. Surg Gynecol Obstet 162: 243–247

Herskovic A, Martz K, Al-Sarraf M et al 1992 Combined chemotherapy and radiotherapy compared with radiotherapy alone in patients with cancer of the oesophagus. N Engl J Med 326: 1593–1598

Hine KR, Atkinson M 1986 The diagnosis and management of perforation of oesophagus and pharynx sustained during intubation of neoplastic strictures. Dig Dis Sci 6: 571–573

Hishikawa Y, Kurisu K, Taniguchi M et al 1991 High dose rate intraluminal brachytherapy for oesophageal cancer: 10 years experience in Hyogo College of Medicine. Radiother Oncol 21: 107–114

Iftikhar SY, Robertson CS, Atkinson M 1989 The outcome of palliative endoscopic intubation for adenocarcinoma of the oesophagus and cardia compared with that for squamous carcinoma. Eur J Gastroenterol Hepatol 1: 113–116

Jensen DM, Machilado G, Randall G et al 1988 Comparison of low power YAG laser and Bicap tumour probe for palliation of oesophageal cancer strictures. Gastroenterology 6: 1263–1270

Johnston JH, Fleischer D, Petrini J et al 1987 Palliative bipolar electrocoagulation therapy of obstructing oesophageal cancer. Gastrointest Endosc 33: 349–353

Kato H, Kawaguchi M, Konaka C et al 1986 Evaluation of photodynamic therapy in early gastric cancer. Lasers Med Sci 1: 67–74

Kavanagh B, Anscher M, Leopold K et al 1992 Patterns of failure following combined modality therapy for oesophageal cancer. Int J Radiat Oncol Biol Phys 24: 633–642

Knyrim K, Wagner HJ, Pausch J et al 1991 Expandable metal stents for the palliative treatment of oesophageal obstruction. Gastrointest Endosc 37: A17

Kozarek RA, Ball TU, Patterson DJ 1992 Metallic self-expanding stent application in the upper gastrointestinal tract: caveats and concerns. Gastrointest Endosc 38: 1–6

Krasner N, Barr H, Skidmore C et al 1987 Palliative laser therapy for malignant dysphagia. Gut 28: 792–798

Lambert R 1992 Endoscopic therapy of oesophagogastric tumours. Endoscopy 24: 24–33

Lightdale CJ 1992 Self-expanding metal stents for oesophageal and gastric cancer – a new opening. Gastrointest Endosc 38: 86–87

Loizou LA, Grigg D, Atkinson M et al 1991 A prospective comparison of laser therapy and intubation in endoscopic palliation for malignant dysphagia. Gastroenterology 100: 1303–1310

Loizou LA, Rampton D, Atkinson M et al 1992 A prospective assessment of quality of life after endoscopic intubation and laser therapy for malignant dysphagia. Cancer 70: 386–391

Lund O, Hasenkam JM, Aagaard MT et al 1989 Time-related changes in characteristics of prognostic significance in carcinomas of the oesophagus and cardia. Br J Surg 76: 1301–1307

Lux GD, Wilson J, Wilson L et al 1987 A cuffed tube for the treatment of oesophagobrochial fistula. Endoscopy 19: 28

McIntyre AS, Morris DL, Sloan RL et al 1989 Palliative therapy of malignant oesophageal stricture with the bipolar tumour probe and prosthetic tube. Gastrointest Endosc 35: 531–535

Marcon NE 1993 Photodynamic therapy and cancer of the oesophagus. Acta Gastroenterol Belg 56: 184–191

Montemaggi P, Smaniotto D, Luzi S et al 1991 Combined external radiotherapy and intracavitary radiotherapy in oesophageal carcinoma. Rays 16: 36–41

Muller JM, Erasmi H, Stelzner M et al 1990 Surgical therapy of oesophageal carcinoma. Br J Surg 77: 845–857

Ogilvie AL, Dronfield MW, Ferguson R et al 1992 Palliative intubation of oesophagogastric neoplasms at fibreoptic endoscopy. Gut 23: 1060–1067

Oliver SE, Robertson CS, Logan RFA et al 1990 What does radiotherapy add to survival over endoscopic intubation alone in inoperable squamous cell oesophageal cancer? Gut 31: 750–752

Overholt BF 1992 Laser and photodynamic therapy of oesophageal cancer. Sem in Surg Oncol 8: 191–203

Payne-James JJ, Spiller RC, Misiewicz JJ et al 1990 Use of ethanol induced tumour necrosis to palliate dysphagia in patients with oesophagogastric cancer. Gastrointest Endosc 36: 43–46

Pearson JG 1966 The radiotherapy of carcinoma of the oesophagus and post cricoid region in South East Scotland. Clin Radiol 17: 242–257

Radford C, Ahlquist D, Gostout C et al 1989 Prospective comparison of contact with non-contact Nd:YAG laser therapy for palliation of oesophageal carcinoma. Gastrointest Endosc 35: 394–397

Reilly HF, Fleischer DE 1991 Palliative treatment of oesophageal carcinoma using laser and tumour probe therapy. Gastroenterol Clin North Am 20: 731–742

Robertson CS, Atkinson M 1986 A modified prosthetic oesophageal tube to manage malignant oesophagorespiratory fistulae. Lancet 2: 949–950

Robertson CS, Morris DL 1989 Palliation of malignant upper-third oesophageal stricture by bipolar diathermy probe. Surg Endosc 3: 70–72

Rowland G, Pagliero KM 1985 Intracavitary irradiation in palliation of carcinoma of oesophagus and cardia. Lancet 2: 981–983

Sargeant IR, Loizou LA, Tobias JS et al 1992 Radiation enhancement of laser palliation for malignant dysphagia: a pilot study. Gut 33: 1597–1601

Schaer J, Katon RM, Ivancev K et al 1992 Treatment of malignant oesophageal obstruction with silicone-coated metallic self-expanding stents. Gastrointest Endosc 38: 7–11

Slevin NJ, Stour R 1989 Carcinoma of oesophagus — a review of 108 cases treated by radical radiotherapy. Clin Radiol 40: 200–203

Symonds CJ 1887 The treatment of malignant stricture of the oesophagus by tubage or permanent catheterism. Br Med J 1: 870–878

Tytgat GNJ 1990 Endoscopic therapy of oesophageal cancer: possibilities and limitations. Endoscopy 22: 263–277

Wara WM, Nauch PM, Thomas AN et al 1976 Palliation for carcinoma of the oesophagus Radiology 121: 717–720

Watson A 1988 Surgery for carcinoma of the oesophagus. Postgrad Med J 64: 860–864

Wright RA, O'Conner KW 1990 A pilot study of endoscopic injection chemo-sclerotherapy of oesophageal carcinoma. Gastrointest Endosc 36: 47–48

4

Screening for colorectal cancer

D. H. Bennett   J. D. Hardcastle

The incidence of colorectal carcinoma in England and Wales is increasing, with approximately 18 000 deaths reported in 1992 (Office of Population Censuses and Surveys 1993). Although there has been a 10% improvement in overall survival during the last 20 years (Stower & Hardcastle 1985), prognosis is still chiefly related to the extent of spread of the tumour at the time of diagnosis (Deans et al 1994). The cause of colorectal carcinoma is likely to be multifactorial, and associations have been reported with family history, diet, alcohol and sedentary habits (Weisburger 1991). Failure to define a major primary cause has prevented primary prevention programmes being developed, and attention has therefore focused on screening. The screening process aims, by investigating selected asymptomatic individuals, to detect large adenomas and less advanced cancers, their treatment leading both to a reduction in mortality from colorectal cancer and a decrease in its incidence.

The biology and natural history of the disease form the basis for screening. It is now widely accepted that the majority of colorectal cancers arise from adenomas which, in turn, develop from normal mucosa. Until recently, epidemiological evidence formed the basis of this hypothesis (Burkitt 1974, Morson 1974, Cancer Research Campaign 1988, Pollock & Quirke 1991). However, the advances in molecular biology have now defined many of the genetic mutations associated with each step in the progression from normal mucosa to metastatic carcinoma (Vogelstein et al 1988, Hamilton 1992) and have raised the possibility of genetic screening for individuals at increased risk (Mulcahy & O'Donoghue 1993).

For a screening programme to be successful, (1) the disease in question must be common, (2) a simple, acceptable, sensitive, specific, safe and effective screening test should be available, and (3) accurate and effective investigation and treatment of positive test results should be possible.

TARGET POPULATION

For screening to be effective, it must be offered to those at risk of developing the disease. The incidence of colorectal cancer increases exponentially with age, those over 50 years old making up only 37% of the population yet accounting for 95% of cases and 96% of deaths (Office of Population Censuses and Surveys 1990). Calculations show that a 50-year-old person has a 5% risk of developing colorectal cancer by the age of 80 years and 2.5% risk of dying from it (Boring et al 1993). Therefore, to be cost effective, population screening should be offered to individuals over the age of 50 years.

Ulcerative colitis

Persons at high risk of developing colorectal cancer are shown in Table 4.1.

Table 4.1   Risk factors for colorectal cancer

Chronic ulcerative colitis
Familial adenomatous polyposis
Gardner's syndrome
Turcot syndrome
Hereditary non-polyposis colorectal cancer
Family history
   Colorectal adenomas
   Colorectal cancer
Personal history
   Colorectal adenomas
   Colorectal cancer

The risk of patients with ulcerative colitis developing colorectal carcinoma increases with the duration of the disease and is greater in patience with total or extensive colitis (Greenstein et al 1979). The magnitude of the risk has been difficult to quantify but has been estimated as 7% at 20 years of disease (Lennard-Jones et al 1990), 7–14% at 25 years of disease (Lofberg et al 1990), and as high as 30% after 35 years (Ekbom et al 1990). Colonic surveillance for dysphagia once a year or every 2 years with random biopsies is advocated for this group although the effectiveness of these screening programmes has been questioned recently (Lynch et al 1993a, Sachar 1993).

Inherited risk

Familial adenomatous polyposis (FAP) is an autosomal dominantly inherited syndrome with a near 100% lifetime risk of its carriers developing colorectal cancer. It accounts for approximately 1% of all observed colorectal cancer cases and has a prevalence of 1 in 10 000. The gene responsible for FAP has been identified and is known as the APC gene (adenomatous polyposis coli gene) (Groden et al 1991). Prior to the characterization of this gene, screening affected relatives had entailed annual sigmoidoscopy from puberty to at least 40 years of age before a family member could be considered unaffected. In addition, phenotypic markers such as congenital hypertrophy of the retinal pigment epithelium and mandibular osteomas are also common in this condition and have been used to identify subjects at increased risk of developing FAP. However, genetic probes for the APC gene are now available and genetic screening can exclude the presence of the APC gene in the majority of family members, those with the gene undergoing prophylactic surgery by the age of 20 years.

A second form of hereditary colorectal cancer has been described, hereditary non-polyposis colon cancer (HNPCC) or Lynch syndrome, which accounts for 5–6% of all colorectal cancers (Lynch et al 1993b). Unlike FAP, kindreds have a mean age of diagnosis of 48 years, 67% of first colorectal cancers are proximal to the splenic flexure and metachronous lesions are common (40% at 10 years after the first colorectal cancer diagnosed). Screening in HNPCC kindreds involves colonoscopy of all first-degree relatives, commencing at age 25 years, or 5 years earlier than the earliest colorectal cancer occurrence in that specific family. Colonoscopy is repeated at 2–3-year intervals in patients without neoplasia, whereas those with adenomas undergo annual colonoscopy (Lynch et al 1993b). However, the discovery of the HNPCC gene, hMSH2 (Leach et al 1993), and the development of specific DNA probes means that genetic screening may soon be available for this condition.

Family history

Exclduing the very high risk conditions discussed, the overall relative risk of colorectal cancer for first-degree relatives of patients is between 2 and 4 (Stephenson et al 1991). The risk is greatest for those whose first-degree relatives developed colorectal cancer under the age of 45 years (St John et al 1993a). There is also a threefold increased risk of adenomas developing in relatives of patients with colorectal adenoma or carcinoma (Cannon-Albright et al 1988). As a high proportion of colorectal cancers arising in those with FAP or HNPCC occur in the right colon (Orrom et al 1990), flexible sigmoidoscopy is not appropriate as a screening investigation. However, for those with a familial predisposition at intermediate risk, it is better than faecal occult blood testing alone. A screening protocol has been devised by St Mark's Hospital based on personal risk, calculated according to the family history (Houlston et al 1990). Those with a lifetime risk of 1:10 or greater are offered colonoscopy while lower risk individuals receive annual faecal occult blood tests.

Previous neoplasia

A history of previous colorectal neoplasia increases the risk of developing colorectal cancer. Patients with adenomas have a two- to threefold increased risk of developing malignancy while the risk of metachronous colorectal cancer is 5%. Recent evidence suggests that polypectomy is effective in reducing the incidence of colorectal cancer. The National Polyp Study found a significant reduction in the number of cancers detected amongst a group of

1422 subjects undergoing polypectomy and subsequent colonoscopic follow-up compared with three reference populations (Winawer et al 1993). The Funen Adenoma Follow-up Study, a prospective randomized study of 1056 patients, reported both a reduced incidence and a reduced mortality from colorectal cancer following polypectomy (Jorgensen et al 1993). However, no randomized trials comparing polypectomy with leaving the polyp in situ have been performed and trials comparing their results to reference populations should be interpreted with caution due to the possible introduction of selection bias.

Colonoscopic follow-up after adenoma removal has demonstrated a rate of metachronous lesions of between 20% and 60%, depending on length of follow-up. The timing and frequency of follow-up following polypectomy remains the subject of debate: evidence suggests a recurrence rate of 25–30% with only small polyps, showing mild atypia, recurring at 2-year intervals (Wegener et al 1986). Winawer et al (1993) prospectively compared colonoscopic follow-up at 1 and 3 years with follow-up at 3 years only, and reported that the percentage of patients with adenomas with advanced pathological features (defined as those >1 cm in diameter and those with high-grade dysplasia or invasive cancer) was the same in both groups (3.3%). Risk factors for recurrent polyps are male sex, size of the index polyp, multiple polyps, villous architecture and the presence of severe dysplasia (Stein & Coller 1993).

The current recommendations of the King's Fund Consensus Symposium (King's Fund Centre 1990) are that colonoscopy should be performed every 3–5 years for those under the age of 75 years with large (>1 cm) or multiple adenomas or those exhibiting severe dysplasia. Similar recommendations have recently been published by the American Society for Gastrointestinal Endoscopy and the American Gastroenterological Association (Bond 1993) recommending initial follow-up to be performed at 3 years. After one negative result of a 3-year examination, the interval can be increased to 5 years.

SCREENING TECHNIQUES

Stool tests

Faecal occult blood tests

Although the concept of occult blood detection has existed since 1864, Greegor reintroduced the guaiac test for occult blood in the stool in 1967. While on a high-fibre, meat-free diet, patients were asked to smear two samples of stool per day for 3 days onto a paper slide impregnated with guaiac. Colorectal cancers were detected in several patients at an early pathological stage and this method formed the basis of all future faecal occult blood test studies. The guaiac paper slide test consists of filter paper impregnated with guaiac which undergoes phenolic oxidation in the presence of haemoglobin in the stool and hydrogen peroxide in the test reagent (the most commonly employed test being Haemoccult (Rohm Pharma)).

The basis of the positive reaction is the pseudoperoxidase activity of haematin; haematin interacts with hydrogen peroxide, resulting in phenolic oxidation of the guaiac, changing it to blue. Anything with peroxidase activity — for example, fresh fruit such a bananas and uncooked vegetables such as horseradish and cauliflower — can produce a positive reaction. Agents (such as ascorbic acid) that interfere with the oxidation reaction may produce a false-negative reaction in the presence of haemoglobin. A positive test, therefore, can be the result of: non-haemoglobin peroxidases; animal haemoglobin present in foods such as meat, human haemoglobin lost from benign lesions such as angiodysplasia and diverticular disease or normal conditions, or from neoplastic lesions such as adenomas and cancers. Sufficient quantitites of blood anywhere in the gastrointestinal tract can lead to a positive test.

Total gastrointestinal blood loss in normal individuals is 0.5 ± 0.4 ml/day, quantified by radiochromium labelling (Pierson et al 1961) or haem-porphyrin assay (Schwartz & Ellefson 1985). There is no defined level of bleeding that separates basal from pathological tumour blood loss. Indeed, there is considerable overlap, particularly from left-sided cancers and adenomas (Macrae & St John 1982). Haemoccult will detect losses of 10 ml/day in 67% of cases (Stroehlein et al 1976) and >20 ml/day in 80–90% of cases (Doran & Hardcastle 1982), allowing reasonable test sensitivity without resulting in large numbers of false-positives.

Alternative faecal occult blood tests have subsequently been developed, including more sensitive peroxidase-based tests, immunochemical tests specific for human haemoglobin, and haemporphyrin assays. The more sensitive peroxidase-based tests improve the detection of neoplasia but suffer from the same drawbacks as Haemoccult in terms of false-positive results and therefore have a much lower specificity (Feneyrou et al 1982, Pye et al 1990). HemoQuant, a haem-porphyrin assay based on the fluorescence of haem-derived porphyrins, is a quantitative measure of total blood loss into the gastrointestinal tract. Its advantage is that pseudoperoxidase activity will not affect the assay, but a strict dietary protocol excluding non-human haem and the fact that blood lost anywhere in the gastrointestinal tract is measured detract from its employment. While provisional studies were encouraging (Ahlquist et al 1985), subsequent reports have indicated that it is not suitable for colorectal cancer screening (St John et al 1992).

Immunological tests have the theoretical advantages of (1) avoiding dietary interference by specifically detecting human haemoglobin and (2) decreasing the likelihood of false-positive reactions from upper gastrointestinal bleeding, as the immunologically reactive site will have been lost by digestion by the time the blood reaches the large bowel. A comparison of Haemoccult with an example of each of these new tests has recently been performed, using HaemoccultSENSA (a new guaiac-based test), HemeSelect (an immunological test) and HemoQuant (St John et al 1993b). The sensitivities for these tests in patients with known colorectal malignancies were 94%, 97% and 71% respectively compared with 89% for Haemoccult. This is a high sensitivity for Haemoccult, possibly due to case selection, the majority of studies reporting a sensitivity of approximately 50%. HemeSelect and HaemoccultSENSA were also assessed in 1355 screened subjects, positivity rates being 3% and 5% respectively. Sensitivity data are not available for these cases as follow-up is still too short, but estimated specificities are 97.8% and 96.1% respectively. While these results appear encouraging, it should be noted that small changes in specificity drastically alter the performance of screening tests. A reduction of specificity of 1% may reduce positive predictivity as much as twofold (Morrison 1985) (specificity for Haemoccult is approximately 98%). The study concludes: 'the immunochemical test HemeSelect provides the best combination of specificity and sensitivity'.

Further support for immunological faecal occult blood tests is derived from a study comparing Haemoccult and HemeSelect directly in an asymptomatic population (Robinson et al 1994a). Both tests were completed by 1489 subjects with positivity rates of 1.1% for Haemoccult and 9.7% for HemeSelect. Nine cancers were detected by HemeSelect of which only one was Haemoccult-positive. Similarly, 49 patients with adenomas were identified: 48 were HemeSelect-positive compared to only eight Haemoccult-positive. When Haemoccult and HemeSelect were compared in a high-risk population undergoing colonic surveillance by colonsocopy, the positivity rate was 3.8% and 18.5% respectively (Robinson et al 1994b). While the sensitivity of Haemoccult for cancer was 25% and for neoplasia ≥ 1 cm was 33%, the respective values for HemeSelect were 67% and 45%. While the greater sensitivity of HemeSelect is evident, the much lower specificity results in a considerably increased endoscopic workload. This, together with the greater cost of HemeSelect, means further studies are necessary before the use of either HemeSelect or HaemoccultSENSA can be supported in population screening studies.

Population screening trials using Haemoccult

The first trial to report mortality data was a non-randomized study which systematically assigned participants to screening or control groups (Winawer & Schottenfield 1991). Although there was a 43% reduction in mortality in the screened group after 10 years of follow-up, the study failed to reach statistical significance owing to an inadequate number of deaths from colorectal cancer.

In Germany, a faecal occult blood test was added to the cancer screening programme in 1977, targeted at persons over 45 years of age. A case control analysis of the data compared the percentage of patients who had died of colorectal cancer, and who had completed faecal occult blood tests, with a control group (Wahrendorf 1992). Twenty-nine per cent of women in the control had completed a faecal occult blood test compared to only 16% in the study group, a statistically significant result implying a mortality advantage to those completing a test. However, there was no difference between the two groups for men (13% versus 14%).

Table 4.2   Randomized controlled trials of Haemoccult testing in screening for colorectal cancer. (Reproduced with permission from Bennett & Hardcastle 1994).

	Nottingham England	Goteborg, Sweden	Fuhnen, Denmark	Burgundy, France	New York USA*	Minnesota, USA
Cohort size	155 000	52 000	62 000	94 000	22 000	48 000
Positivity rate (%)	2.1	1.9[†] 5.8[‡]	1.0	2.1	1.7	2.4[†] 9.8[‡]
Compliance (%)	54	65	67	52	75[¶]	90[¶]
Predictive value % for presence of neoplasia	50	22	57	31	30	31
Dukes' A Cancers (%)						
Screened group	52	50	51	52	43	34
Test group	30	30	27	n/a	35	n/a
Control group	13	12	9	n/a	27	35

*Trial included rigid sigmoidoscopy in both arms of trial.
[†]Non-rehydrated Haemoccult slides.
[‡]Rehydrated Haemoccult slides.
[¶]Subjects recruited were volunteers rather than identified from Practice lists and then randomized.

Six prospective randomized trials have been instigated (Table 4.2), of which one has now reported. Three of the European studies have reported interim results. The Swedish trial (Kewenter et al 1988) targeted participants aged 60–64 years and rescreened the test group after a mean interval of 20 months. The test group was further divided such that half the tests were rehydrated. The effect of rehydrating the Haemoccult slides was to increase the positivity rate from 1.9% to 5.8% and to reduce the positive predictive value of the test from 32% to 22%. Of 322 subjects with a positive test, investigation revealed 16 cancers and 58 individuals with one or more adenomas. Rescreening, with a compliance of 58%, revealed 19 cancers and 92 adenomas. In the interim period, 26 cancers presented symptomatically in the screened group and 16 in the control group. Although there was a greater proportion of Dukes' stage A tumours in those screened, there was no statistical difference between the test group as a whole and the control group in the stage of tumour detected, 46% of the test group having stage A or B tumours compared to 40% in the control group. The trial has been extended to 52 000 participants and is due to report in 1995.

The Danish study (Kronborg et al 1989) targeted 45–47 year olds with a mean rescreening interval of 2 years, 93% of those initially screened completing the second test. The first screen detected 37 cancers and 86 adenomas during the investigation of 215 positive tests compared with 13 cancers and 76 adenomas at the rescreen. During the follow-up, 40 interval cases and 39 non-responders presented with a cancer compared with a total of 115 cancers in the control group. The screened group showed a statistically significant earlier Dukes' stage than the controls (59% Dukes' stage A or B compared to 45% respectively). Although there was a trend towards a colorectal cancer-specific reduction in mortality in the screened group, this did not reach statistical significance. The trial is still in progress and further results are awaited.

Table 4.3 Results of the Nottingham screening study

	Initial screen	First rescreen	Second rescreen	Third rescreen	Fourth rescreen
Number offered screening	77 226	46 371	43 727	36 570	10 113
Acceptors	41 114 (54.5%)	32 191 (69%)	26 425 (60%)	18 589 (51%)	5159 (51%)
Tests positive	843 (2.0%)	415 (1.3%)	271 (1.0%)	256 (1.4%)	80 (1.5%)
Neoplastic disease detected					
Carcinomas	89 (2.2/1000)	55 (1.7/1000)	32 (1.2/1000)	38 (2.0/1000)	9 (1.7/1000)
Adenomas	461	199	125	93	61

The largest of the randomized trials is taking place in Nottingham (Hardcastle et al 1989) where 155 034 persons aged 50–74 years have been randomly allocated to test and control groups. Rescreening has been carried out at 2-yearly intervals. The results of the initial screen and subsqent rescreen are shown in Table 4.3. The relatively low compliance rates from the second rescreen onwards reflect the fact that previous non-responders were re-invited to complete Haemoccult tests at this time. For example, compliance with the second rescreen was 88% in previous responders compared to only 13.5% in previous refusers, with an average compliance of 60%.

There were a significantly greater number of screened persons with less advanced tumours than among the controls (56% Dukes'. A or B compared with 46%) and this wa also found to be the case on rescreening (62% Dukes' A or B). This difference in the proportion of less advanced cancers between the screen-detected and control groups accords with the findings of the Danish trial. The Nottingham study also reported fewer emergency procedures, unresectable tumours and fixed tumours in the screened group.

The Minnesota Colon Cancer Control Study (Mandel et al 1993) has reported the first statistically significant reduction in mortality from colorectal cancer by faecal occult blood test screening. The study recruited 48 000 volunteers and assigned them to screening annually, biannually or to a control group. Compliance was higher than in the European studies, attributable to the fact that volunteers rather than the general population were studied. There were 1002 cases of colorectal cancer detected over the 13-year follow-up period and 320 cancer-specific deaths, with a cumulative mortality of 5.88 per 1000 in the annually screened group and 8.33 per 1000 in the biannially screened group compared with the control group rate of 8.83 per 1000. There is thus a statistically significant 33% reduction in mortality in the annually screened group compared with the control gorup. While there is a trend towards a reduction in the biannially screened group, this does not reach statistical significance.

This study is very encouraging for proponents of screening by faecal occult blood testing, but a word of caution is necessary. This study utilized rehydrated Haemoccult slides which, while increasing the sensitivity (92.2%), resulted in a very low specificity (90.4%) relative to non-rehydrated slides (98–99%). The practical effect, as discussed earlier, was a much higher rate of colonoscopy: 38% of the annually and 28% of the biannially screened participants underwent at least one colonoscopy. The financial implications for population screening make it unlikely to be economically feasible at the present time.

The positive predictive value falls significantly if rehydrated Haemoccult slides are used (Table 4.2), with further implications for the cost of diagnostic investigations. Interestingly, using this very sensitive test, there was no significant difference between the number of Dukes' stage A and B tumours detected in the annually screened group compared to the control group and the percentage of Dukes' stage A tumours detected was the lowest of all the trials (Table 4.2).

Albumin

Albumin has been suggested as an alternative faecal marker of colorectal neoplasia, the hypothesis being that, as a relatively low molecular weight protein, it is lost into the gut in situations of tissue or capillary damage. Using filter paper smears of stool, Nakayama et al (1987) described significant differences between faecal albumin concentrations in 45 normal subjects and in ten patients known to have colorectal cancer.

In another study (Thomas 1991), faecal albumin concentrations were determined in 144 asymptomatic subjects prior to colonoscopic investigation of positive faecal occult blood tests. Using a predetermined upper limit of normal (95th percentile), a significantly greater proportion of subjects with cancer or an adenoma were positive for faecal albumin than were normal subjects. Cancer stage and tumour site did not significantly affect the amount of faecal albumin detected. However, it should be noted that by defining the upper limits of normal as the 95th percentile, one implies a 95% specificity which would result in an unacceptable false-positive rate in a screening situation. This may be partly due to selection bias: all the specimens examined had come from patients with a positive faecal occult blood test and it is possible that some of those with false-positive tests are bleeding at the upper range of normal, levels known to encroach into the range of pathological blood loss and to result in positive Haemoccult tests. Alternative plasma proteins, such as α_1 antitrypsin, are presently being evaluated to define their specificity in detecting asymptomatic colorectal neoplasia.

Carcinoembryonic antigen

Evidence in the 1970s (Gold et al 1970) suggested that carcinoembryonic antigen (CEA) was a tumour-specific antigen localized to the colonic cancer cell surface. Faecal expression of CEA might be expected to be raised in patients with colonic neoplasia given the rapid turnover of tumour cells, the surface localization of the antigen and the probability that cells are eroded from the surface of tumours by the passage of stool.

Studies have confirmed that faecal CEA is indeed elevated in patients suffering from colorectal cancer and that the elevated faecal levels do not correlate with either Dukes' stage or serum CEA levels (Elias et al 1973, Fujimoto et al 1979). Thomas (1991) measured faecal antigen levels in 149 asymptomatic subjects and reported that, although absolute levels of faecal CEA were higher in subjects with neoplasia, when a discriminating value (95th percentile) was used to determine the sensitivity of the test, the proportions of subjects with rasied levels was similar in those with cancers, adenomas or normal colons. It seems probable that the normal colonic expression of CEA is responsible for the high levels seen in some individuals and that the normal faecal expression of CEA makes this approach too non-specific to be of value in screening.

Our increasing understanding of the genetic basis of colorectal cancer opens exciting prospects for the future. The demonstration by Sidransky et al (1992) that ki-*ras* mutations can be detected in the stool of patients with colorectal cancer suggests that future stool tets may be directed at detecting the underlying genetic mutations associated with carcinogenesis. Not all colorectal carcinomas and adenomas bleed, a fact which reduces the sensitivity of all occult blood tests, whereas all neoplasms shed cells into the bowel lumen, which should theoretically increase the potential sensitivity of stool genetic tests.

Endoscopy

Rigid sigmoidoscopy

This has not been a popular screening technique due partly to the medical input required and partly to the patient inconvenience and discomfort. In 1960, the results of a uniphase screening programme initiated by the Memorial Sloan-Kettering Hospital were reported (Hertz et al 1960). Cancers were diagnosed in 58 patients out of 26 126 individuals who underwent sigmoidoscopy, a detection rate at the initial screen of 2.2 per 1000. The majority of these tumours were at an early stage and 5-year patient survival was reported as 88%.

In another uncontrolled study, annual proctosigmoidscopic surveillance was performed on 21 000 subjects following a 'clearing' proctosigmoidoscopy (Gilbertson & Nelms 1978). After a mean of 4 years of follow-up, only 13 rectal cancers had been diagnosed compared with an expected 90. The authors concluded that 85% of the expected cancers had been prevented by polypectomy although others have calculated a more modest reduction in incidence (60%) (Neugut & Pita 1988).

More recently, the Kaiser Permanente study of multiphasic health checks reported its results for screening sigmoidoscopy (Selby et al 1988). Existing members of the health care programme were randomized either to receive encouragement to schedule annual health check-ups or to a group who were not so encouraged. For colorectal cancers arising within the reach of the sigmoidoscopy, the actively encouraged group had both a lower cumulative incidence (4.3 versus 6.7 cases per 1000 persons) and a better stage distribution (86% versus 54% stage B or better) than the non-encouraged controls. These results should be interpreted with caution, however, as all those involved were already part of a health care programme and the results may not be extrapolatable to the general population. In addition, there was only a 5% difference between the two groups in their exposure to sigmoidoscopy, too small a difference to account for the variation noted in incidence.

Previous exposure to sigmoidoscopy was also examined in a retrospective case-controlled study (Selby et al 1992) in which patients who had died of colorectal cancer were compared to a general population sample. Over 24% of the control group had undergone sigmoidoscopy in the preceding 10 years compared to only 8.8% of those who had died of colorectal cancer, suggesting screening by rigid sigmoidoscopy reduces the risk of developing colorectal cancer within the reach of the sigmoidoscope within the next 10 years by over two-thirds. The design of this study has been criticized, with selection bias of the case group argued to account for the difference. However, the study contains its own control in that tumours above the reach of the sigmoidoscope were also reported and they occurred with equal frequency in the two groups.

Additional evidence for the benefit of proctosigmoidoscopy was provided by St Mark's Hospital, London (Atkin et al 1992). The long-term risk of colorectal cancer in 1618 men and women who had had adenomas removed via the sigmoidoscope was analyzed and, although more than half the patients had either died or reached the upper age limit for the study of 86 years, only 14 (0.9%) had developed rectal cancer. It was calculated that a minimum of 80 rectal cancers were expected, suggesting that at least 85% of rectal cancers had been prevented by adenoma removal.

Flexible sigmoidoscopy

The rigid instrument is limited by its length, average depth of insertion being only 17 cm (Wilking et al 1986), allowing, at best, visualization of 40% of all colorectal cancers. The development of the 65 cm flexible sigmoidoscope has focused attention on this technique as a possible alternative to either rigid sigmoidoscopy or faecal occult blood testing. Following a simple enema, it enables examination of the distal 60 cm of the colon, where 70% of cancers and large adenomas are found (Kronborg et al 1989, Hardcastle et al 1989). Furthermore, Gillespie et al (1979) reported that 94% of polyps containing malignancy were located distal to the splenic flexure, within reach of the flexible endoscope. It is better tolerated than rigid sigmoidoscopy (Wilking et al 1986) although it is also more expensive. The logistic problem of population screening by this technique may be overcome by training nurses or general practitioners as endoscopists, and a European randomized trial of flexible sigmoidoscopic screening is currently in progress to assess the additional benefit of adding sigmoidoscopy to faecal occult blood testing alone.

It has been suggested that combining flexible sigmoidoscopy with a faecal occult blood test would result in a more realistic sensitivity for the detection of colorectal neoplasia in a screening programme. Indeed, 15 or 22 interval cancers presenting in the Nottingham screening study were in the rectum and sigmoid colon; if these cases had been detected by flexible sigmoidoscopy at the time of screening, the sensitivity of combined faecal blood testing and sigmoidoscopic screening would have been 93% — a gain of 18% over the sensitivity of Haemoccult alone.

An alternative suggestion for population screening is for a single flexible sigmoidoscopy examination at age 55–60 years with appropriate colonic surveillance for the 3–5% found to have high-risk adenomas (Atkin et al 1993). The authors calculated that a single flexible sigmoidoscopy at 55–60 years would prevent 70% of distal colorectal cancers occurring up to age 75 years and 50% of cancers occurring between 75 and 79 years. This would equate to prevention of about 3500 colorectal cancer deaths per year and an increase in life-expectancy of 7 years for each case prevented. It is likely that a prospective randomized trial will be instigated based on these calculations although mortality data would not be available from such a trial for approximately 15 years.

Colonoscopy

Colonoscopic investigation of the large bowel is the most sensitive technique of evaluation. However, it is labour-intensive, expensive and has a serious complication rate (perforation and haemorrhage) of 0.2% (Macrae et al 1993), precluding its use as a population screening test. It remains the surveillence technique of choice in high-risk individuals, particularly those with FAP,

HNPCC or chronic ulcerative colitis. It is also becoming increasingly the method of choice in relatives of patients, particularly when more than one first-degree relative is affected. The ability to perform snare polypectomy or biopsy at the same time as diagnosis makes it particularly suited for the investigation of individuals with a positive faecal occult blood test.

KEY POINTS FOR CLINICAL PRACTICE

- A significant amount of time and money has been spent evaluating screening programme for colorectal cancer. The results show that screening by Haemoccult is feasible and interim results are encouraging. For the first time a randomized trial has shown a reduced mortality by faecal occult blood test screening and the reports of the European trials are anticipated in the near future. However, Haemoccult testing remains relatively insensitive and detects well below the estimated prevalence of neoplasms.
- The newer faecal occult blood tests suggest that the sensitivity can be improved, but it remains to be seen whether the results of the small studies performed to date can be duplicated on a larger scale. The incorporation of flexible sigmoidoscopy is attractive due to its high sensitivity, but screening is a delicate balance between, amongst other factors, test sensitivity and patient compliance. Whether the introduction of sigmoidoscopy into the screening protocol will result in an unacceptable decrease in compliance is still to be evaluated.
- The way forward lies in developing a test which is more sensitive yet as specific as Haemoccult, investigating methods of improving patient compliance and calculating the cost as well as the benefits of population screening.

REFERENCES

Ahlquist DA, McGill DB, Fleming JL et al 1985 Fecal blood levels in health and disease: a study using HemoQuant. N Engl J Med 312: 1422–1428

Atkin WS, Morson BC, Cuzick J 1992 Long-term risk of colorectal cancer after excision of rectosigmoid adenomas. N Engl J Med 326: 658–662

Atkin WS, Cuzick J, Northover JMA et al 1993 Prevention of colorectal cancer by once-only sigmoidoscopy. Lancet 341: 736–740

Bond JH 1993 Polyp guideline: diagnosis, treatment and surveillance for patients with nonfamilial colorectal polyps. Ann Intern Med 199: 836–843

Bennett DH, Hardcastle JD 1994 Screening for Colorectal Cancer. Postgrad Med J 70: 470

Boring CC, Squires TS, Tong T 1993 Cancer statistics, 1993. CA 43: 7–26

Burkitt DP 1974 Epidemiology of cancer of the colon and rectum. Cancer 28: 3–13

Cancer Research Campaign 1988 Facts on cancer. Mortality in the UK Cancer Research Campaign, London

Cannon-Albright LA, Skolnick MH, Bishop DT et al 1988 Common inheritance of susceptibility to colonic adenomatous polyps and associated colorectal cancers. N Engl J Med 319: 533–537

Deans GT, Patterson CC, Parks TG et al 1994 Colorectal carcinoma: importance of clinical and pathological factors in survival. Ann R Coll Surg Engl 76: 59–64

Doran J, Hardcastle JD 1982 Bleeding patterns in colorectal cancer: the effect of aspirin and implications for faecal occult blood testing. Br J Surg 69: 711–713

Ekbom A, Helmick C, Zack M et al 1990 Ulcerative colitis and colorectal cancer: a population based study. N Engl J Med 323: 1288–1293

Elias EG, Holyoke ED, Ming Chu T 1973 Carcinoembryonic antigen in faeces and plasma of normal subjects and patients with colorectal cancer. Disc Colon Rectum 17: 38–41

Feneyrou B, Bories P, Pomier-Layrargues G et al 1982 Discrepancy in results from three guaiacum resin tests. Br Med J 284: 235–236

Fujimoto S, Kitsukawa Y, Itoh K 1979 Carcinoembryonic antigen in gastric juice or faeces as an aid in the diagnosis of gastrointestinal cancer. Ann Surg 189: 34–38

Gilbertson VA, Nelms JM 1978 The prevention of invasive cancer of the rectum. Cancer 41: 1137–1139

Gillespie PE, Chambers TJ, Chan K et al 1979 Colonic adenomas: a colonoscopic survey. Gut 20: 240–245

Gold P, Krupev J, Ansari H 1970 Position of the carcinoembryonic antigen of the human digestive system in ultrastructure of tumour cell surface. J Natl Cancer Inst 45: 219–225

Greegor DH 1967 Diagnosis of large bowel cancer in the asymptomatic patient. JAMA 201: 943–945

Greenstein AJ, Sachar DB, Smith H et al 1979 Cancer in universal and left-sided ulcerative colitis: factors determining risk. Gastroenterology 77: 290–294

Groden J, Thliveris A, Samowitz W et al 1991 Identification and characterisation of the familial adenomatous polyposis coli gene. Cell 66: 589–600

Hamilton SR 1992 Molecular genetics of colorectal carcinoma. Cancer 70: 1216–1221

Hardcastle JD, Thomas WM, Chamberlain J et al 1989 Randomised, control trial of faecal occult blood screening for colorectal cancer: results for first 107,349 subjects. Lancet 1: 1160–1164

Hertz REL. Deddish MR, Day E 1960 Value of periodic examinations in detecting cancer of the colon and rectum. Postgrad Med 27: 290–294

Houlston RS, Murday V, Harocopos C et al 1990 Screening and genetic counselling for relatives of patients with colorectal cancer in a family history clinic. Br Med J 301: 366–368

Jorgensen OD, Kronborg O, Fenger C 1993 The Funen Adenoma Follow-up Study. Incidence and death from colorectal carcinoma in an adenoma surveillence program. Scand J Gastroenterol 28: 869–874

Kewenter J, Bjork S, Haglind E et al 1988 Screening and rescreening for colorectal cancer. Cancer 62: 645–651

King's Fund Centre 1990 Cancer of the colon and rectum; the seventh King's Fund consensus statement. Br J Surg 77: 1063–1065

Kronborg O, Fenger C, Olsen J et al 1989 Repeated screening for colorectal cancer with faecal occult blood test. Scand J Gastroenterol 24: 599–606

Leach FS, Nicolaides NC, Papadopoulos N et al 1993 Mutations of a *mutS* homolog in hereditary nonpolyposis colorectal cancer. Cell 75: 1215–1225

Lennard-Jones JE, Nelville DM, Morson BC et al 1990 Precancer and cancer in extensive ulcerative colitis: findings among 401 patients over 22 years. Gut 31: 800–806

Lofberg R, Brostrom O, Karlen P et al 1990 Colonoscopic surveillance in long-standing total ulcerative colitis: a 15 year follow-up study. Gastroenterology 99: 1021–1031

Lynch DAF, Lobo AJ, Sobala GM et al 1993a Failure of colonoscopic surveillance in ulcerative colitis. Gut 34: 1075–1080

Lynch HT, Symrk TC, Watson P et al 1993b Genetics, natural history, tumour spectrum and pathology of hereditary nonpolyposis colorectal cancer: an updated review. Gastroenterology 104: 1535–1549

Macrae FA, St John DJB. 1982 Relationship between patterns of bleeding and Haemoccult sensitivity in patients with colorectal cancers or adenomas. Gastroenterology 82: 891–898

Macrae FA, Tan KG, Williams CB 1983 Towards safer colonoscopy: a report on the complications of 5000 diagnostic or therapeutic colonoscopies. Gut 24: 376–383

Mandel JS, Bond JH, Church TR et al 1993 Reducing mortality from colorectal cancer by screening for faecal occult blood. N Engl J Med 328: 1365–1371

Morrison AS 1985 Screening in chronic disease. Oxford University Press, New York

Morson BC 1974 Evolution of cancer of the colon and rectum. Cancer 34: 845–849

Mulcahy HE, O'Donoghue DP 1993 Molecular biology. Setting the stage in colorectal cancer? Gut 34: 1476–1477

Nakayama T, Yasuoka H, Kishino T 1987 Enzyme linked immunosorbent assay of human faecal occult albumin. Lancet 1: 1368–1369

Neugut AI, Pita S 1988 Role of sigmoidoscopy in screening for colorectal cancer: a critical review. Gastroenterology 95: 492–499

Office of Population Censuses and Surveys 1990 Mortality statistics 1988, Series DH2, 15. HMSO, London

Office of Population Censuses and Surveys 1993 Mortality statistics 1992. Personal communication

Orrom WJ, Brzezinski WS, Weins EW 1990 Hereditary and colorectal cancer: a prospective, community-based, endoscopic study. Dis Colon Rectum 33: 490–493

Pierson RN, Holt PR, Watson RM et al 1961 Aspirin and gastrointestinal bleeding: chromate 51 blood loss studies. Am. J Med 31: 259–265

Pollock AM, Quirke P 1991 Adenoma screening and colorectal cancer. Br Med J 303: 3–4

Pye G, Jackson J, Thomas WM et al 1990 Comparison of Coloscreen Self-test and Haemoccult faecal occult blood tests in the detection of colorectal cancer in symptomatic patients. Br J Surg 77: 630–631

Robinson MHE, Marks CG, Farrands PA et al 1994a Population screening for colorectal cancer: Comparison between a guaiac and immunological faecal occult blood test. Br J Surg 81: 448–451

Robinson WHE, Williams CB, Hardcastle JD 1994b Surveillance of those at high risk of colorectal cancer using an immunological faecal occult blood test. (in press)

Sachar DB 1993 Clinical and colonoscopic surveillance in ulcerative colitis: are we saving colons or saving lives? Gastroenterology 105: 588–597.

St John DJB, Young GP. McHutchison JG et al 1992 Comparison of the specificity and sensitivity of Haemoccult and HemoQuant in screening for colorectal neoplasia. Ann Intern Med 117: 376–382

St John DJB, McDermott FT, Hopper JL et al 1993a Cancer risk in relatives of patients with common colorectal cancer. Ann Intern Med 118: 785–790

St John DJB, Young GP, Alexeyeff MA et al 1993b Evaluation of new occult blood tests for detection of colorectal neoplasia. Gastroenterology 104: 1661–1668

Schwartz S, Ellefson M 1985 Quantitative faecal recovery of ingested haemoglobin-heme in blood: comparison by HemoQuant assay with ingested fish and meat. Gastroenterology 89: 19–26

Selby JV, Friedman GD, Collen MF 1988 Sigmoidoscopy and mortality from colorectal cancer: the Kaiser Permanente multiphasic evaluation study. J Clin Epidemiol 41: 427–434

Selby JV, Friedman GD, Quesenberry CP et al 1992 A case-control study of screening sigmoidoscopy and mortality from colorectal cancer. N Engl J Med 326: 653–657

Sidransky D, Tokino T, Hamilton SR et al 1992 Identification of *ras* oncogene mutations in the stool of patients with curable colorectal timours. Science 256: 102–105

Stephenson BM, Finan PJ, Gascoyne J et al 1991 Frequency of familial colorectal cancer. Br J Surg 78: 1162–1166

Stein BL, Coller JA 1993 Management of malignant colorectal polyps. Surg Clin North Am 73: 47–66

Stower MJ, Hardcastle JD 1985 The results of 1115 patients with colorectal cancer treated over an 8-year period in a single hospital. Eur J Surg Oncol 11: 119–123

Stroehlein JR, Fairbanks VF, McGill BD et al 1976 Haemoccult detection of faecal occult blood quantitated by radioassay. Am J Dig Dis 21: 841–844

Thomas WM 1991 Faecal screening tests for colorectal carcinoma. University of Nottingham, UK DM Thesis

Vogelstein B, Fearon ER, Hamilton SR et al 1988 Genetic alterations during colorectal-tumour development. N Engl J Med 319: 525–532

Wahrendorf J, Robra BP, Wiebelt H et al 1993 Effectiveness of colorectal cancer screening: results from a population-based case-control evaluation in Saarland, Germany. Euro J Cancer Prev 2: 221–227

Wegener M, Borsh G, Schmidt G 1986 Colorectal adenomas: distribution, incidence of malignant transformation and rate of recurrence. Dis Colon Rectum 29: 383–387

Weisburger JH 1991 Causes, relevant mechanisms and prevention of large bowel cancer. Semin Oncol 18: 316–336

Wilking N, Petrelli NJ, Herrera-Ornelas L et al 1986 A comparison of the rigid proctosigmoidoscope with the 65 cm flexible endoscope in the screening of patients for colorectal cancer. Cancer 57: 669–671

Winawer SJ, Schottenfeld BJ 1991 Colorectal cancer screening. J Natl Cancer Inst 83: 243–253

Winawer SJ, Zauber AG, Ho MM et al 1993 Prevention of colorectal cancer by coloroscopic polypectomy. N Engl J Med 329: 1977–1981

Winawer SJ, Zauber AG, O'Brien MJ et al 1993 Randomized comparison of surveillance intervals after colonoscopic removal of newly diagnosed adenomatous polyps. N Engl J Med 328: 901–906

5

Penetrating chest injury

S. S. Ashraf, G. Grötte

Penetrating chest injury (PCI) can be defined as trauma in which the primary injury produces an open communication between the intrathoracic contents and the environment.

It is important after basic resuscitative measures to determine the mode of injury (stab or missile wound), the location (central wound or peripheral wound) and the degree of haemodynamic instability. Patients present with a wide spectrum of cardiopulmonary instability, from those requiring simple observation to those requiring life-saving thoracotomy. The management of such patients starts at the scene of the incident where basic resuscitative measures are undertaken, including securing an airway, intravenous access and fluid replacement if, and as, required. The patient must then be rapidly transported to a nearby hospital. En route, the two major complications that must be addressed immediately are a 'sucking chest wound' and 'tension pneumothorax' (Jacobs et al 1984). Sucking chest wounds are hazardous if they are greater than two-thirds of the tracheal diameter, since air will preferentially enter the wound and the pleural space instead of the trachea. As a result, ventilation can be severely compromised. Such a wound should be sealed off with an airtight occlusive dressing.

Tension pneumothorax should be decompressed by means of a large bore (14 gauge) intravenous cannula in the affected side at the second intercostal space, midclavicular line, or in the fourth or fifth interspace, between the mid- and anterior axillary lines.

Modes of PCI

These can be divided into stab wounds, free missile wounds, impalement.

Stab wounds

These are more commonly seen and tend to be less severe. The damage is due to the disruption of tissues in the path of the blade. The penetrating object should not be removed until the patient is in the operating theatre.

Missile wounds

These can be subdivided as follows:

Gunshot wounds.   These tend to be more severe than stab wounds. The mechanism of injury depends upon the velocity of the bullet:

- < 300 m/s (e.g. plastic bullets). These crush and lacerate tissue in the pathway. Their pathway may be erratic and may be deflected off bone.
- > 300 m/s causes cavitation of tissues surrounding the tract of the bullet. The cavitation may be 10–30 times the size of the bullet.
- > 770 m/s causes shock waves upon impact, thus imparting a 'blast-like' injury.

The kinetic energy (KE) of the bullet transferred to the body is given by

$$KE = m(V1 - V2)^2$$

where m is mass of the bullet, $V1$ is impact velocity and $V2$ is exit velocity. Thus the kinetic energy of a hunting rifle is more than that of a magnum, which in turn is more than that of a 38 calibre handgun.

The amount of destruction is determined by a variety of other factors:

- Flight pattern of the bullet.
- Surface area of impact: a large surface area causes a quicker deceleration and thus a quicker loss of entry.
- Type of tissue injured. The specific gravity of a tissue, if high, implies an increased energy of absorption and thus more damage. The specific gravity of bone, liver and muscle is more than that of the lung.
- The distance between the assailant and victim. It is worth remembering that, as a bullet goes through a tissue, foreign material may get sucked into the tract.

Shotgun wounds.   These generally behave like low-velocity handgun wounds of less than 3 yards. They cause massive soft tissue destruction. A chest X-ray can identify the position of the pellets.

Fragments of bomb casing and shrapnel.

Fragments from structures nearby in a blast injury.   These require early surgical debridement. If the missile is small enough, it may penetrate vessels and can embolize (Shannon 1987).

Impalements

These fall into two categories: true impalements, where a patient is attached to a relatively immovable or non-transportable object, and retained foreign bodies such as a knife. In cases of true impalement, part of the object must be detached to allow patient transport (Hyde et al 1987). More commonly, the patient arrives with a knife or other object still protruding from the chest.

Unless the patient is in cardiorespiratory arrest and the object precludes resuscitation, removal should take place in the operating room. If the patient's condition permits, a radiograph should be obtained before transferring the patient to the operating theatre. This can be helpful in defining organ proximity or penetration and thus the best surgical approach for removal (McGill 1986).

ASSESSMENT OF THE PATIENT

In general, assessment and management should proceed simultaneously.

Penetrating chest injury may be just one component of multiple injury. What has to be decided is if any additional injuries (abdominal, head) are more life-threatening than those to the chest. The patient should be disrobed and a survey made. The mode of PCI should be established, looking for the position, direction and exit points. The size of the wound is important.

The organ affected in PCI is most rapidly assessed by the position of the entry/exit point which can be central or peripheral. Central injuries are bounded superiorly by the sternal notch and clavicles, laterally by midclavicular lines and inferiorly by the central margin and xiphisternum. Peripheral injuries lie either side of these boundaries. It must be remembered, however, that the trajectory of the penetrating object can extend from central to peripheral areas and vice versa. The peripheral and central areas can be further subdivided into superior and inferior regions by a line running between the nipples and below the tip of the scapula, which delineates the position of the diaphragm and thus the position of the abdominal and thoracic cavities. Centrally located injuries are likely to result in serious injury since they involve the mediastinal structures. Thoracic injuries at the level of the diaphragm may extend into the liver, stomach and the spleen and vice versa.

GENERAL PRINCIPLES OF MANAGEMENT

After a swift assessment of the patient, basic resuscitative measures of airway, breathing and circulation maintenance must be implemented as, and when, required. One should have a high index of suspicion of complicating pneumothorax (especially tension pneumothorax), haemothorax and pericardial tamponade, and treat these accordingly. A chest X-ray and arterial blood gases should be performed as soon as possible. Ideally, the chest X-rays should be erect posteroanterior and lateral views, but in many cases this is impractical, and so an anteroposterior supine film will suffice. However, an anteroposterior view may cause apparent mediastinal widening and obscure haemothoraces.

Most cases (80–85%) of PCI are dealt with by fluid resuscitation, insertion of a chest drain, adequate analgesia and physiotherapy, whilst under stringent observation. However, 15–20% of PCI will require surgical intervention

(Ivatury et al 1987), be it life-saving resuscitative thoracotomy in the accident and emergency department or later in the operating theatre.

Management of the stable patient

Stable patients with central penetrating chest injury may provide additional time for diagnostic investigations. The patient's clinical condition and wound location will guide the mode and extent of investigation (Mandal & Oparah 1989, Richardson et al 1981).

In the author's opinion, two-dimensional bedside echocardiography is a good tool for diagnosing or excluding pericardial tamponade, or valvular and septal injuries of the heart (Reid et al 1987). Suspected injuries to the great vessels should be confirmed or excluded by means of angiography. Whenever there is clinical and radiological evidence of major airway injury, bronchoscopy is indicated. In penetrating central chest injury, CT (computed tomography) scan of the thorax has proved to be fruitless unless there is associated head or abdominal injury (Brooks & Olson 1989). It must be stressed that, during these investigations, the stable patient may rapidly deteriorate and necessitate urgent surgical intervention. Mattox et al (1989) advocate a median sternotomy in all cases of central penetrating chest trauma with suspected vascular injury, without prior diagnostic evaluation. This is because they have experienced some false negative angiograms. However, the author believes that whilst investigating one should have a low threshold for surgical intervention of penetrating central chest injury.

Management of unstable patient

Unstable patients are those who remain moribund despite elementary resuscitative measures. They may require urgent resuscitative thoracotomy in the emergency department. This procedure most benefits those who arrive at the hospital with some sign of life.

Patients who arrest at the scene of the incident, or en route, have a very poor prognosis (Feliciano et al 1986, Baxter et al 1988, Borlase et al 1989, Ivatury et al 1991). The following are indications for emergency department resuscitative thoracotomy:

1. Acute pericardial tamponade which is unresponsive to external cardiac massage.
2. Exsanguinating, uncontrollable, intrathoracic haemorrhage.
3. Massive intraabdominal haemorrhage, where aortic cross-clamping and intraaortic transfusion facilitates preferential resuscitation of the brain and myocardium and arrest abdominal bleeding.
4. Unresponsive, external cardiopulmonary resuscitation, necessitating internal cardiac massage.

Mortality is quite high in emergency room thoracotomy. Different authors have quoted different figures: e.g. Mandal & Oparah (1989) report 70% mortality.

There is a further group of patients who, after basic resuscitative measures, become stable but deteriorate during observation. These patients require elective thoracotomy in the sterile atmosphere of the operating theatre. Indications for elective thoracotomy are as follows:

1. If initial chest drain insertion yields 1500 ml of blood immediately, or there is loss of blood of more than 200 ml/h for the next 4 h. However, these criteria are subject to much variation from author to author and no universal algorithm has yet been developed.
2. Large unevacuated clotted haemothorax (to expand the underlying lung and prevent empyema or fibrothorax) (Coselli et al 1984, Milfield et al 1978). Enzymatic breakdown of the clot has not always been successful.
3. Developing cardiac tamponade.
4. Chest wall defects in which there has been loss of chest wall substance produced by high-velocity missile, close-range shotgun and blast injury.
5. Massive air leak when pneumothorax persists despite adequate drainage. This suggests major bronchial or tracheal injury. Bronchoscopy should precede the thoracotomy to confirm the diagnosis.
6. Proven great vessel injury by means of arteriography.
7. Proven oesophageal injury.
8. Lacerated diaphragmatic injury.
9. Traumatic septal and/or valvular injury of the heart. These injuries can present insidiously and should be confirmed by echocardiography and cardiac catheterization.

COMPLICATIONS IN THE MANAGEMENT OF PCI

There are four common complications which need to be addressed immediately in the management of the PCI: hypovolaemic shock, pneumothorax, haemothorax and pericardial tamponade.

Pneumothorax and haemothorax

In a penetrating chest injury coexisting pneumothorax and haemothorax are the most common complications. The chest wall usually seals small objects such as stab wounds and most bullet wounds, but this is frequently not the case with large defects such as shotgun blasts which is the true example of sucking chest, or open chest injury. An open chest wound which exceeds the laryngeal cross-sectional area will produce complete collapse of the lung and shifting of the mediastinum with each respiratory effort. This will result in hypoventilation and diminished cardiac output. Management is by occlusive dressing and chest drainage. This is followed by reconstruction.

Tension pneumothorax

This is produced when the injury to the lung results in a continuing air leak which progressively allows air to accumulate in the pleural space. After the involved lung has completely collapsed, further accumulation of air results in positive intrapleural pressure. This will shift the mediastinal structures away from the involved side and produce partial collapse of the contralateral lung. Clinical features include weak pulse, low blood pressure, displaced trachea, severe inspiratory distress and elevated jugular venous pressure (unless the patient is hypovolaemic). Tension pneumothorax is a true surgical emergency, which requires immediate relief with a 16 gauge needle before confirmation by chest X-ray.

Haemothorax

This is a common sequela of both penetrating and blunt chest trauma. In both types of injury, the incidence of isolated haemothorax is 20–30% (Weill 1982, Trunkey & Lewis 1985). The pleural cavity has a potential volume of 2–3 litres. On a plain erect X-ray a haemothorax of 250–400 ml is indicated by blunting of the costophrenic angle, whereas on a supine chest X-ray a collection of up to 1 litre may be missed. Slightly increased opacity of one lung field may be the only clue. Opacification is more obvious on lateral decubitus films.

In 90–95% of cases the source of bleeding is systemic vessels (intercostal or internal mammary). Pulmonary vasculature is involved in 5–10% of cases (Trunkey & Lewis 1985). Blood loss from a pulmonary laceration normally stops when the lung re-expands; in contrast, bleeding from the aorta and hilar vessels is usually massive and rapidly fatal. In the majority of cases, insertion of a chest drain is the only treatment required (Swan 1980, Weill 1982). This encourages lung expansion which helps arrest the bleeding, and decreases the chances of empyema formation. Chest drainage is an important determinant of the patient's progress and the need for surgery. Indications for thoracotomy have already been mentioned.

Technique of chest drain insertion (Fig. 5.1)

Since the insertion of a chest drain plays a central role in the management of penetrating chest trauma, it is important that we review the principle of the procedure. Unless tension pneumothorax is suspected, a chest X-ray should be performed prior to its insertion. The site of insertion is at the midaxillary line, between the fourth and sixth intercostal spaces, with the corresponding arm abducted to widen the intercostal spaces. The skin, intercostal muscles and parietal pleura are infiltrated with 20 ml of 1% lignocaine.

A 2-cm incision in the skin and subcutaneous fat is made, using blunt dissection with forceps and finger to make a tract through the intercostal

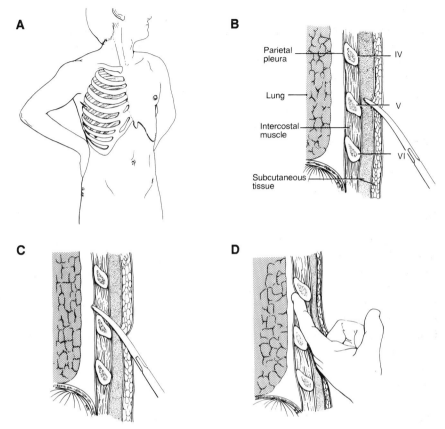

Fig. 5.1 Insertion of a chest drain. **A** Incision over intercostal space. **B** Development of subcutaneous tract. **C** Penetration of parietal pleura. **D** Digital confirmation that the lung is not adherent to chest wall at puncture site.

muscles, along the upper border of the rib and through the parietal pleura. A chest drain of at least size 28 is inserted, ensuring that the sharp metal point of the trocar is not used to cut or separate the tissue. It is a fallacy that the drain must be in a basal position to drain blood and in an apical position to drain air. Always apply negative pressure of 15–20 cm H_2O to the chest drain to ensure evacuation of continued haemorrhage or air leak. The position and effect of the drain must be reassessed by repeat chest X-ray.

Autotransfusion

A brief discussion of autotransfusion seems appropriate in conjunction with the topic of haemothorax. Autotransfusion is an excellent alternative to homologous blood for many reasons. The problems of delay in transfusion, incompatibility of blood, spread of communicable diseases and hypothermia are solved. Salvaged blood has higher levels of 2,3-Diphosphoglycerate (Young and Purcell 1983) and the labile coagulation factors (Jacobs & Hsich 1984). It also has some disadvantages: lower fibrinogen level, increased risk of haemolysis and subsequent renal failure. There are two basic types of autotransfusion. The simplest type captures shed blood in a device that can serve as a transfusion vehicle, allowing reinfusion of the blood.

The other device, which is more complex, washes and concentrates the blood. This requires a set-up time and a technician to operate. Compared to a simple device, the complex one is more expensive to purchase and can only be used in the operating room, whereas the simple device can be deployed in the accident and emergency department.

Pericardial tamponade

This is one of the major complications of penetrating chest trauma, affecting the central area, in which there is a haemopericardium of sufficient degree to compromise passive filling during diastole, resulting in diminished cardiac output. In this syndrome, the classical signs may not always be present: hypotension, venous distension and muffled heart sounds (collectively known as Beck's triad — seen in only 40% of cases) and pulsus paradoxus. However, hypovolaemia may mask any increase in central venous pressure.

The initial chest X-ray may show a classical 'globular heart'. One should be wary of apparent mediastinal widening due to anterior–posterior magnification. Management of tamponade depends upon the haemodynamic stability of the patient. The unstable patient may require urgent emergency room thoracotomy, whereas a stable patient may provide further time for diagnostic confirmation. In the emergency setting, pericardiocentesis as a diagnostic procedure is diminishing in popularity, due to over 33% false negative or false positive results (Trinkle 1979).

Two-dimensional bedside echocardiography is reported to have 96% accuracy, 97% specificity and 90% sensitivity (Reid 1987) in the diagnosis of tamponade secondary to cardiac injury in a stable patient. In these patients diagnosis of cardiac injuries must be made expeditiously to prevent sudden deterioration. It has the advantage of being non-invasive, can be performed in the accident and emergency department and is easily interpreted by trained staff.

Subxiphoid pericardiotomy, as both a diagnostic and a therapeutic technique, has been recommended by many authors (Trinkle 1979, Arom 1977). Through a small subxiphoid incision, the diaphragm is elevated, the diaphragm and pericardium are entered in the midline and the tamponade is decompressed. This procedure should only be performed when facilities for immediate median sternotomy are available, since relief of a tamponade may be followed by rapid exsanguination. Subxyphoid pericardiotomy has its greatest value as a diagnostic procedure in the patient who does not have any actual intrapericardial injury.

Cardiac injury

The fraction of patients reaching hospital alive has been subject to much variation, ranging from 15% to 50% (Attar 1991). The determinants appear to be: mode of penetrating chest injury, speed of hospitalization, and early implementation of life-support measures.

The incidence of penetrating cardiac injuries appears to be rising, presumably because of an increase in civilian violence (Symbas 1976). Improvements in the prehospital phase of trauma management and more rapid transport of patients from the scene of injury may have contributed to a greater number of patients reaching hospital alive.

The most common sites of cardiac penetration, in order of prevalence, are: right ventricle, left ventricle, right atrium (McGill et al 1986, Mandal & Oparah 1989). The consequences of penetrating trauma to the heart naturally depend on the structure involved: damage to the chamber of the heart or coronary vessels will result in a spectrum in which the extremes are tamponade or haemorrhage. Tamponade is more likely to occur in small vents such as stab wounds, since this results in the pericardial laceration sealing up with clots and adjacent fat. Rapid haemorrhage is more likely to occur if the pericardial wound is so large that it cannot seal, e.g. shotgun wounds. Generally speaking, tamponade carries a better prognosis than frank haemorrhage (Attar 1991). Less commonly the valves and septum can be involved.

Surgical treatment of cardiac injuries

The incision of choice in relatively unstable patients is left anterolateral thoracotomy, through the fifth intercostal space (Fig. 5.2). This incision can be extended to the right pleural cavity transternally.

After opening the pericardium anterior to the phrenic nerve, a tamponade may be relieved and if necessary internal cardiac massage commenced. To maximize perfusion to the brain and myocardium, the descending thoracic aorta can be cross-clamped. Recently, median sternotomy has become more favoured since this provides excellent exposure of the heart and great vessels. This incision can be extended into a midline laparotomy for suspected abdominal damage. However, median sternotomy does not provide good exposure for posterior mediastinal structures. All active haemorrhage should be controlled by digital pressure. Atrial, aortic and pulmonary artery lacerations are clamped, and the defect is closed by buttressed sutures, with or without Teflon pledgets (Figs 5.3, 5.4). For ventricular laceration, horizontal buttressed mattress sutures using Teflon pledgets are most useful (Fig. 5.6). Sutures should extend 5–8 mm from the laceration and should be tight enough to control bleeding and yet not cut through the myocardium. Large wounds may need digital pressure to the inferior or superior vena cava to control input to the heart, thus decompressing it whilst one or two mattress

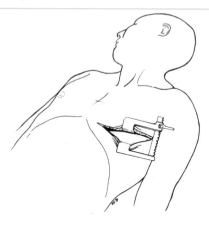

Fig. 5.2   Emergency room thoracotomy through the fifth intercostal space.

sutures are placed. These cardiac and vascular repairs are best carried out whilst the patient is slightly hypotensive since increasing the blood pressure will worsen the bleeding. Lacerated major coronary arteries should be ligated at both ends followed by coronary artery bypass graft with extra circulation.

Once the patient is haemodynamically stable, the chest should not be closed until one is satisfied that there is no further bleeding and the threat of valvular or septal defect has been excluded.

Tracheobronchial injury

Penetrating trauma to major airways can be the result of a central chest wound and more commonly neck wound involving the cervical trachea (Pate & Casini 1989). One must exclude injury to related structures, particularly the oesophagus. The non-specific presentation includes cough, haemoptysis, dyspnoea, stridor, voice impairment and frothy bleeding at the site of the wound. Other manifestations of injury distal to the main bronchi include pneumothorax (if the pleura is torn), pneumomediastinum (if the pleura is intact) and subcutaneous emphysema. The most common presentation of major airway injury is persistent air leak and failure in lung re-expansion, despite the insertion of a chest drain. The unstable patient with intratracheobronchial haemorrhage will require immediate endotracheal

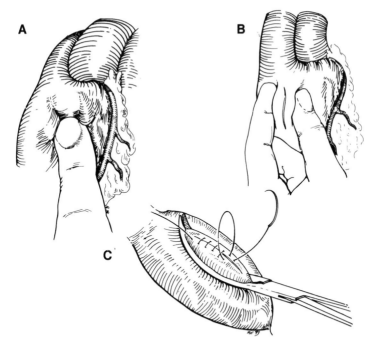

Fig. 5.3 Control of haemorrhage from an injury to the right atrium. **A** Control of haemorrhage by digital pressure. **B** Control of haemorrhage by pinching right atrium between index finger and thumb. **C** Application of curved vascular clamp.

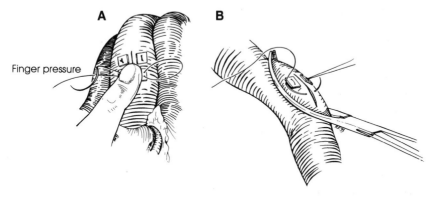

Fig. 5.4 Control of haemorrhage and repair of injured aorta. **A** Temporary control of bleeding from a penetrating injury to aorta. Buttressed sutures are used to close defect. **B** Application of curved vascular clamp. Closure as in **A**.

intubation with direct visualization of the vocal cords. If this is not feasible, one should proceed to tracheostomy. The site and extent of the airway injury can cautiously be assessed by fibreoptic bronchoscopy, bearing in mind that it does carry a risk of a false negative result.

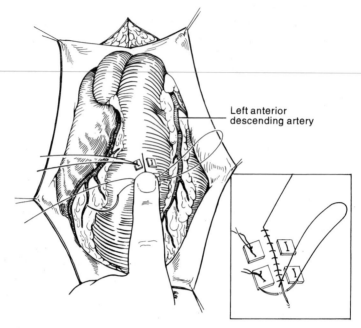

Left anterior
descending artery

Fig. 5.5   Digital control of bleeding and repair of right ventricular wall. Plegeted sutures in buttressed form are used.

If the patient's general condition allows, rigid bronchoscopy is preferable. Anterior tracheal wounds of less than half the tracheal circumference are treated by direct primary closure. Larger anterior wounds and all posterior wounds require debridement prior to repair. Extensive tracheal injury may be managed by resection of two to four rings and re-anastomosis with absorbable sutures. The mortality of cervical tracheal injury is greater than that of intrathoracic injury (Kelly et al 1985, 1987). The overall mortality of tracheobronchial injury is around 30%.

Pulmonary parenchymal injury

The major problems of pulmonary parenchymal injury are haemopneumothorax and haemorrhage. The management depends largely upon the mode of penetrating chest injury: 90% of stab wounds (Mandal & Oparah 1989) and 70% of low-velocity missile wounds can be dealt with by insertion of a chest drain and analgesia. High-velocity (770 m/s) penetrating chest injury requires exploration with resection of lacerated areas of lung and vascular repair, particularly of the hilar structure (which occurs in 20% of penetrating chest injuries).

One of the most dramatic but rarer complications of pulmonary and tracheobronchial injury is air embolism (Graham 1977). It occurs when airway and vascular injury coexist, giving rise to neurological signs (loss of consciousness, seizures, confusion) and cardiovascular features (due to air in the coronary artery). Treatment consists of cardiopulmonary resuscitation, positioning the head lower than the trunk and the injured lung below the left atrium. Surgical intervention to control the source of air embolism is the ultimate treatment.

Oesophageal injuries

Recently, the increased use of firearms has caused an increase in oesophageal injury, particularly cervical. Almost always there is associated injury to neighbouring vascular and tracheobronchial structures. Presentation is usually insidious and non-specific, including subcutaneous emphysema, pneumomediastinum and pleural effusion, which later becomes empyemic. Food particles may be noticed in the chest drain. Diagnosis is confirmed by a combination of gastrograffin oesophagography and oesophagoscopy, since individually they give false negative results (White 1992). Once the diagnosis is made, insertion of a chest drain is mandatory to limit empyema formation. A wide variety of surgical techniques are the definitive treatment. Prognostically, treatment within 12-16 h yields the most favourable result (Nesbitt 1987). Overall mortality is approximately 15–30%.

Great vessel injuries

Victims of major thoracic vascular injury usually exsanguinate at the scene. Penetrating injuries to the innominate subclavian system that do not sustain prehospital arrest have a good prognosis, with a survival rate of up to 85% (Mandal 1989).

Many patients with profound vascular injury will require immediate thoracotomy; those who are in a stable condition with equivocal features will need confirmatory angiography. Most intrathoracic great vessel injuries can be surgically approached through a median sternotomy, except for those of the descending thoracic aorta which necessitate left posterolateral thoracotomy.

KEY POINTS FOR CLINICAL PRACTICE

- There is an increasing incidence of penetrating chest injury as society becomes more violent.
- Recent guidelines described in ATLS (Advance Trauma Life Support) have resulted in a significant improvement in the understanding of penetrating chest injury.
- In patients with central chest injury, the threshold for immediate surgical intervention should be lower than for those with peripheral chest injury.
- Emergency room thoracotomy can be a life-saving procedure in unstable patients.

- All attendant medical staff should feel confident in carrying out thoracotomy if, and when, indicated.

ACKNOWLEDGEMENT

I am indebted toMr T. Malik for the careful preparation of the manuscript.

REFERENCES

Arom KV, Richardson VD, Webb G et al 1977 Subxyphoid poicardial window in patient with suspected traumatic pericardial tamponade. Ann Thorac Surg 23: 545

Attar S, Suter CM, Hankins JR et al 1991 Penetrating cardiac injuries. Ann Thorac Surg 51: 711–716

Baxter BT, Moore EE, Moor JB 1988 Emergency department thoracotomy following injury. Critical determinants for patient salvage. World J Surg 12: 671–675

Borlase BC, Moore EE, Moore FA 1989 Penetrating wound to the posterior chest. Analysis of urgent thoracotomy and laparotomy. J Emerg Med 7: 445–447

Brooks AP, Olson LK 1989 Computed tomography of the chest in the trauma patient. Clin Radiol 40: 127–132

Coselli JS, Mattox KL, Beal AC Jr 1984 Re-evaluation of early evacuation of clotted haemothorax. Ann J Surg 184: 786–790

Feliciano DV, Bitondo CG, Cuse PA 1986 Liberal use of emergency center thoracotomy. Ann J Surg 152: 654–657

Graham JM, Beal AC Jr, Mattox KL et al 1977 Systemic air embolism following penetrating trauma to the lung. Chest 72: 449–454

Hyde MR, Schmidt CA, Jacobson JG 1987 Impalement injuries to the thorax as a result of motor vehicle accidents. Ann Thorac Surg 43: 189–190

Ivatury RR, Nallathambi MN, Roberge RJ et al 1987 Penetrating thoracic injuries. Infield stabilization vs prompt transport. J Trauma 27: 1066–1073

Ivatury RR, Kazigo J, Rohman M et al 1991 Directed emergency from thoracotomy: a prognostic requisite for survival. J Trauma 31: 1076–1081

Jacobs LM, Hsich JWA 1984 A clinical review of autotransfusion and its role in trauma. JAMA 251: 3283–3287

Jacobs LM, Sinclair A, Beiser A 1984 Prehospital advanced life support: benefits in trauma. J Trauma 24: 8–13

Kelly JP, Webb WR, Moulder PV et al 1985 Management of airway trauma I: Tracheobronchial injuries. Ann Thorac Surg 40: 551–553

Kelly JP, Webb WR, Moulder PV et al 1987 Management of airway trauma. II: Combined injuries of trachea and oesophagus. Ann Thorac Surg 43: 160–164

McGill JW, Moore EE, Marx JA 1986 Successful management of cardiac impalement. The result of an integrated EMS-trauma system. J Trauma 26: 702–705

Mandal AK, Oparah SS 1989 Unusually low mortality of penetrating wounds of the chest. J Thorac Cardiovasc Surg 97: 119–125

Mattox KL, Bickell WH, Pep PE et al 1989 Prospective MAST study in 911 patients. J Trauma 29: 1104–1112

Milfield DJ, Mattox KL, Beal ACJ 1978 Early evacuation of clotted haemothorax. Ann J Surg 136: 686–692

Nesbitt JC, Sawyers JL 1987 Surgical management of oesophageal perforation Am Surg 53: 183–91

Pate JW, Casini MC 1989 Penetrating wounds of the neck: Explore or not? Ann Surg 46: 38

Reid CL, Kawaniski DT, Rahimtoola SH 1987 Chest trauma: evaluation by two-dimensional echocardiography. Ann Heart J 113: 971–976

Richardson JD, Flint LM, Snow NJ 1981 Management of trans-mediastinal gun shot wounds. Surgery 90: 671–676

Shannon JJ, Rich NM, Stanton PE Jr 1987 Peripheral arterial missile embolization: a case report and 22 years literature review. J Vasc Surg 5: 773–778

Swan KC, Swan RC 1980 Gunshot wounds. Physiology and management. Little, Maine PSG, Publishing

Symbas PN 1976 Cardiac trauma Am Heart J 92: 387

Trinkle JK, Richardson JD, Fraz JL et al 1979 Management of affairs of the wounded heart: penetrating cardiac wounds. J Trauma 19: 467–471

Trunkey DD, Lewis FR (eds) 1985 Current therapy of trauma, 1984–1985. BC Decker, Philadelphia

Weill PH 1982 The management of traumatic haemothorax. Wien Klin Wochenschr 94: 176–177

White RK, Morris DM 1992 Diagnosis and management of oesophageal perforations Am Surg 58: 112–119

Young GP, Purcell TB 1983 Emergency autotransfusion. Ann Emerg Med 12: 180–186

6

Management of advanced breast cancer

I. S. Fentiman

Benign breast problems and operable cancers form most of the workload for surgeons with an interest in breast diseases. However, there is still a significant number of women who present with advanced breast cancer or who relapse after primary treatment. For these patients treatment is often multidisciplinary, but there are certain important contributions a surgeon can make to their management.

It would be hoped that breast screening would reduce the proportion of patients with advanced disease, but unfortunately those who decline the offer of screening are also those more likely to present with advanced breast cancer. In the Edinburgh breast cancer screening pilot project it was found that of those women who declined the offer of screening and who subsequently went on to develop breast cancer, 50% of these had either stage III or stage IV disease (Roberts et al 1990).

As more women are given appropriate adjuvant therapy so there will be fewer cases which relapse, although those who do relapse may have more aggressive disease which is less likely to be responsive to treatment and thus carry a worse prognosis (Rubens et al 1994).

The aim of treatment in early breast cancer is to maximize the chances of cure of the disease. For patients with advanced or relapsed breast cancer cure is not a realistic hope at present and thus the intention would be to palliate the patient's symptoms, balancing efficacy of treatment with toxicity in order to attain optimal quality of life.

Patients with locally advanced breast cancer comprise a heterogeneous group, some of whom have rapidly evolving inflammatory disease with diffuse enlargement, peau d'orange and erythema, and others who have, for a variety of reasons, delayed before seeking medical help. Thus some of these may have relatively indolent disease. Other unlucky women may be those who did not present with localized hard lumps and thus were not aware of the presence of diffuse carcinoma until it was beyond hope of local treatment.

STAGING OF ADVANCED BREAST CANCER

A variety of systems have been derived for the staging of locally advanced breast carcinoma, but the main ones now in use are the Manchester, Columbia Clinical Classification and UICC/AJC systems. These are illustrated in Fig. 6.1. In the Manchester system stage III carcinoma is divided into 3A in which there is skin involvement by the primary tumour, and 3B in which the tumour is fixed to the chest. The Columbia Clinical Classification has five criteria of inoperability: peau d'orange, skin ulceration, chest wall fixation, axillary nodes >2.5 cm in diameter or fixed axillary lymph nodes. In the UICC/AJC classification stage 3A is based on size of primary tumour and/or nodal involvement, whereas stage 3B comprises any patient with T4 disease (tumour >5 cm diameter) but without metastases or those with fixed nodal involvement with or without T4.

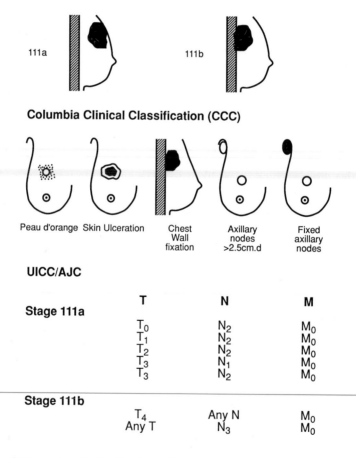

Fig. 6.1 Staging systems for locally advanced breast cancer.

Inflammatory breast cancer

This particular aggressive disease variant was first described by Lee & Tannenbaum in 1924 and since that time has been recognized as carrying a particularly poor prognosis. The diagnosis is clinical and the signs are an increase in size of the affected breast, diffuse induration, skin erythema and peau d'orange. Not all of these features will necessarily be present. Haagensen reported in his series of patients with inflammatory breast carcinoma that 57% had a breast mass, 57% had skin erythema, 48% breast enlargement, 29% pain in breast/nipple, 16% breast tenderness, 16% generalized breast hardness, 13% nipple retraction, 13% skin oedema, 9% axillary mass, 8% warmness of the skin (Haagensen 1971). The mean duration of symptoms in such cases was 2.5 months.

Because these signs may be mimicked by non-malignant inflammatory conditions, it is essential that a cytological or histological diagnosis be made to confirm the nature of the lesion before instigating treatment. Although a skin biopsy may show the presence of dermal lymphatic obstruction by tumour this is not invariable and thus breast rather than skin biopsy is usually the best way of making the diagnosis.

A recent review of treatment of modalities for inflammatory breast carcinoma showed that the 5-year survival after either radical or simple mastectomy was less than 10% (Jaiyesimi et al 1992). The addition of radiotherapy to surgery reduced the rate of local relapse, but did not have any impact on survival, the mean survival time being 18 months. This type of disease tends not to be hormonally sensitive and in a series of five patients with inflammatory breast carcinoma, treated with tamoxifen, none responded (Veronesi et al 1981). For these reasons combined management with chemotherapy and local treatment is now usually recommended. Usually anthracycline-containing chemotherapy is given in an attempt to induce a response which is then followed by radiotherapy or occasionally surgery. With such approaches a 5-year disease-free survival of 22–48% has been reported (Jaiyesimi et al 1992).

Non-inflammatory stage III breast carcinoma

The mainstay of treatment for locally advanced breast cancer has been external radiotherapy. Data are now available from prospective randomized trials which have examined the value of additional systemic therapy. The EORTC Breast Cancer Cooperative Group conducted a trial, EORTC 10792, in which patients with locally advanced carcinoma of the breast were randomized to either radiotherapy alone, radiotherapy and endocrine therapy, radiotherapy and chemotherapy, or radiotherapy chemotherapy and endocrine therapy (Rubens et al 1989). Chemotherapy comprised cyclophosphamide, methotrexate and fluorouracil (CMF); endocrine therapy was ovarian ablation in the premenopausal women and tamoxifen in post-menopausal women.

There were 363 evaluable patients in this factorial 2×2 trial and it was found that time to first progression was delayed significantly by either endocrine or chemotherapy with the greatest effect in those who received both endocrine and chemotherapy. However, the major impact of therapy was on local control with only a non-significant trend towards a reduction in distant metastases in those receiving systemic therapy. A recent analysis of this trial reveals that endocrine therapy, but not chemotherapy, has had a significant effect on prolonging survival (Rubens, 1994).

In an Austrian trial patients with T3 and T4 disease were treated by either pre- and postoperative chemotherapy or pre- and postoperative radiotherapy (Rainer 1993). Those who did not respond to preoperative chemotherapy were then crossed over to postoperative radiotherapy. Chemotherapy consisted of fluorouracil, methotrexate, cyclophosphamide, vincristine and mitozantrone plus tamoxifen. There was a similar remission rate of 60% for both treatment arms. Relapse-free survival and overall survival were improved significantly among those who received chemotherapy. For those who responded to chemotherapy the overall survival was 79% compared with only 24% for the non-responders. Among those who were treated with radiotherapy the overall survival was only 25%. Wound healing was impaired after mastectomy in 36% of those who received preoperative chemotherapy and in 47% of those who had preoperative radiotherapy.

Thus it would appear that local treatment alone with surgery and radiotherapy is inadequate and to improve local control and have some impact on distant recurrence it is necessary to use systemic therapy. Balancing toxicity of this treatment against benefits in terms of local relapse-free survival and distant relapse-free survival will require further investigation in prospective randomized trials.

For some patients who have troublesome local relapse of disease after combined chemotherapy and radiotherapy the surgeon may be able to salvage the local problem by performing a mastectomy. Because of skin involvement it can be necessary to take an extensive area of skin so that primary closure, even after undercutting the edges, may be impossible; under these circumstances skin cover can be achieved with either a split skin graft or with a rotational myocutaneous flap.

The better option is a rotational flap either based on latissimus dorsi and subscapular vessels (which is almost invariably viable), or using transverse rectus abdominis and the superior epigastric pedicle, which is more precarious and likely to lead to complications.

As a second best a split skin graft may be used. This is more problematic, does not achieve a good cosmetic result and does not withstand subsequent radiation, if necessary. Nevertheless, where there is doubt about the margins of excision, or for the surgeon who has not been trained to perform rotational flaps, it will provide some, albeit suboptional, skin cover.

RELAPSE AFTER ADJUVANT TREATMENT

Meta-analysis of trials of adjuvant therapy has shown that in women given tamoxifen there is a greater effect on local relapse (8.3%) than on mortality (3.6%) at 5 years. However, by 10 years the effects are almost equal (6.6% versus 6.2%) (EBCTG 1992). Similarly, for premenopausal women given adjuvant chemotherapy the 5-year effect was greater on relapse than survival (9.2% versus 3.3%), but similar at 10 years (8.4% versus 6.3%).

Recently, the International Breast Cancer Study Group reanalysed first relapse data from a series of adjuvant trials which they had conducted (Goldhirsch et al 1994). Treatments were divided into those that were more effective and less effective. When women who received the more effective treatments were compared with those given less effective therapy the relapse rate fell from 36% to 18% at 10 years. However, bone and visceral deposits occurred with equal frequency (18%) in those given either more effective or less effective treatments. Thus the major impact of adjuvant therapy appears to be improvement of local control with little impact on development of metastatic disease in bone or viscera, which had been present either at the time of diagnosis or possibly as the result of manipulations at the time of first treatment.

Prior adjuvant systemic therapy may also have an impact on response to subsequent systemic therapy after relapse has occurred (Rubens et al 1994). Thus when patients given adjuvant CMF were compared with untreated controls the response to subsequent CMF was 23% in the former group compared with 47% among those who had received no prior adjuvant chemotherapy (Houston et al 1993). Similarly, in trials comparing tamoxifen with no treatment and giving tamoxifen at the time of relapse there was a reduced response rate in those given prior tamoxifen (14% versus 54%) (Fornander et al 1987). However, prior treatment with tamoxifen does not appear to influence response to chemotherapy at the time of relapse (Rubens et al 1994).

A scheme for the management of relapse after adjuvant chemotherapy is given in Fig. 6.2. If the relapse is locoregional the first treatment would usually be tumour excision when technically possible followed by radiotherapy if there is doubt about the completeness of excision and when the area has not been irradiated previously. For those who develop distant recurrences the disease-free interval is an important indicator of the aggressiveness of the disease. If the disease-free interval is 2 years or more, and providing the disease is not life-threatening, it is worthwhile giving a trial of endocrine therapy which would comprise ovarian radiation or oophorectomy for those still menstruating and tamoxifen for the postmenopausal. Gonadotrophin releasing hormone analogues or tamoxifen are also reasonable alternatives for premenopausal patients. Should the interval be less than 2 years it is unlikely that there will be response to endocrine therapy, but this may still be tried in those in whom there is no life-threatening disease present. If the recurrence is imminently

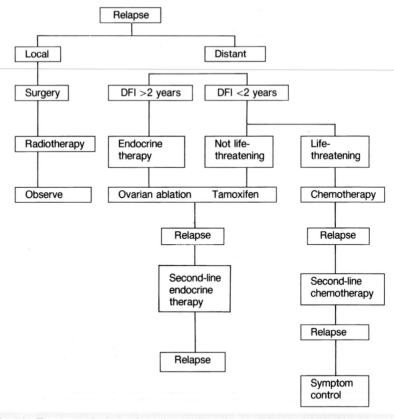

Fig. 6.2   Treatment of relapse after adjuvant chemotherapy. DFI, disease-free interval.

life-threatening, such as lymphangitis carcinomatosa, liver metastases or brain secondaries, such patients are usually given chemotherapy.

The majority of patients who relapse after adjuvant therapy will have received or been taking tamoxifen; a management scheme for these patients is given in Fig. 6.3. If the relapse occurs more than 1 year after stopping adjuvant tamoxifen, providing it is not life-threatening, tamoxifen may be given again or alternatively second-line endocrine therapy such as aminoglutethimide, formestane (4-hydroxyandrostenedione), megoestrol, or medroxyprogesterone acetate.

If the disease has recurred in less than 1 year or while taking tamoxifen, second-line endocrine therapy should be tried in those who do not have life-threatening metastases. However, if hepatic or lymphangitic pulmonary disease is present, chemotherapy should be instigated and providing that there is a response then second-line chemotherapy can be given when subsequent relapse occurs. Non-responders to first- or second-line chemotherapy will have disease whose behaviour is unlikely to be affected by remaining toxic chemotherapy regimens. Under these circumstances the main aim of

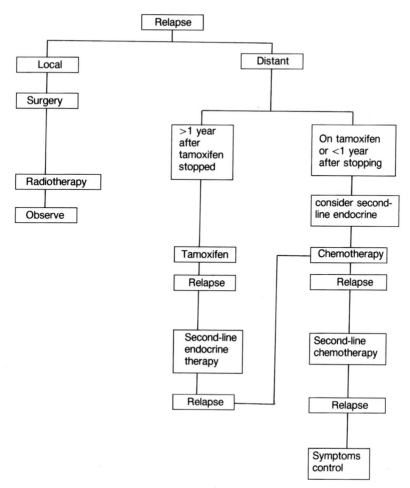

Fig. 6.3   Treatment of relapse after adjuvant tamoxifen.

treatment should be the palliation of symptoms rather than attempting to destroy tumour cells.

In patients whose advanced disease responds to chemotherapy the optimal duration of treatment is unknown, but 6 months is reasonable. Prolonging the course of chemotherapy leads to more toxicity, but has no impact on survival (Harris et al 1990). Thus there is no place for maintenance chemotherapy in those who have had a complete remission of disease.

SPECIFIC PROBLEMS IN ADVANCED DISEASE

Bone metastases

Up to 30% of patients who develop a relapse of breast carcinoma will have bone metastases. For women with metastatic disease this will eventually affect the bone in up to 70% of cases (Coleman et al 1987). Some of these metastases will be asymptomatic; bone secondaries can produce pain, pathological fracture, spinal cord compression and hypercalcaemia.

There is no value in carrying out routine bone scans on asymptomatic women being followed-up after treatment for breast cancer (Kagan et al 1991). However, patients complaining of skeletal symptoms should have these areas X-rayed together with a radioisotopic bone scan to determine the extent of metastases, if present. Treatment of localized painful lesions is usually by external radiotherapy in order to relieve pain and prevent further bone destruction.

Lytic bone metastases in weight-bearing bones such as the femur require careful evaluation to determine how extensive the cortical damage is since some will benefit from prophylactic pinning followed by radiotherapy in order to prevent pathological fractures. In women with only a few bone secondaries, after pain relief has been achieved and reversal of osteolysis has been obtained by radiotherapy, there is little evidence to support changing systemic treatment.

However, there is evidence that subsequent progression of bone metastases can be reduced with bisphosphonates. In a Finnish study 34 women with multiple metastases and who were normocalcaemic were randomized to receive either disodium dichloromethylene diphosphonate (clodronate) 1600 mg/day, or placebo for between 3 and 9 months (Elomaa et al 1983). Hypercalcaemia developed in four of the placebo group and in only one of the treated patients. New bone metastases occurred in 11 out of 17 (65%) of those given placebo and three out of 17 (18%) of the group treated with clodronate.

In a larger study, 173 patients who had bone metastases from breast cancer were treated with oral clodronate (85 patients) at a dose of 1600 mg/day, or given placebo (88 patients) (Paterson et al 1993). Those given clodronate had significantly fewer hypercalcaemic episodes (33% versus 59%). Additionally, vertebral fractures were less common in the treated group (84 versus 124 per 100 women years). Furthermore, the total number of skeletal events, new metastases or fractures was reduced by clodronate from 252 down to 168 per 100 women years. There were no differences in terms of side-effects and no significant differences in survival of the two groups.

Thus there is a place for clodronate in the palliation of women with bone metastases, or in those who have relapsed and are at increased risk of development of bone secondaries from breast cancer.

Brain metastases

This type of relapse can be particularly distressing and usually carries a poor prognosis. Presenting symptoms include headache, nausea and vomiting fits, paresis and incoordination. Clinical examinations may reveal evidence of papilloedema with localized central nervous system signs. Immediate treatment is reduction in cerebral oedema using steroids (dexamethasone 4 mg four times daily). Confirmation of the diagnosis and extent of intracranial disease is usually by computed tomographic scan.

Treatment is by cranial irradiation and a short course is as good as more prolonged treatment. Only under very exceptional circumstances is surgery indicated to remove an isolated cerebral metastasis. Occasionally, carcinomatous meningitis may occur, causing symptoms of confusion, headache and either nerve root pain or cranial nerve palsies. Such cases respond to radiotherapy but the place for intrathecal chemotherapy is controversial.

Vertebral bone metastases may cause spinal cord compression giving rise to back pain, girdle pain and either limb weakness or bladder dysfunction. The diagnosis can be confirmed by magnetic resonance imaging. After initial steroids, radiotherapy is the main treatment, although surgical decompression and spinal stabilization may be indicated for limited deposits.

Pleural effusions

Pleural effusions are a common problem in patients with metastatic breast cancer. In a series of 105 patients treated at Guy's Hospital the mean interval between diagnosis of the primary tumour and presentation with a pleural effusion was 42 months and the mean survival after diagnosis of effusion was 16 months (Fentiman et al 1981). Thus effective treatment can greatly improve the quality of life of patients since this is the first evidence of recurrence in almost 50% of the cases with pleural effusion.

Patients with pleura effusions usually complain of shortness of breath, sometimes associated with a cough. There may be a dull chest pain and occasionally pleuritic pain (Fentiman 1987). Clinical examination reveals dullness to percussion and reduced air intake over the lung base on the affected side. This manifests as an opacity on a chest X-ray with a shift of the fluid on lateral decubitis view. Confirmation of the diagnosis is made by needle thoracentesis, taking enough fluid for cytological evaluation.

A management plan for patients with pleural effusions is given in Fig. 6.4. After aspiration, there will be cytological evidence of malignant cells in approximately 60% of patients in whom the effusion is due to metastatic disease. If a pleural biopsy is performed, a few (7%) more cases will be confirmed as having metastatic disease (Salyer et al 1975).

Thoracoscopy may sometimes be of value in confirming the presence of metastases with parenchymal deposits being identified in up to 60% of patients with negative fluid cytology (Fentiman et al 1982). For patients with cytologically negative effusions, other causes such as cardiac failure, infection and pulmonary embolus should be excluded.

For patients with metastatic disease elsewhere and for whom systemic therapy is needed, drainage to dryness may be sufficient. However, the majority of patients will develop a recurrence of the effusion and for this it is

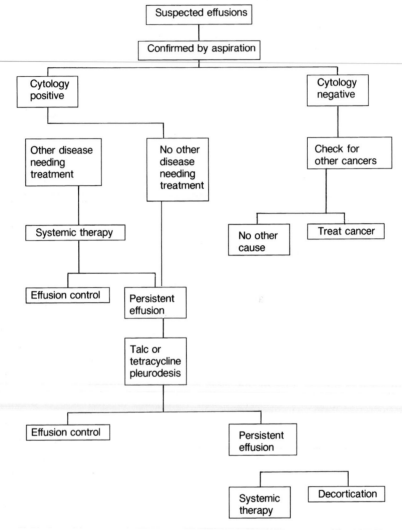

Fig. 6.4 Management of pleural effusions in patients with breast cancer.

best to carry out a definitive pleurodesis. For this to be effective three criteria have to be met; first, the effusion should be drained to dryness; secondly, an effective agent should be instilled; finally, the parietal and visceral pleura must be apposed so that a fibrous reaction can occur.

Numerous agents have been tested for achieving pleurodesis and those that have been evaluated in clinical trials are given in Table 6.1. All agents act in a similar manner to sclerosants and there is no advantage in giving intracavity chemotherapy, particularly since there may be systemic absorption giving rise to side-effects and possibly compromising subsequent chemotherapy. The

Table 6.1 Results of trials of intracavitary agents for pleurodesis in women with breast cancer

Author	Trial agents	Control rate (%)
Izbicki et al 1975	Drainage alone	50
	^{32}P	54
Mejer 1977	Drainage alone	33
	Quinacrine	75
Bayly et al 1978	Tetracycline	71
	Quinacrine	67
Fentiman et al 1983a	Mustine	53
	Talc	90
Fentiman et al 1986	Tetracycline	48
	Talc	92
Hamed et al 1989	Bleomycin	67
	Talc	100

agent which emerges as the most effective is talc. If this is insufflated after drainage to dryness and an intercostal drain is left in place for 5 days, control of the effusion will occur in more than 90% of patients. Talc insufflation is usually performed under general anaesthesia, and the opportunity is taken to perform a thoracoscopy to assess the extent of metastatic disease within the lungs and pleura.

If the patient is too ill to undergo general anaesthesia, tetracyline (500 mg) can be instilled under local anaesthesia, but this should be mixed with a local anaesthetic since it can be very painful. Because of loculation of effusion, pleurodesis may occasionally fail and such patients, provided they are fit enough, may benefit from decortication (pleurectomy) but this does carry a 5% operative mortality rate (Martini et al 1975).

The most difficult decision is not what to do for pleurodesis but when to do it. At present prognostic indices for patients with pleural effusions are not in use. Some patients develop effusions are preterminal events and in the trials that have been conducted up to 20% of those taking part died within 1 month of attempted pleurodesis. If in doubt it is best to go ahead since effective symptomatic relief can greatly improve the patient's quality of life.

Ascites

Development of ascites is a relatively uncommon event and the prognosis depends upon whether this is a result of hepatic metastases or of peritoneal seedlings (Fentiman et al 1983b). In a series of 56 patients who developed ascites secondary to breast cancer, it was found that those dying within 3 months of diagnosis were significantly more likely to have hepatomegaly and jaundice than those who survived for longer periods.

For symptomatic relief in the absence of hepatic metastases, first-line diuretics should be tried, and only if these do not relieve symptoms should local measures such as paracentesis be performed. For selected patients insertion of a peritoneovenous shunt of the LeVeen or Denver type may be of help in relieving abdominal distension (Fentiman 1994).

PALLIATIVE CARE

Patients may derive more benefit from effective palliation of symptoms than from therapy designed to kill cancer cells. In particular, pain relief must be a prime aim in patients with the earlier symptoms of advanced breast cancer. Analgesics should be given as appropriate according to the World Health Organization (1990) analgesic ladder given in Table 6.2.

Table 6.2   World Health Organization three-step analgesia ladder

Pain severity	Drug type	Examples
Mild	Simple analgesic	Paracetamol Aspirin
Moderate	NSAID Weak opioid	Co-proxamol Dihydrocodeine
Severe	Strong opioid	Morphine Diamorphine

NSAID, non-steroidal anti-inflammatory drug.

Simple analgesics such as paracetamol and aspirin should be given to those with mild pain, whereas moderate pain will require non-steroidal anti-inflammatory drugs such as dextropropoxyphene and diclofenac. If such agents do not control the pain, morphine sulphate slow-release tablets should be given together with antiemetics and laxatives. Diamorphine as a continuous infusion can be valuable in the terminal stages of the disease.

It is important that patients with pain from cancer are seen by pain-relief specialists and when possible referred to Macmillan nurses whose training is based on the alleviation of symptoms from terminal malignancy. Many hospices run outpatient clinics and their calm and empathetic atmosphere may be of great psychological and physical benefit to the patient with advanced breast cancer.

KEY POINTS FOR CLINICAL PRACTICE

- For patients with advanced breast cancer the aim of treatment is palliation, not cure.
- Locally advanced disease responds better to a combination of systemic and local therapy than to local treatment alone, and endocrine therapy may prolong survival.
- Symptomatic chest wall recurrence in selected patients can be controlled by extensive surgery, usually with a rotational flap to achieve skin closure.

- Early relapse after systemic adjuvant therapy can be less responsive to subsequent treatment.
- Patients with bone metastases may benefit from disphosphonate both in terms of inhibition of subsequent bone metastases and reduction of hypercalcaemic episodes.
- Symptomatic pleural effusions can be palliated effectively by talc pleurodesis.
- Selected patients with abdominal ascites benefit from peritoneovenous shunts.
- Experts in pain relief and symptom control should be involved in the management of terminal patients to allow them death with dignity.

REFERENCES

Bayly TC, Kisner DL, Sybert A et al 1978 Tetracycline and quinacrine in the control of malignant pleural effusions. A randomised trial. Cancer 41: 1188–1192
Coleman RE, Rubens RD 1987 The clinical course of bone metastases from breast cancer. Br J Cancer 55: 61–66
Early Breast Cancer Trialists' Collaborative Group 1992 Systemic treatment of early breast cancer by homonal, cytoxic or immune therapy. Lancet 339: 1–15
Elomaa I, Blumquist C, Grohn P et al 1983 Long-term controlled trial with diphosphonate in patients with osteolytic bone metastases. Lancet 1: 146–149
Fentiman IS 1987 Diagnosis and treatment of malignant pleural effusions. Cancer Treat Rev 14: 107–118
Fentiman IS 1995 Serous effusions. In: eds Oxford textbook of oncology. Peckham M, Pinedo R, Veronesi V. Oxford University Press, Oxford (in press)
Fentiman IS, Millis RR, Sexton S et al 1981 Pleural effusion in breast cancer: a review of 105 cases. Cancer 47: 2087–2092
Fentiman IS, Rubens RD, Hayward JL 1982 The pattern of metastatic disease in patients with pleural effusions secondary to breast cancer. Br J Surg 69: 193–194
Fentiman IS, Rubens RD, Hayward JJ 1983a Control of pleural effusions in patients with breast cancer. A randomised trial. Cancer 52: 737–739
Fentiman IS, Rubens RD, Hayward JL 1983b Ascites in breast cancer. Br Med J 287: 1023.
Fentiman, IS, Rubens RD, Hayward JL 1986 A comparison of intracavitary talc and tetracycline for the control of pleural effusions secondary to breast cancer. Eur J Cancer Clin Oncol 22: 1079–1081
Fornander T, Rutqvist LE, Glas V 1987 Response to tamoxifen and fluoxymesterone in a group of breast cancer patients with disease recurrence after cessation of adjuvant tamoxifen Cancer Treat Rep 71: 685–686
Goldhirsch A, Gelber RD, Price UN et al 1994 Effect of systemic adjuvant treatment on first sites of breast cancer relapse. Lancet 343: 377–381
Haagensen CD 1971 Diseases of the breast, 2nd edn. Saunders WB, Philadelphia, pp 576–584
Hamed H, Fentiman IS, Chaudary MA et al 1989 Comparison of intracavitary bleomycin and talc for control of pleural effusions secondary to carcinoma of the breast. Br J Surg 76: 1266–1267
Harris AL, Cantwell BMJ, Carmichael J et al 1990 Comparison of short-term and continuous chemotherapy (mitozantrone) for advanced breast cancer. Lancet 1: 186–190
Houston SJ, Richards MA, Bentley AE et al 1993 The influence of adjuvant chemotherapy on outcome after relapse for patients with breast cancer. Eur J Cancer 29A: 1513–1518
Izbicki R, Weyhing BT, Baker L et al 1975 Pleural effusions in cancer patients. Cancer 36: 1511–1518
Jaiyesimi IA, Buzdar AV, Hortobagyi G 1992 Inflammatory breast cancer: a review. J Clin Oncol 10: 1014–1024
Kagan R, Steckel RJ 1991 Routine imaging studies for the post-treatment surveillance of

breast and colorectal carcinoma. J Clin Oncol 9: 837–842

Lee B, Tannenbaum N 1924 Inflammatory carcinoma of the breast: a report of twenty-eight cases from the breast clinic of Memorial Hospital. Surg Gynecol Obstet 39: 580–598

Martini N, Bains MS, Beattie EJ 1975 Indications for pleurectomy in malignant effusions. Cancer 35: 734–738

Mejer J, Mortensen KM, Hansen HM 1977 Mepacrine hydrochloride in the treatment of malignant pleural effusion: a controlled randomised trial. Scand J Resp Dis 58: 319–323

Paterson AHG, Powles TJ, Kanis JA et al 1993 Double-blind controlled trial of oral clodronate in patients with bone metastases from breast cancer. J Clin Oncol 11: 59–65

Rainer H 1993 Prospective randomised clinical trial of primary treatment in breast cancer stages T3/4 N + MO. Chemotherapy versus radiotherapy. Anticancer Res 13: 1917–1924

Roberts MM, Alexander FE, Anderson TJ et al 1990 Edinburgh trial of screening for breast cancer: mortality at seven years. Lancet 335: 241–246

Rubens RD 1994 Personal communication

Rubens RD, Bartelink H, Engelsman E et al 1989 Locally advanced breast cancer: the contribution of cytotoxic and endocrine treatment to radiotherapy. Eur J Cancer Clin Oncol 25: 667–678

Rubens RD, Bajetta E, Bonneterre J et al 1994 Treatment of relapse of breast cancer after adjuvant systemic therapy — review and guidelines for future research. Eur J Cancer 30A: 106–111

Salyer WR, Eggleston JC, Erozan YS 1975 Efficacy of pleural biopsy and pleural fluid cytopathology in the diagnosis of malignant neoplasm involving the pleura. Chest 67: 536–539

Veronesi A, Frustaci S, Tirelli V et al 1993 Tamoxifen therapy in post-menopausal advanced breast cancer: efficacy at the primary site in 46 evaluable patients. Tumori 67: 235–238

World Health Organization 1990. Cancer pain relief and palliative care. World Health Organization, Geneva.

7

Parathyroid surgery

A. W. Goode

Herr Albert J had been discharged from the Austrian Army with tuberculosis during the Great War. He became a tramcar conductor in Vienna and in 1921 at the age of 34 developed pain in his leg, felt tired and was unable to work. X-rays in 1923 showed transparent bones containing cysts and the next year he fractured his femur. He was admitted to the Hocheregg Clinic under the care of Felix Mandl. His blood calcium and urinary calcium excretion were found to be very high and in July 1925 neck exploration yielded a grossly enlarged parathyroid gland, excised with dramatic results both biochemically and clinically. (Welbourn 1990)

Since that day, hyperparathyroidism has become recognized as one of the most common of the endocrinopathies with an incidence of approximately 1 per 1000 of the population, while in women older than 45 years the incidence increases to 1 per 500 (Heath et al 1980). Since the advent of serum autoanalysers in the 1960s, elevations of serum calcium are routinely detected even in asymptomatic patients. In recent years, improved parathyroid hormone radioimmunoassays and parathyroid localization procedures have simplified the diagnosis of patients with hyperparathyroidism by documenting the simultaneous elevation of both serum calcium and parathyroid hormone levels (Duh et al 1986).

ANATOMY AND PATHOPHYSIOLOGY

The parathyroid glands derive from the endoderm of pharyngeal pouches III and IV, and symmetry of position in relation to the thyroid gland is found in 80% of patients. A fourth gland may be absent in 3% and supernumerary glands may be found in 13%, usually in the thymus (Ankerström et al 1984); however, in hyperparathyroidism the described anatomical relationship may not be present.

Parathyroid hormone (PTH) is an 84 amino acid peptide with a molecular weight of 9500. It has a short half-life of minutes in the circulation before fragmenting into an amino-terminal fragment consisting of amino acids 1–34 which retains biological activity with a half-life of minutes and a carboxy-terminal fragment with a half-life of hours. Assays are available to measure either the intact hormone or the fragments. PTH binds to specific receptors on kidney, bone and intestine and mediates its action by stimulating adenylate cyclase and hence the production of cyclic AMP in the target tissues (Canterbury et al 1973).

Excess production of PTH results in hypercalcaemia and is termed hyperparathyroidism. The excess hormone acts directly on bone and kidney. Bone remodelling is increased with the release of calcium into the extracellular fluid. Production of 1,25-dihydroxyvitamin D by the kidney is also increased, thus stimulating intestinal absorption of calcium. The net effect is to increase the movement of calcium into the extracellular fluid and to promote the dissolution of bone mineral. Hyperparathyroidism is the result of a single parathyroid adenoma in up to 85% of patients, multigland disease — hyperplasia or multiple adenomata — in up to 15% and, rarely, carcinoma of the parathyroid in 1%.

Primary hyperparathyroidism is the abnormal secretion of PTH with normal or elevated serum calcium levels. In most patients, the cause of neoplastic transformation of the parathyroid glands is unknown. It has been shown that, in patients with both adenomas and hyperplasia, there is a multicellular origin of these neoplasms (Fialkon et al 1977) and low-dose ionizing radiation to the neck has been associated with some cases (Prinz et al 1977). Chronic stimulation of the parathyroid glands may occur with low-calcium high-phosphate diets and long-term frusemide (Lasix) administration.

Secondary PTH excretion is an attempt to compensate for a chronic low serum calcium level. This most commonly occurs in chronic renal failure and is the consequence of phosphate retention; however, decreased conversion of vitamin D to its active metabolite 1,25-dihydroxyvitamin D and a decrease in the metabolic clearance of PTH also contribute. Other clinical causes include malabsorption, osteomalacia and rickets. When the stimulus for parathyroid hypersecretion is corrected, most patients with secondary hyperparathyroidism will correct their PTH level within 6 months (David 1975). Some patients have, however, developed relatively autonomous parathyroid function which does not respond to the correction; this is termed tertiary hyperparathyroidism.

DIFFERENTIAL DIAGNOSIS OF HYPERCALCAEMIA

Serum calcium occurs as calcium ions complexed to citrate and bound to albumin. Thus to obtain the corrected serum calcium value, serum albumin concentration should be measured and the following formula applied:

$$\text{Corrected serum calcium (mmol/l)} = \left[\text{Measured serum calcium (mmol/l)} + (40 - A) \right] \times 0.02$$

where A is serum albumin (g/l).

The differential diagnosis of hypercalcaemia is a classical diagnostic problem and the common causes are listed in Table 7.1. Most of the clinical

Table 7.1 Causes of hypercalcaemia

Primary hyperparathyroidism
Malignancy
Granulomatous disease
    Sarcoidosis
    Tuberculosis
Medication
    Thiazide diuretics
    Vitamin D toxicity
    Lithium
    Hormone treatment of carcinoma of the breast
    Milk alkali syndrome
Familial hypercalciuric hypercalcaemia
Endocrine
    Thyrotoxicosis
    Adrenal crisis
    Phaeochromocytoma
Immobilization
Renal failure
Diuretic phase of acute renal failure
Post-transplantation or dialysis
Aluminium intoxication

manifestations of hyperparathyroidism are caused by hypercalcaemia and may be diffuse with apparently trivial symptoms being overlooked; thus the key to diagnosis is awareness of the protean manifestations. The common symptoms are listed in Table 7.2, and the relative frequency of their presentation in Table 7.3.

Table 7.2 Symptoms of hyperparathyroidism

General	Polydipsia and weight loss
Renal	Colic, haematuria, back pain, polyuria
Cardiovascular	Hypertension, heart block
Musculoskeletal	Non-specific aches and pains, bone pain, pathological fractures, arthritis
Gastrointestinal	Anorexia, nausea, dyspepsia, constipation, abdominal pain
Neurological	Depression, lethargy, apathy, weakness, confusion, neurosis, psychosis

Table 7.3 Incidence of clinical presentation of hyperparathyroidism

	%
Asymptomatic hypercalcaemia	50
Renal stones	28
Polyuria, polydipsia, weakness, lethargy, constipation	5
Peptic ulcer	4
Hypertension	4
Bone disease	3
Multiple endocrine adenopathys type I (MEA I)	1
Thyroid disease	0.5
Neonatal tetany	0.5

Renal calculi, once the hallmark of primary hyperparathyroidism, are now found in only a minority of patients. Although the mechanism is unclear, elevated circulating concentration of 1,25-dihydroxyvitamin D and hypercalcuria are thought to be contributing factors.

Functional abnormalities of the kidney are more common, with decreased renal tubular reabsorption of bicarbonate producing a tendency to hyperchloraemic acidosis.

Osteitis fibrosa cystica, the classical skeletal lesion of patients with hyperparathyroidism, is characterized by bone pain, tenderness and susceptibility to fracture. Serum alkaline phosphate is mildly elevated and radiography of the hands may show subperiostial resorption of the phalanges or even resorption of the tufts of the distal phalanges (Fig. 7.1).

Peptic ulcer disease occurs with increased frequency in the presence of primary hyperparathyroidism due to gastric acid and pepsin secretion stimulated by calcium ions. Gastrinoma and milk alkali syndrome should be excluded.

Hypertension occurs with increasing frequency in primary hyperparathyroidism but whether a causal relationship exists is unclear. Elevation of blood pressure is usually mild and is not related to the level of serum calcium or creatinine. It may, in the initial period after successful surgery, return to normal values but in the longer term may rise again (Britton et al 1973).

Neuromuscular complications include mild proximal muscle weakness despite normal levels of muscle enzymes. Rheumatic complications include calcification of articular cartilage and episodes of painful joint effusions with

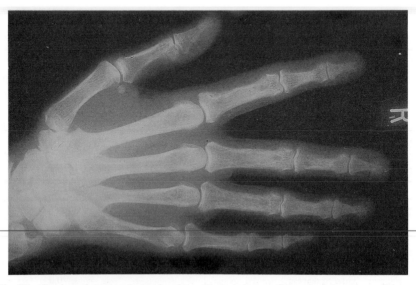

Fig. 7.1   Erosion of the terminal tufts of the distal phalanges. Subperiostial erosions of the radial aspect of the middle phalanges.

deposition of calcium pyrophosphate crystals, while gout and periarthritis occur with increased frequency. The role of primary hyperparathyroidism in osteoporosis is unclear, although cortical bone density is reduced at the time of diagnosis compared with control subjects; trabecular bone is spared and the bone loss is not progressive (Wilson et al 1988). In pregnancy, maternal hypercalcaemia may induce functional apathy of the fetal parathyroid glands with the advent of neonatal tetany within hours after delivery.

Acute hypercalcaemic crisis may develop when the serum level of calcium exceeds 3 mmol/l. This is accompanied by anorexia, nausea, vomiting, dehydration, fatigue, confusion and eventually coma. This constitutes an emergency as untreated it will proceed to oliguric renal failure, cardiac arrythmias and death. Treatment is urgent, with particular attention directed towards rehydration.

Despite this complexity of clinical presentations, the majority of patients appear to be asymptomatic at the time of diagnosis. The disease would not have been recognized but for the routine measurement of the serum calcium by laboratory autoanalysers. Care must be exercised before a patient is identified as asymptomatic since some complications are indeed subtle, and a careful history may reveal that many 'asymptomatic' patients may have symptoms (Purnell et al 1971). Untreated asymptomatic patients followed-up for 10 years were found to deteriorate; 26% developed specific indications for surgery, 24% died, while 16% failed to return for follow-up (Scholz & Purnell 1981).

BIOCHEMICAL INVESTIGATION

Biochemical investigation of suspected hyperparathyroidism is the reference point upon which all hinges. An elevated corrected serum calcium level is almost essential for the diagnosis but rarely normocalcaemic hyper-parathyroidism may present. Approximately three-quarters of patients with hypercalcaemia have hypercalcuria, i.e. a daily urinary calcium excretion in excess of 10 nmol. PTH measurement is fundamental in making the diagnosis with the mid-region and carboxy-terminal assays being the best, but in renal failure the carboxy-terminal fragment may give falsely high levels. In hyperparathyroidism an infusion of sodium EDTA (ethylerediaminetetracetic acid) or an intramuscular injection of calcitonin induces a fall in serum calcium but the EDTA always, and the calcitonin invariably, causes a rise in the mid-region intact PTH fragment; this is unique and does not occur in a raised calcium due to other underlying causes (Ljungham et al 1988). In suspected hypercalcaemia due to malignancy, the PTH level may be normal while the calcium elevation has been induced by tumour-derived PTH related protein for which a specific assay is now available (Bundred et al 1990).

Hypophosphataemia is found in half the patients as PTH decreases renal tubular resorption of phosphate and increases urinary phosphate loss. When hypophosphataemia is found in a patient with hypercalcaemia, hyperparathyroidism is by far the most likely diagnosis. Similarly, in the presence of hypercalcaemia, an elevated serum chloride concentration suggests the diagnosis as PTH decreases the resorption of bicarbonate in the proximal renal tubule. This leads to an increased resorption of chloride and mild hyperchloraemic renal tubular acidosis; in other causes of hypercalcaemia the serum chloride is normal. The ratio of serum chloride to phosphate suggests hyperparathyroidism if it exceeds 33 in a patient with hypercalcaemia (Reeves et al 1975).

Our studies have suggested that the β_2-microglobulins may be a particularly sensitive test of renal tubular dysfunction in primary hyperparathyroidism, being disturbed even in asymptomatic patients with normal serum creatinine and creatinine clearance (Goode et al 1987). Curative surgery results in return to normal values, suggesting that the asymptomatic patient does have subtle changes not found on conventional testing. Current studies are directed to the possible prognostic use of preoperative β_2-microglobulin measurements as a predictor of the long-term development of hypertension (Nader-Sepathi et al 1992).

A chest X-ray is valuable in eliminating carcinoma of the lung as a cause of hypercalcaemia. Abdominal films revealing nephrolithiasis or nephrocalcinosis suggest chronic hypercalcaemia, while overt skeletal changes such as periostial erosions are found in only 10% of patients. Angiotensin-converting enzyme is useful in identifying a patient suspected of having active sarcoidosis but it is not specific to the disorder (Lufkin et al 1983).

Familial hypocalciuric hypercalcaemia

This is an autosomal dominant disorder with a high penetrence which is found in less than 1% of patients with hypercalcaemia (Law & Heath 1985). It is characterized by lifelong moderate hypercalcaemia, apparently the result of a cellular defect causing increased renal tubular reabsorption of calcium. The urine level of calcium is less than 2.5 nmol/day in three-quarters of patients and the ratio of calcium clearance to creatinine clearance is less than 0.01; the serum PTH is normal or only very slightly elevated. The condition is almost always benign and its identification is important as parathyroid surgery is contraindicated. The presence of hypercalcaemia in two generations of a family suggests the possibility of the diagnosis especially when one member has had unsuccessful parathyroid surgery.

Normocalcaemic hypercalciuria

The incidence of normocalcaemic hypercalciuria in patients with hypercalciuria is not known. Patients with hyperparathyroidism benefit from parathyroidectomy whereas patients with idiopathic hypercalciuria due to hyperabsorption of calcium from the bowel or primary renal tubular calcium leak do not. All patients thought to have a normocalcaemic hypercalciuria should be assessed by at least three separate serum calcium estimations to exclude intermittent hypercalcaemia. The serum ionized calcium should be determined as some patients may have a normal total serum calcium. Elevation of both the PTH and ionized calcium levels with a normal total calcium concentration is diagnostic of normocalcaemic hyperparathyroidism. A phosphate deprivation test is useful in differentiating normocalcaemic hyperparathyroidism from idiopathic hypercalcuria. A 3-day diet of normal calorie content and calcium but restricted to 350 mg of phosphate is provided; 60 ml aluminium hydroxide gel are given four times daily and serum calcium phosphate and protein concentrations obtained daily. Patients whose serum calcium rises above normal or those with persistent hypercalcuria have hyperparathyroidism (Nichols & Flanagan 1967).

Acute hypercalcaemic crisis

Life-threatening hypercalcaemia with a corrected serum calcium concentration greater than 4 mmol/l may present acutely in patients who were previously asymptomatic or with chronic disease. Symptoms vary but include weakness, nausea, vomiting, drowsiness, stupor and tachycardia.

The immediate management is rehydration, correction of the electrolyte imbalance and maintenance of a high urine output with a diuretic (frusemide). Mild hypercalcaemia is treated by rehydration and diuresis but thiazide diuretics should not be used as they decrease calcium excretion. Severe hypercalcaemia which persists following rehydration should be actively treated with drugs which stop the mobilization of calcium from bone. The bisphosphonates are particularly effective and safe. Disodium pamidronate (Aredia) is probably most effective given by slow intravenous infusion according to the plasma calcium concentration; 15–60 mg may be given either as a single infusion or over 2–4 days with a maximum dose of 90 mg over the complete course of treatment. Nausea, diarrhoea, asymptomatic hypocalcaemia, a transient rise in body temperature and lymphocytaemia are all reported side-effects. Corticosteroids are often given but may only be of value when the hypercalcaemia is due to sarcoidosis or vitamin D intoxication and their action is slow over several days. Calcitonin is non-toxic but expensive and its effect is of short duration — perhaps 2 days; further, it is rarely effective when biophophonates have failed. Intravenous chelating drugs such as trisodium edetate are rarely used since they cause pain in the infusion limb and possible renal damage. Similarly, sodium cellulose phosphate which binds calcium in the gut is rarely helpful and the induced rise in serum phosphate may be dangerous.

PREOPERATIVE PARATHYROID LOCALIZATION

Although an experienced parathyroid surgeon may be expected to find up to

95% of the parathyroid glands at the time of surgery, it is useful if he knows where the problem is located and whether the gland is in a primary anatomical site (as will occur in three-quarters of cases (Winzelberg 1987)).

Opinion is divided about the use of preoperative localization of parathyroid glands in primary disease when no previous exploration has been undertaken and rather an awareness of the possible sites and their systematic exploration is considered the key to success. However, many other experienced parathyroid surgeons subscribe to the view that non-invasive preoperative localization is invaluable.

Clinical examination, barium swallow and thermography are of little value. However, more recent techniques such as ultrasonography, computed tomography (CT), magnetic resonance imaging and thallium/technetium scanning have proved helpful. Selective venous catherization to measure PTH levels is reserved for patients with persistent or recurrent disease.

Ultrasonography

Sample et al (1978) showed that traditional static grey-scale ultrasonography using a 5 MHz transducer was able to identify abnormal parathyroid glands with a sensitivity of 87%. Ultrasonography, like other cross-sectional imaging modalities, is operator-dependent and accuracy rates vary. It does have the capability of identifying very small glands and those situated within the thyroid gland. It does not, however, image glands situated behind the sternum, trachea or oesophagus and may miss lesions situated deep within the neck (Clark et al 1985). In the majority of patients, ultrasonography will not detect normal parathyroid glands. An adenoma is seen as a discrete sharply marginated soft tissue mass with a reduced echogenicity compared to the adjacent thyroid tissue (Winzelberg 1987), but the shape, size and echogenicity are variable. Hyperplastic glands have been described as being less echogenic than adenomas; however, the variable appearance of the latter makes this evaluation subjective and of limited use in differentiation.

Computed tomography

CT of the neck is a non-invasive method of localization which has been developed since the late 1970s. In the neck, there are problems with clarity of definition, especially of the area just caudal to the thyroid gland where oblique or tortuous vessels may be misinterpreted as parathyroid adenomas. Technical improvements in scanning have helped but tumour size is more of a limitation for detection by CT than for ultrasonography. Stark et al (1983), however, have concluded that CT can equal the accuracy of ultrasound. CT is particularly useful for identifying ectopic glands but not good at imaging glands between the thyroid and clavicles, which is a common site. The use of

CT in evaluating patients with persistent or recurrent disease varies in different centres and may be best employed in conjunction with other localizing modalities.

Magnetic resonance imaging

Although the role of magnetic resonance imaging is still being defined it is potentially the most useful. Improved resolution from neck surface coils has resulted in high-contrast images of soft tissues, blood vessels, thyroid and parathyroid glands. Initial studies suggest an 83% detection rate with lesions rather smaller than 0.5 cm being identified (Peck et al 1987, Spritler et al 1987). Factors which appear to limit resolution are the similarity of the parathyroid signal with that of the thyroid gland, respiration-induced artefact and the confusion of a thyroid adenoma with that of a parathyroid adenoma. Initial studies suggest that T_2 sequence weighted images may show the best resolution between a parathyroid adenoma and the surrounding tissues.

Scintigraphy

A second technique which has been extensively developed in the last decade is that of scintigraphic imaging, a method akin to that of a thyroid scan. The combined use of ^{99m}Tc (as pertechnate) and ^{201}Tlcl (thallium chloride) with an appropriate subtraction technique has become the radionucleotide imaging technique of choice. The method is based upon the fact that the thyroid gland will accumulate both ^{99m}Tc pertechnate and ^{201}Tlcl, while the parathyroid gland will accumulate thallium-201 pertechnate only. A computer is then employed to substract the ^{99m}Tc image from the ^{201}Tl image, which leaves only the parathyroid uptake (Fig. 7.2). Preliminary studies (Wheeler et al 1984, Young et al 1983) have localized up to 85% of abnormal glands.

The specificity of the technique is adversely affected by ^{201}Tl uptake in thyroid abnormalities such as multinodular goitre, thyroiditis and thyroid adenoma, while metastatic cervical lymph nodes, lymphoma and sarcoidosis are causes of false-positive results. Recent developments have been directed to reversal of the order of administration of the isotopes, to obtain improved sensitivity, and three-dimensional imaging (Jenkins et al 1990). This has correctly localized glands weighing as little as 100 mg.

A new scanning agent, ^{99}Tc sestamibi, is being studied. It has differential clearance rates for the solid structures of the neck, and initial studies show improved results particularly in the localization of hyperplastic glands. In our unit, thallium–technetium subtraction has proved the best single method of preoperative gland localization, but others advocate a multimodal approach combining ultrasonography and magnetic resonance imaging techniques. Further studies are indicated to identify the optimal approach.

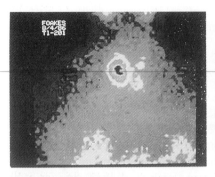
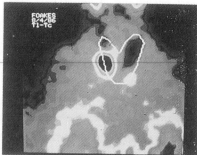
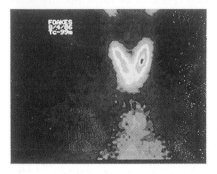

Fig. 7.2 Two-dimensional thallium–technetium scan with thallium image of the thyroid and parathyroid and a technetium image of the thyroid gland. The third image (right) is the subtraction image with the single focus of activity representing a parathyroid adenoma shown in relation to the outline of the parathyroid gland.

Preoperative methylene blue

Methylene blue dye given intravenously preoperatively in a dose of 3.5 mg/kg body weight dissolved in 500 ml of dextrose and infused over 1 h will selectively stain parathyroid glands. Normal glands stain pale green and pathological glands dark blue or black. The method has varying degrees of acceptance in different centres where enthusiasts regard is as invaluable and detractors do not resort to it.

Selective venous catherization

Selective venous catherization is an invasive procedure in which blood from multiple sampling sites in cervical and mediastinal neck veins is assayed for PTH levels, and is the most sensitive of the invasive methods. A PTH level that is twice the peripheral venous level is considered significant. An adenoma is associated with a unilateral elevation and hyperplasia usually with a bilateral elevated level. It is principally a lateralizing procedure rather than a localizing procedure and, although initially used as an investigative procedure at the first presentation, it is now almost exclusively reserved for patients who have had previous parathyroid surgery in whom non-invasive localizing procedures have proven to be unsatisfactory.

THE SURGICAL MANAGEMENT OF HYPERPARATHYROIDISM

When a definitive clinical and biochemical diagnosis of hyperparathyroidism has been made, a strategy for future management has emerged in two of the three major clinical presentations.

If the biochemical changes are minimal and the patient elderly with few symptoms then surgery is not indicated, unless on follow-up there is clear evidence of deterioration of the condition. By contrast, those patients with symptoms and a corrected serum calcium greater than 2.8 mmol/l or complications arising from the elevated calcium level require surgical exploration. However, a 'grey' area occurs in mild asymptomatic patients where opinion is divided between conservative management, since some follow-up studies suggest the condition is static without deleterious effects, and surgery, based on the suggestion that these patients exhibit subtle pathological changes which may deteriorate and that they have improved quality of life after surgery. Most clinicians adopt a pragmatic approach with each patient assessed on merit — but the debate continues.

Patients who require parathyroidectomy must have their vocal cords inspected by preoperative laryngoscopy to rule out any pre-existing abnormality. There is no substitute for surgical expertise in parathyroid surgery and no place for the occasional parathyroid surgeon.

Under a general anaesthetic the patient is placed on the operating table in a supine position. A sandbag is placed under the shoulders and the head placed on a padded ring, thus gently extending the neck; simultaneously the patient is in a position where the head is higher than the feet. A collar incision is made and skin flaps dissected.

Absolute haemostasis is a basic requirement because blood-stained tissue can make identification of parathyroid tissue difficult. The exploration may be characterized by a number of technical steps:

I. Exposure and dissection of the posterior thyroid capsule. The middle thyroid vein is divided bilaterally and the lobes of the thyroid are mobilized posteriorly.

II. Dissection of the superior mediastinum, identifying the lower poles of the thyroid, delivery of the thymus and its exploration. Superior parathyroid glands should be looked for in their normal location at the superior aspect of the recurrent laryngeal nerves and the inferior glands in their normal location near the inferior pole of the thyroid and then within the thymus.

III. Dissection of the paraoesophageal, pharyngeal, retro-oesophageal and retropharyngeal spaces when abnormal glands have not been located.

IV. Total thyroid lobectomy on the side without normal parathyroid anatomy. Up to 2% of all glands may be intrathyroidal.
V. Incision of the carotid sheath as glands may be located in or adjacent to the sheath up to the carotid bifurcation.
VI. Mediastinotomy and mediastinal dissection are usually reserved for a second operation. This may be required in up to 2% of patients.
VII. At the end of surgery, two suction drains are inserted, one on each side of the neck. The vocal cords are routinely examined for appropriate movement by the anaesthetist at the end of surgery. The drains are removed on the first or second postoperative day when drainage has ceased and the skin clips on the third and fourth postoperative days.

Normal gland? Hyperplasia? Adenoma?

Intraoperative frozen section facilities are mandatory to answer these questions and it is precisely from these answers that the next phase of the operative strategy can be planned.

When all four glands have been visualized, the largest is excised for pathological diagnosis. About 80% of patients with primary hyperparathyroidism will have a single adenoma as the cause (Barnes 1984), hyperplasia in about 15% and a double adenoma is about 2%. Intraoperative histological proof of an adenoma and one normal gland will, in most patients, suffice. It has recently been suggested that simultaneous intraoperative sampling of intact PTH levels will show if an adenoma has been completely excised by a fall to normal values within 15 min (Robertson et al 1992). A recent international survey of surgical strategy in the management of a solitary adenoma suggests that intraoperative frozen section histology is employed in most centres, that excision of the adenoma is preferred to multigland biopsy and that with the aid of modern localization techniques preoperatively unilateral neck dissection is finding favour (Tibblin et al 1991).

Hyperplasia

With histological proof of hyperplasia, excision of all four glands is performed and a fragment of one is autotransplanted into a market pocket of forearm muscle tissue. Future overactivity of the gland is thus simplified by exploration of the implant and partial excision. This avoids the technically demanding requirement for a re-exploration of the neck. In secondary and tertiary hyperparathyroidism, all four glands are likely to be uniformly hyperplasia. Again, excision of all four glands and autotransplantation of a gland fragment to a selected forearm site is the treatment of choice.

The overall success rate in the management of patients with primary hyperparathyroidism in the hands of an experienced surgeon is between 95% and 97% (Purnell et al 1977). In patients with multigland disease due to hyperplasia the success rate is about 90% and up to 70% in multiple endocrine adenopathy type I (MEA I) (Prinz et al 1981).

Postoperative complications

Possible postoperative complications include bleeding which is dealt with in a similar manner to that following thyroidectomy. Hypocalcaemia may occur in the postoperative period. Serum calcium levels should be monitored daily. Mild hypocalcaemia may not need treatment but symptomatic patients who develop tetany require relief; 10% calcium gluconate infusion given slowly intravenously over a 5-min interval is prompt in relieving symptoms while, if longer term supplementation is required, oral calcium salts and vitamin D are effective, and serum calcium levels should be monitored.

HYPERPARATHYROIDISM AND MULTIPLE ENDOCRINE NEOPLASIA (MEN) SYNDROME

Overactivity of the parathyroid glands may be associated with other endocrine tumours. The cells involved irrespective of the site have the common chemical characteristics of amine precursor uptake and decarboxylation and are thus known as APUD cells.

Hyperparathyroidism is a central companion for these syndromes, being characterized by parathyroid hyperplasia (Majenski & Wilson 1979). The age of clinical presentation and the presentation of other manifestation of the syndromes vary greatly. MEN 1 syndrome is composed of hyper-parathyroidism, pancreatic gastrinoma (although some may be located in the duodenum) and pituitary adenomas, usually a prolactinoma. Variants of the syndrome include an insulinoma in place of a gastrinoma, lipoma, thymoma and Cushing's syndrome.

Surgical correction of the hyperparathyroidism in MEN 1 syndrome is usually required because of the degree of hypercalcaemia and gastric hyperacidity associated with the high calcium levels. A high recurrence rate of hyperparathyroidism is found after both total parathyroidectomy with autotransplantation and subtotal parathyroidectomy (Malmaeus et al 1986). Because of this high recurrence rate and the relative ease of re-exploration of an autotransplantation forearm site of parathyroid tissue, this procedure has gained favour. Future regular monitoring of serum calcium levels is mandatory as a rise is a possible indication for further surgery.

The MEN II syndrome comprises parathyroid hyperplasia, bilateral medullary carcinoma of the thyroid and phaechromocytomas. The MEN IIb syndrome in addition comprises characteristic mucosal neuromas, present earlier in life; the parathyroid disease may be mild or absent. Progress has been made in identifying a genetic basis for MEN II syndrome with the gene located on chromosome 10 (Pounder 1990). The lethal consequences of a phaeochromocytoma make this lesion a priority for treatment superseding surgery to the thyroid or parathyroid glands. Again total parathyroidectomy and autotransplantation is the treatment of choice for those patients with clinical hyperparathyroidism. Total thyroidectomy is the definitive treatment for medullary carcinoma of the thyroid. Serum gastrin, calcitonin and prolactin are not of value as MEN syndrome markers in patient with primary hyperparathyroidism (Farndon et al 1987).

Carcinoid tumour of the foregut may be associated with hyperparathyroidism in a familial condition (Duh et al 1987). The carcinoids produce a wide variety of hormones with the predominant hormones determining the clinical presentation. The parathyroid glands are hyperplastic and total parathyroidectomy and autotransplantation are indicated.

The sporadic association of hyperparathyroidism with almost all known endocrine neoplasms has been described (Vair et al 1987). The raised calcium is usually the consequence of a single enlarged parathyroid gland and, if the gland is hyperplastic, it is vital to screen family members for endocrine neoplasms including hyperparathyroidism.

PERSISTENT OR RECURRENT HYPERPARATHYROIDISM

Persistent primary hyperparathyroidism is hypercalcaemia documented within 6 months of the initial surgery usually from a missed adenoma, while recurrent disease occurs more than 6 months after surgery with an interval when the serum calcium reverted to normal, and is particularly associated with inadequate surgery for hyperplasia.

Patients with persistent or recurrent primary hyperparathyroidism are a difficult management problem for, when the initial surgery fails, reoperation is associated with a higher morbidity and greater chance of failure (Brennan et al 1985). The most common cause of a failed initial operation is an unrecognized parathyroid adenoma.

A thorough assessment of the patient's history, operation notes and pathology is an essential first step to plan future management. In particular, a family history of MEN syndrome should be sought and excluded. The documented pathology findings should be reviewed in conjunction with the operation notes to identify the sites explored. An important distinction in the pathology report is the identification of the parathyroid tissue excised as normal, hyperplasia or an adenoma. The persistence of hyperparathyroidism should be proven biochemically and reoperation should be considered for symptomatic patients when the corrected serum calcium is greater than 3 mmol/l. Preoperative localization studies are of vital importance as precise localization may reduce the tissue dissection required in an operative area deformed from the initial surgery.

Non-invasive localization studies are performed first: neck ultrasonography, CT and thallium–technetium scintigraphy have a combined sensitivity of 78% for adenoma localization when performed in combination, while magnetic resonance imaging has a claimed 75% sensitivity and 4% false-positive incidence. The most sensitive invasive study which in our practice is reserved for localization of recurrent or persistent hyperparathyroidism is selective PTH venous sampling. It has an 80% sensitivity and is of particular value in identifying thoracic lesions and providing lateralizing information.

A planned operative strategy is then followed based on the preoperative localization studies. Reoperation is initially directed to the indicated site. When localization studies are negative, the neck is explored initially and then the thorax if no lesion has been found. If an adenoma is excised and confirmed on histology, surgery is complete, but hyperplasia requires excision of all four glands and autotransplantation.

In reported series of reoperation findings (Wang 1977, Grant et al 1986) most adenomas are found in the neck, one-third in the usual location for an upper gland, 20% in the usual lower gland location, 16% intrathyroidal and 14% in a paraoesophageal location. Parathyroid tumours at reoperation are often enclosed in scar tissue and intraoperative ultrasonography may be of value to identify abnormal glands. This technique is claimed to be more sensitive than any preoperative localization study (Kern et al 1987).

Routine dissection and removal of the thymus is advocated. In the chest, areas along the aortic arch, innominate vein and pericardium are searched. A survey of the world literature suggests that, in an experienced centre, the operative success for reoperation is about 90%. There was a 6% incidence of recurrent laryngeal nerve damage and a 14% incidence of permanent hypoparathyroidism requiring treatment.

HYPERPARATHYROIDISM AND PREGNANCY

The management of a patient with primary hyperparathyroidism during pregnancy should be decided according to the individual need. In most pregnant women primary hyperparathyroidism is not detected and there is an uncomplicated pregnancy. If there is mild asymptomatic hyperparathyroidism the mother should be regularly monitored and treated using oral bisphosphonates if required. After delivery the baby must be closely monitored as there is a real risk of tetany and hypoglycaemia. If the serum calcium is greatly elevated then surgery should be considered during the second trimester (Croom & Thomas 1984) but only if there is no response to oral bisphosphonates.

Definitive surgical treatment should be advised for any women with an elevated serum calcium if she is contemplating future pregnancy.

LONG-TERM FOLLOW-UP

There have been a number of long-term studies (Reonni-Sivula 1984, Palmer et al 1987) which suggest that patients successfully operated on for primary hyperparathyroidism run an increased risk of death compared to age- and sex-matched controls. A recent study of 896 patients followed for a mean time of 12.9 years confirms this view (Hedback et al 1990). The risk of premature death remained significantly increased, with the principal causes being cardiovascular and malignant disease. These studies suggest that primary hyperparathyroidism may cause damage which is not reversed by surgery, and long-term postoperative follow-up should be instituted. It is uncertain whether early surgical intervention in asymptomatic patients will influence this trend.

PARATHYROID CARCINOMA

Parathyroid carcinoma is rare and a difficult diagnosis to make. This rare condition should be considered when a high serum calcium is associated with a palpable lump in the neck. At surgery, it has a characteristic grey-white colour and may be adherent with local invasion.

However, both macroscopic and microscopic appearances may be ambiguous and a diagnosis only possible with unequivocal evidence of local infiltration of surrounding tissues or metastases. Aggressive surgical management should include an ipsilateral thyroid lobectomy and surgical clips used to outline the tumour bed for subsequent radiotherapy. The postoperative clinical course is characterized by recurrent episodes of hypercalcaemia and cervical recurrence or lung metastases. Patients treated with extensive surgery — tumour resection and unilateral or bilateral thyroidectomy — have both a longer survival and disease-free interval. Age is an important factor for survival and an aberrant DNA content is an important factor for early recurrence (Sandelin et al 1992).

KEY POINTS FOR CLINICAL PRACTICE

- Hyperparathyroidism is a more common condition than had been previously believed.
- The commonest clinical presentation is the 'asymptomatic' patient, while the symptomatic presentation may vary.
- The diagnosis is based upon the biochemical findings of a corrected serum calcium level above the upper limit of normal with the simultaneous elevation of the serum parathyroid hormone level.
- Preoperative localization studies may be of value.
- It is mandatory that the surgery should be performed by an experienced parathyroid surgeon.
- Long-term postoperative follow-up is desirable.

REFERENCES

Ankerstrom G, Malmaeus J, Bergstrom R, 1984 Surgical anatomy of human parathyroid glands. Surgery 95: 14–21
Barnes AD 1984 The changing face of parathyroid surgery. Ann R Coll Surg Engl 66: 77–80

Brennan MF, Norton JA 1985 Reoperation for persistent or recurrent hyperparathyroidism. Ann Surg, 201: 40–44

Britton DC, Johnston IDA, Thompson MH, Fleming LB, 1973 The outcome of treatment and changes in presentation of primary hyperparathyroidism. Br J Surg 60: 782–785

Bundred NJ, Ratcliffe WA, Walker RA et al 1990 Parathyroid hormone related protein and hypercalcaemia in breast cancer. Br J Med 303: 1506–1509

Canterbury JM, Levey GS, Reiss E 1973 Activation of renal cortical adenylate cyclase by circulating immunoreactive parathyroid hormone. J Clin Invest 52: 524–528

Clark OH, Okerlund MD, Moss AA 1985 Localisation studies in patients with persistent or recurrent hyperparathyroidism. Surgery 98: 1083–1094

Croom RD, Thomas CG 1984 Primary hyperparathyroidism during pregnancy. Surgery 96: 1109–1118

David DS 1975 Calcium metabolism in renal failure. Am J Med 58: 48–51

Duh Q-Y, Arnaud CD, Levin KE et al 1986 Parathyroid hormone: before and after parathyroidectomy. Surgery 100: 1021–1024

Duh Q-Y, Hybarger CP, Geist R et al 1987 Carcinoids associated with multiple endocrine neoplasia syndromes. Am J Surg 154: 142–148

Farndon JR, Geraghty TM, Dilley WG et al 1987 Serum gastrin calcitonin and prolactin as markers of multiple endocrine neoplasia syndrome in patients with primary hyperparathyroidism. World J Surg 11: 252–257

Failkon PJ, Jackson CE, Block MA et al 1977 Multicellular origin of parathyroid 'adenomas'. N Engl J Med 297: 696–698

Goode A, Jenkins B, Sprague D et al 1987 The beta 2 microglobulin urine to serum ratio: an early marker of renal dysfunction in primary hyperparathyroidism. Surgery 102: 914–916

Grant CS, van Heerden JA, Charbonear JW et al 1986 Clinical management of persistent and/or recurrent primary hyperparathyroidism. World J Surg 10: 555–565

Heath H, Hodgson SF, Kennedy MA 1980 Primary hyperparathyroidism: incidence, morbidity and potential economic impact in a community. N Engl J Med 302: 189–193

Hedback G, Tisell L, Bengisson B et al 1990 Premature deaths in patients operated on for primary hyperparathyroidism. World J Surg 14: 829–836

Jenkins BJ, Newell M, Goode AW et al 1990 The pre-operative localisation of parathyroid tissue using thallium-201 and technetium 99^m subtraction scintigraphy. J R Soc Med 83: 427–430

Kern KA, Shanker TH, Doppmann JL 1987 The use of high resolution ultrasound to locate parathyroid tumours during reoperations for primary hyperparathyroidism. World J Surg 11: 579–585

Law WM, Heath H 1985 Familial benign hypercalcaemia (hypocalciuric hypercalcaemia): clinical and pathogenetic studies in 21 families. Ann Intern Med 102: 511–519

Ljungham S, Benson L, Wide L et al 1988 Improved differential diagnosis of hypercalcaemia by hypocalcaemia stimulation of parathyroid hormone secretion. World J Surg 12: 496–501

Lufkin EG, De Remee RA, Rohrbach MS 1983 The predictive value of serum angiotensin converting enzyme activity in the differential diagnosis of hypercalcaemia. Mayo Clin Proc 58: 447–451

Majenski JT, Wilson SD 1979 The MEA I syndrome: an all or none phenomenon? Surgery 101: 738–745

Malmaeus J, Benson L, Johansson H et al 1986 Parathyroid surgery in multiple endocrine neoplasia type I syndrome: choice of surgical procedure. World J Surg 10: 668–672

Nader-Sepathi A, Goode A, Jenkins B et al 1992 Association between degree of β2 microglobulinaemia and long term outcome following curative surgery of primary hyperparathyroidism. Clin Sci 84: 12p

Nichols G, Flanagan B 1967 Normocalcaemic hyperparathyroidism. Trans Assoc Am Physicians 80: 314–318

Palmer H, Adams HO, Bergstrom R et al 1987 Mortality after surgery for primary hyperparathyroidism: a follow up of 441 patients operated on from 1956 to 1979. Surgery 102: 1–8

Peck WW, Higgins CB, Fisher MR 1987 Hyperparathyroidism: comparison of MR imaging with radionucleotide scanning. Radiology 163: 415–420

Pounder B 1990 Multiple endocrine neoplasia type 2: the search for the gene continues. Br

Med J 300: 484–485

Prinz RA, Payolan E, Lawrence AM et al 1977 Radiation associated hyperparathyroidism: a new syndrome? Surgery 82: 296–302

Prinz RA, Gamvros OI, Sellu D et al 1981 Subtotal parathyroidectomy for primary chief cell hyperplasia of multiple endocrine neoplasia type I syndromes. Ann Surg 193: 26–29

Purnell DC, Scholz DA, Beahrs OH 1977 Hyperparathyroidism due to single gland enlargement: prospective preoperative study. Arch Surg 112: 369–372

Purnell DC, Smith LH, Scholz DA et al 1971 Primary hyperparathyroidism: a prospective clinical study. Am J Med 50: 670–674

Reeves CD, Palmer F, Bacchus H et al 1975 Differential diagnosis of hypercalcaemia by the chloride/phosphate ratio. Am J Surg 130: 166–170

Robertson GSM, Iqbal S, Bell PRF et al 1992 Intraoperative parathyroid hormone estimation: a valuable adjunct to parathyroid surgery. Ann R Coll Surg Engl 74: 19–22

Reonni-Sivula H 1984 Causes of death in patients previously operated on for primary hyperparathyroidism. Ann Chir Gynaecol 74: 13–18

Sample W, Mitchell S, Bleaste R 1978 Parathyroid ultrasonography. Radiology 127: 485–490

Sandelin K, Aver G, Bondeson L et al 1992 Prognostic factors in parathyroid cancer: a review of 95 cases. World J Surg 16: 724–731

Scholz DA, Purnell DC 1981 Asymptomatic primary hyperparathyroidism. Am J Pathol 50: 549–554

Spritler CE, Geeter WB, Hamilton R 1987 Abnormal parathyroid glands: high resolution MR imaging. Radiology 162: 487–491

Stark DD, Moss AA, Gooding GA et al 1983 Parathyroid scanning by computed tomography. Radiology 162: 487–491

Tibblin S, Bondesson A-G, Uden P 1991 Current trends in the surgical treatment of solitary parathyroid adenoma. Eur J Surg 157: 103–107

Vair DB, Boudreau SF, Reid EL 1987 Pancreatic islet-cell neoplasia with secretion of a parathyroid-like substance and hypercalcaemia. Can J Surg 30: 108–110

Wang C 1977 Parathyroid re-exploration. A clinical and pathological study of 112 cases. Ann Surg 186: 140–145

Welbourn RB 1990 The history of endocrine surgery. Praeger, New York

Wheeler MH, Harrison BJ, French AP et al 1984 Preliminary results of thallium 201 and technetium 99 subtraction scanning of parathyroid glands. Surgery 96: 1078–1082

Wilson RO, Rao DS, Ellis B et al 1988 Mild asymptomatic primary hyperparathyroidism is not a risk factor vertebral fractures. Ann Intern Med 109: 959–962

Winzelberg GG 1987 Parathyroid imaging. Ann Int Med 107: 64–70

Young AE, Gaunt JI, Croft DN et al 1983 Localisation of parathyroid adenomas by thallium 201 and technetium -99m subtraction scanning. BMJ 286: 1184–1186

8

The critically ischaemic limb

W. G. Tennant   C. V. Ruckley

Critical limb ischaemia (CLI) is a major cause of morbidity in developed countries. This chapter will summarize the most recent developments in determining the pathophysiology and incidence of CLI. It will go on to deal with innovations in therapy and the results of treatment of both acute and chronic CLI.

DEFINITION OF CRITICAL LIMB ISCHAEMIA

To arrive at an accepted definition of CLI is one of the most difficult problems in vascular surgery, but it is increasingly necessary as treatment options grow in number and effectiveness so that studies dealing with results of different treatments may be seen to compare similar groups, and so that improvement can be objectively assessed.

Previous definitions have been clinical. The Fontaine Classification, used for many years, is unsatisfactory because it lacks objectivity (Table 8.1). More recently the European Working Group on Critical Leg Ischaemia (1991) produced the European Consensus Document. This defines CLI as 'persistently recurring ischaemic rest pain requiring regular, adequate analgesia for more than 2 weeks, or ulceration or gangrene of the foot or toes, with an ankle systolic pressure of <50 mmHg or a toe systolic pressure of <30 mmHg'. This is now the most frequently used definition and applies to diabetic and non-diabetic patients.

Table 8.1 The Fontaine Classification of limb ischaemia. Type 1 is sometimes subdivided into types 2a (well compensated) and 2b (poorly compensated), but these are impossible to define accurately and add to the confusion

Stage 1	No clinical symptoms
Stage 2	Intermittent claudication
Stage 3	Ischaemic rest pain
Stage 4	Ischaemic ulcer, gangrene

INCIDENCE

The true incidence of CLI and its trends with time are unknown because of the varying definitions applied to CLI over the years. Amputation rates give an indirect indication of the incidence, but a more reliable method is to follow the course of cohorts of claudicants to detect early predictors of eventual CLI. The total expected number of CLI patients can then be extrapolated from the total number of existing claudicants with those predictors.

The prevalence of asymptomatic vascular occlusive disease is estimated at some five times the incidence of claudication (Criqui et al 1985). At the present time, the prevalence of claudication in males over 50 years is approximately 5%, increasing with age. There is agreement between American and British series (Dormandy et al 1989, Fowkes et al 1991). It is thought that progression from claudication to CLI occurs in about 5% in the first year, with a further 2–3% per year in succeeding years (Criqui et al 1992).

Among claudicants followed-up for over 5 years, the amputation rate is approximately 11% in those continuing to smoke (Couch 1986), while in critical ischaemia the incidence is approximately 50% in those surviving 5 years (Widmer et al 1985, Kannel & McGee 1985, Bohlin et al 1988). The main cause of death in both groups is myocardial infarction (Dormandy et al 1989, O'Riordain & O'Donnell 1991). The 5-year mortality in patients with critical ischaemia is approximately 50%, compared to 15–20% among claudicants.

AETIOLOGY AND PATHOPHYSIOLOGY

Symptoms of CLI occur when the arterial supply is insufficient to meet the nutritional requirement of the resting limb. Chronic CLI is caused by atheromatous stenosis or occlusion in major arteries, and may be compounded by cardiac insufficiency caused by dysrhythmias, drugs, valvular disease or ischaemia. In addition, there are microcirculatory and haematological changes consequent upon macrovascular occlusion which contribute to the picture of chronic critical limb ischaemia. Acute CLI may occur because of a sudden thrombotic or embolic occlusion in a formerly normal circulation. Because of the paucity of developed collateral vessels in this situation, symptoms are usually sudden and severe. Treatment is urgently required to save the limb. More commonly, acute CLI occurs because of thrombosis or embolism in limbs already compromised by chronic occlusive disease. In this context, the acute event results in a sudden worsening of established chronic CLI, but because of the presence of developed collateral vessels in response to the chronic disease limb loss may not be inevitable, giving more time for accurate assessment and planning of treatment.

Because contributions to the syndromes of acute and chronic CLI may be made by almost any component of the circulation, each will be dealt with in turn.

The heart

The heart may act as a source of emboli to the lower limb. This well-recognized clinical entity is most common in patients who have atrial fibrillation, or who are convalescing from myocardial infarction. Less frequently, vegetations on a diseased or prosthetic heart valve may act as the primary source of emboli. Acute CLI may in these circumstances be treated by urgent embolectomy or, more commonly now, by thrombolysis.

The cardiac output may drop as a result of dysrhythmias, poor contractility, or obstructive disease such as aortic stenosis or pulmonary embolism. Atrial fibrillation can reduce the cardiac output by 10%, and both this and other dysrhythmias can, rarely, reduce the cardiac output sufficiently to produce peripheral gangrene in the presence of an anatomically normal circulation (Bird et al 1954). Most commonly, however, reduction in cardiac output acts in the presence of arterial occlusion to reduce the peripheral circulatory pressure to critical levels.

Low cardiac output sufficient to produce peripheral CLI may result from reduced myocardial contractility found in ischaemic cardiomyopathy, or in the overzealous treatment of hypertension or angina with beta-blocking drugs (Gokal et al 1979).

Arteries

Atherosclerosis of the abdominal aorta or peripheral limb arteries may cause partial or complete occlusion of the vessels. Sudden complete occlusion may be caused by emboli originating from atheromatous plaques in the major vessels, or from within aortic or popliteal aneurysms (Fig. 8.1). More commonly, problems are caused by local changes in atheromatous plaques. Occlusion can be produced when, possibly as a response to high intramural shear stress, haemorrhage occurs within an atheromatous plaque. The plaque ruptures exposing the circulating blood to collagen and causing in situ thrombosis. In cases where intraplaque haemorrhage does not cause rupture, or where rupture produces non-occlusive thrombosis, the plaque enlarges (in the latter case by re-endothelialization).

Critical ischaemia results from occlusion or severe multilevel stenosis affecting end arteries or critical collateral vessels.

The microcirculation

It has always been apparent that the severity of large vessel disease does not correlate well with the onset or severity of rest pain, and in recent years there has been increasing interest in changes in the microcirculation in chronic CLI. This has been due at least partly to advances in physiological measurement techniques used to examine the microvessels, some of which will be discussed later in this article.

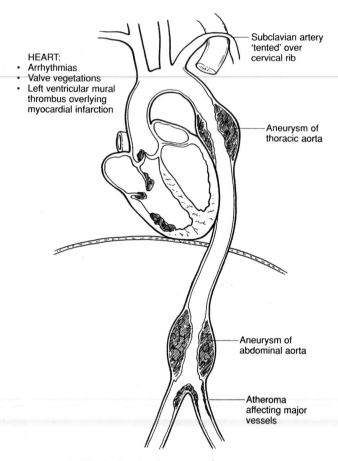

HEART:
• Arrhythmias
• Valve vegetations
• Left ventricular mural thrombus overlying myocardial infarction

Subclavian artery 'tented' over cervical rib

Aneurysm of thoracic aorta

Aneurysm of abdominal aorta

Atheroma affecting major vessels

Fig. 8.1   Sources of emboli in the heart and great vessels.

Redistribution

In the normal lower limb, about 90% of blood supplied passes through non-nutritive, thermoregulatory arteriovenous anastomoses (Conrad 1971). In CLI, the arteriolar beds become maximally vasodilated, probably as a result of locally released metabolites, producing so-called 'vasomotor paralysis'. This is responsible for the sunset red colour of dependent ischaemic feet, and also for the fact that, in some patients with rest pain, the total blood flow to the ischaemic foot is increased over normal levels. It is therefore assumed that the occurrence of ischaemic lesions in the foot is due to maldistribution of flow rather than an overall reduction (McEwan & Ledingham 1971).

Capillary plugging

Simultaneous transcutaneous oxygen tension measurements and fluorescein angiography has shown that ischaemic skin contains normal numbers of capillaries normally distributed, but that there is a functional decrease in the number of capillaries supplying oxygen to the skin in certain areas. This is caused in those affected areas by perfusion of some capillaries with blood of very low haematocrit, and by complete stasis in others (Franzeck et al 1987). The causes of these capillary abnormalities remain unclear, but a number of factors are thought to contribute. These include microthrombosis, collapse of precapillary arterioles because of low perfusion pressure, oedema, endothelial swelling and capillary plugging by blood cells.

Vasomotion

Other studies, using laser Doppler flux measurement, suggest that there is an abnormality of arteriolar vasomotion in ischaemic areas of skin. The normal 3–5 cycles per min 'slow wave' is frequently replaced in ischaemia by a faster oscillation at just over 20 per min. The pattern of vasomotion returns to normal with restoration of the circulation using percutaneous transluminal angioplasty (Seifert et al 1988, Hoffman et al 1989).

Endothelial function

It is likely that endothelial factors also play a part in arterial thrombosis. Normal endothelium produces a number of mediators which prevent thrombosis and promote vasodilation: prostacyclin, tissue-derived plasminogen activator and endothelium-derived relaxing factor. It also degrades some circulating mediators of thrombosis, such as adenosine di- and triphosphate, 5-hydroxytryptamine and thrombin. Little is known about the relevance or contribution of each of these to critical ischaemia, but both diabetes and smoking have been associated with abnormalities in endothelial function.

Veins

Decreased capillary flow may also be caused by venous 'back pressure' secondary to functional or physical reductions in venous return. In congestive cardiac failure, decreased venous return is accompanied by ankle oedema — another potent cause of microcirculatory insufficiency. Deep venous thrombosis may reduce venous flow in a limb to such critical levels as to cause venous gangrene, and subsequent pulmonary embolism can cause right heart failure, exacerbating the problem.

In rare cases of protein C deficiency and purpura fulminans, necrosis of small skin veins may lead directly to skin necrosis.

Haematological factors

Platelets

Several studies have demonstrated changes in platelet numbers or function in CLI. Increased levels of platelet release factors (β-thromboglobulin and 5-hydroxytryptamine), increased platelet numbers and adhesiveness have all been demonstrated in CLI (Lowe et al 1979a, Fitzgerald et al 1984, Zahavi & Zahavi 1985). The role of platelet changes in the pathogenesis of CLI has been uncertain, but recent meta-analyses of the use of platelet inhibitors in vascular disease have demonstrated that significant secondary prevention of atherosclerotic lesions may be obtained (Antiplatelet Trialists Collaboration 1994).

Neutrophils

Neutrophil behaviour has been studied in a number of animal and human models of acute ischaemia. When the blood supply to a limb is occluded, acute ischaemia produces little change in the disposition of neutrophils in the vessels. It is on reperfusion when most of the changes are seen (Goldberg et al 1990, Romanus et al 1978). Venular 'rolling' of neutrophils increases, and neutrophils accumulate in the vessels with simultaneous evidence of endothelial damage. Damage to distant organs, such as pulmonary oedema, may also accompany this so-called 'reperfusion injury' (Klausner et al 1989).

Studies in humans have found that in stable chronic limb ischaemia there is very little evidence of neutrophil activation except when the ischaemic muscle groups are exercised (Neumann et al 1990). It seems that significant prolonged neutrophil activation requires a severe ischaemic insult or reperfusion following severe ischaemia. Thus, neutrophil activation has been demonstrated in severe CLI leading to amputation and in aortic surgery following release of the cross-clamp (Nash et al 1988, Welbourn et al 1991).

The mechanisms by which activated neutrophils cause damage has been the subject of intensive study in the hope that some of these aspects may be open to manipulation. Much of this work has been done in myocardial infarction and stroke, but the principles are now being applied to peripheral ischaemia.

When neutrophils are subjected to severe non-specific insult, such as ischaemia/reperfusion, they become activated and release a number of chemical mediators. These include leukotrienes, oxidizing agents, proteolytic enzymes and thromboxane, all of which cause local endothelial damage and are free to circulate to cause damage at distant sites. Simultaneously, the neutrophils marginate and become adherent to endothelium in peripheral arterioles and capillaries, increasing peripheral resistance and exacerbating tissue ischaemia.

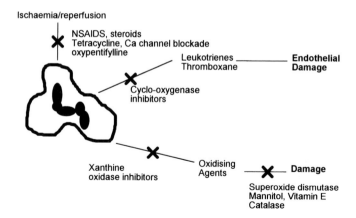

Fig. 8.2 Some of the recognized neutrophil activation products and drugs which may be used to inhibit their action.

Understanding of this mechanism has led to proposals for therapies designed to counteract the causes and consequences of neutrophil activation in the hope that these will limit the damage caused in reperfusion injury. Figure 8.2 shows some neutrophil release products and the agents which have been demonstrated to block or modify their action (Werns & Luccesi 1989, Mullane et al 1987, Altman 1990, Gabler & Creamer 1991).

Fibrinogen

Plasma fibrinogen levels have been linked to peripheral occlusive arterial disease in many ways. Levels are increased in patients who smoke, and it is the most widely available marker of chronic biological damage secondary to smoking. Most of the effects of raised fibrinogen levels are to predispose patients to occlusive vascular disease by raising plasma viscosity (especially in low flow states), increasing red cell and platelet aggregability, and infiltration of the vessel walls (Lowe et al 1991). Raised fibrinogen levels are predictive of coronary disease, stroke, cardiovascular mortality and femoropopliteal graft occlusion (Kannel & D'Agostino 1990, Wiseman et al 1989). In established CLI, the increased viscosity and aggregability lead to microthrombosis, exacerbating ischaemia and tissue hypoxia. Other factors raising fibrinogen levels in established CLI may include cytokine release from activated leukocytes, tissue necrosis and infection.

Because of the apparent importance of fibrinogen in CLI, therapies centring on defibrination with ancrod have been proposed, but have not gained wide acceptance (Lowe et al 1979b). Studies of this agent to date have been few, and have not produced convincing evidence of benefit in critical ischaemia (Lowe et al 1982). Intensive research efforts continue to uncover new mechanisms and mediators which are likely to contribute to the development or progress of CLI. These include studies of endothelial metabolism, fibrinolysis and arachidonate derivatives. While beyond the scope of this article, these may become increasingly relevant to the clinical management of CLI and reperfusion injury in the future.

ASSESSMENT

History

A full clinical history should be taken, including specific inquiry for the presence of risk factors for vascular disease. These include smoking, diabetes, hypertension and familial hyperlipidaemia. The vascular history should not be restricted to the lower limbs, and should include details about myocardial ischaemia, transient hemispheric cerebral ischaemia and amaurosis fugax.

Clinical examinaion

Clinical assessment should include the entire vascular system as well as a thorough general examination. The abdomen should be examined for aortic aneurysm, and both carotids for bruits. Examination of the peripheral circulation should be made using Doppler ultrasound including calculation of the ankle/brachial pressure index.

Non-invasive testing of arterial patency

Further examination of the circulation is usually undertaken in the vascular laboratory. The aims of these more complex non-invasive tests are to make as thorough an assessment of the patient as possible, and to complement invasive radiological investigation.

If bedside Doppler examination has been difficult because of very low pressures, flow in ankle vessels may be detected during augmentation using hyperaemia or dependency. Stenoses may be approximately localized using segmental pressure measurements.

Pulse-generated runoff has been developed as a functional anatomical test of distal arterial patency. Where filling of crural vessels with radiographic contrast is poor owing to proximal occlusions, pulse-generated runoff can reveal the presence of patent vessels. The technique depends upon the production of an artificial pulse wave by a pneumatic cuff inflated and deflated rapidly in succession around the leg just above or just below the knee (Fig. 8.3). The distally travelling arterial pulse wave so produced may be detected at the ankle using a hand-held Doppler probe. There is a well-described 'scoring' system for signal configuration of the derived waveform, and these have been related to angiograms and the success of bypass grafting (Scott et al 1989, 1990).

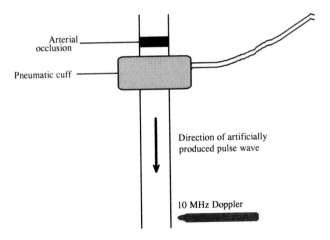

Fig. 8.3 The principle of pulse-generated runoff. A cuff is placed proximally around the limb and inflated and deflated in rapid succession. The pulse wave generated in a patent vessel is detectable distally using an ordinary 10 mHz Doppler probe.

Duplex ultrasound is now used as a preliminary investigation in many cases of lower limb ischaemia. It can be used to judge the position, severity and length of superficial femoral artery stenoses (Pellerito & Taylor 1992). Assessment of the aortoiliac segment with Duplex is possible, but is more difficult. Work is in progress comparing Duplex with other modalities (Currie et al 1994).

A newer option is magnetic resonance angiography (MRA). A variety of techniques, including time of flight and spin echo sequences, can be used to image the aorta and distal vessels. The majority of these do not require the use of radiographic contrast materials, and are of obvious benefit where a history of allergy exists. Although MRA can give highly detailed images of larger vessels, it tends to overestimate the degree of stenosis when there is severely turbulent blood flow. Accuracy is also reduced when attempts are made to image smaller vessels such as the calf arteries where the vessels commonly cross the imaging plane and so produce weak imaging signals (Anderson et al 1990).

To be of clinical value, MRA must compete directly with colour mapped Duplex ultrasound in terms of cost, availability and, above all, accuracy. While MRA equipment continues to fall in price and becomes more widely available the first two goals may soon be achieved. Prospective comparison of MRA and colour Duplex has failed to show that MRA is as accurate as Duplex in clinical use in lower limb vascular disease, although it may be more useful in showing pelvic vessels (Mulligan et al 1991, Fillmore et al 1991). With refinements in technique, MRA may soon give as much, if not more, information than current contrast investigations (Potchen 1992).

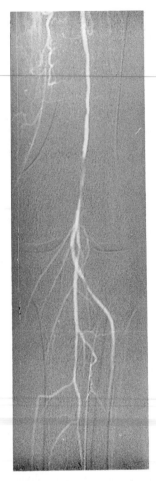

Fig. 8.4 A digital subtraction angiogram. The bone shadows are removed by computer imaging techniques, leaving the angiogram in high contrast. In this case, slight patient movement has allowed the bone shadows to show faintly.

Invasive testing of arterial patency

Conventional arteriography is the reference standard against which other investigations are judged. Digital imaging is a relatively new technique available now in most vascular centres (Fig. 8.4).

This technique has the advantage of requiring smaller doses of intra-arterial contrast agent. It is also more sensitive in imaging small vessels distal to occlusions, where the vessels do not fill well with contrast. In cases where arterial access is difficult or impossible, digital techniques can be used to image the arterial circulation by means of intravenous contrast administration. These images are generally of poorer quality than intra-arterial DSA, but may still provide useful information.

Assessment of the microcirculation

The increasing importance of microcirculatory factors in CLI has been discussed above. Direct examination of the microvessels is possible using vital capillary microscopy, but this technique is little used in the UK. More commonly, indirect measures of the microcirculation are used, and depend on the delivery of oxygen to the skin and the velocity of red blood cells in skin capillaries.

The clinical use of laser doppler flux (LDF) in ischaemia is limited to the measurement of hyperaemic responses and other flow-related characteristics in living tissues (Kvernbo et al 1989, Slagsvold et al 1992, Scheffler & Reiger 1992, Ruth 1993, Lindsberg et al 1992). It has been found useful in assessing the amputation level (Lantsberg & Goldman 1991). Its principal drawback is that it cannot be quantified in relation to blood flow or oxygen delivery.

Transcutaneous oxygen tension measurement quantitatively measures the oxygen flux across intact skin (but not skin tissue oxygen tension). It has had variable success in assessing optimum amputation level; the results have been unreliable and poorly reproducible (Slagsvold et al 1989, Matsen et al 1980). In claudicants, reproducibility has also proved poor. Measurements in this group showed 'considerable variation in individual patients' (Caspary et al 1993) and single readings in patients with claudication are of little value − a finding corroborated by other authors (Svedman et al 1982, Eickhoff & Engel 1981). Neither transcutaneous oxygen pressure measurement nor laser Doppler flux has been related to underlying muscle oxygenation.

Intramuscular oxygen tonometry became possible as a clinical method in the 1960s with the development of needle tonometers. It has been used extensively in experimental physiology (Bylund-Fellenius et al 1981, Soini et al 1992), including that of limb ischaemia (Jussila & Niinikoski 1981). Clinical uses have included monitoring free flap viability in plastic surgery (Mahoney & Lista 1988). It has also been used to determine appropriate amputation level, illustrating too that potential viability of skin may differ from that of muscle at the same anatomical level (Ehrly & Schroeder 1978). No attempts appear to have been made to use muscle oxygen tonometry to assess muscle viability in acute CLI, or to employ it as a clinical monitoring tool.

MANAGEMENT

General measures

Investigation should proceed as quickly as possible, and should be directed at assessing the general state of the patient as well as the ischaemic limb. It should include a thorough general clinical examination, ECG and chest radiograph. Blood should be taken for electrolytes, urea, creatinine, glucose, full blood count and coagulation assays.

Adequate analgesia should be provided for rest pain, and dressings for ulceration. Elevation of the head of the bed can provide 'gravity assistance' for limb blood flow, but care must be taken that this does not produce oedema. Severe hypertension and cardiac failure should be vigorously treated, and diabetes closely controlled.

Specific measures

Investigation generally begins with examination of the pulses of the affected limb. Doppler ankle pressures are measured at the bedside, and the ankle brachial index calculated. Accurate records are made of the site and size of ulcerated lesions, and antibiotics prescribed if appropriate for infected lesions. In acute CLI, movement and sensation in the affected limb must be accurately recorded. The muscles themselves should be palpated for the 'doughy' feel and/or tenderness of irreversible ischaemia and an assay of urine myoglobin should be performed.

Most patients then proceed to angiography, but this may be contraindicated in cases of contrast allergy, or if biochemical investigation demonstrates significant renal impairment. In these cases, Duplex ultrasound and pulse-generated runoff may be of some use, as may MRA if available. Patients with severe cardiac failure resistant to treatment may be unable to lie flat for angiography or insertion of thrombolysis catheters, and in such cases operative treatment is unlikely to be possible. In extremely urgent cases of acute CLI it is occasionally necessary to take the patient immediately to theatre without the benefit of angiograms or other arterial investigation.

Patients with CLI require active treatment if lives are to be made bearable or limbs saved. If tissue necrosis is not too far advanced, the aim is restoration of blood flow. Some, who have advanced disease or whose concomitant medical conditions preclude this type of treatment, must be managed conservatively until amputation becomes necessary. For these patients, the current options are drug therapy or sympathectomy.

All patients presenting with acute ischaemia are commenced on intravenous heparin therapy pending investigation and more specific measures.

Thrombolysis

This is an option in cases of acute or acute-on-chronic ischaemia, and can be successfully employed for both embolism and thrombosis (Fig. 8.5A,B). There are many reports of restoration of patency in occlusions of several weeks' duration and success may even be achieved up to a year after occlusion (Lammer et al 1986).

A catheter is passed percutaneously into the blocked vessel and embedded in the occluding thrombus. An enzyme solution is then infused to dissolve the clot. Streptokinase or recombinant tissue plasminogen activator (rTPA) are the most frequently used enzymes in the UK, although urokinase is

A

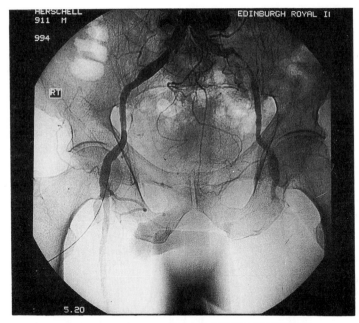

B

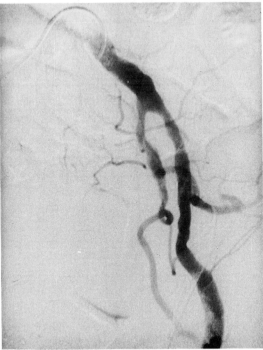

Fig. 8.5   A This patient had a thrombosis of the left common iliac artery deemed suitable for thrombolysis on clinical and radiological grounds. **B** This shows a detailed view of the left common iliac artery following successful thrombolysis. The lumen has been restored, and the internal iliac artery can be seen to fill.

commonly used in North America. In most cases, streptokinase infused at a rate of 5000 i.u. in 10 ml per hour is sufficient to re-open the vessel lumen in 12–24 h. rTPA is twenty times more expensive, and is usually reserved for patients who have been previously treated with streptokinase (e.g. for myocardial infarction). Other indications for the use of rTPA include its reputedly faster action, although this property has not been conclusively proven to be clinically useful (Earnshaw et al 1993, Comerota & Cohen 1993). During thrombolytic therapy, heparin is administered through the sheath of the delivery catheter to prevent pericatheter thrombosis. Fig. 8.6 illustrates the procedure for thrombolysis.

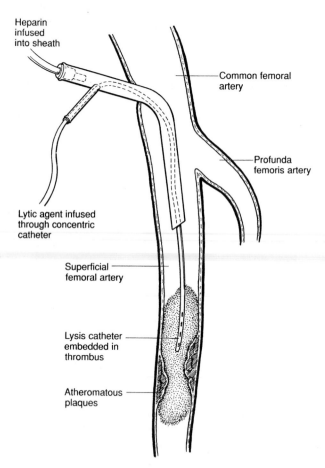

Fig. 8.6 The principle of thrombolysis. A sheath is introduced into the common femoral artery over a guidewire using the Seldinger technique. Heparin is infused through the lumen of the sheath to prevent pericatheter thrombosis. A fine lysis catheter is passed through the sheath and advanced into the thrombus. Lytic agent (normally streptokinase in the UK) is infused through the catheter to lyse the thrombus. Periodic check angiograms are taken to assess the progress of lysis and allow the catheter to be repositioned to continue to lie within the thrombus.

More recently, the pulse-spray delivery system has been developed for thrombolysis (Bookstein & Valji 1992). This forces lytic agent through a multi-holed catheter embedded in the thrombus, but instead of a steady infusion rate the infusion is pulsed, to add mechanical disruption to the action of the enzyme. This considerably speeds up the process of dissolution. Thrombolysis can also be employed intraoperatively if, following mechanical thromboembolectomy, on-table angiography shows residual thrombosis in distal vessels; 100 000 units of streptokinase in 50 ml is infused over 20 min into the occluded vessels, and followed by further attempts at embolectomy and angiography (Beard et al 1992).

Pre-treatment full blood count and coagulation screen are advisable but, given normal values, haematological monitoring is not normally required since thrombolytic agents at these dose levels do not affect systemic parameters unless continued for several days.

Relative contraindications to the use of thrombolysis are recent operation (including intra-abdominal aortic grafts), recent cerebral infarction or haemorrhage, gastrointestinal ulceration, or bleeding diatheses. Complications are rare, but include defibrination and bleeding from the puncture site or gastrointestinal tract and stroke.

Angioplasty

Introduced in 1964, percutaneous transluminal angioplasty (PTA) became more common after the invention of the balloon catheter in 1974. It should now be available in all centres undertaking the treatment of vascular disease. Obliterative lesions giving rise to CLI are usually too extensive to be treated solely by PTA, but the latter may be valuable in combination with bypass surgery to improve inflow to or outflow from a graft. PTA in Britain is performed almost exclusively by radiologists.

The balloon catheter is introduced percutaneously over a guidewire which crosses the stenosis or occlusion to be treated (Fig. 8.7). The most suitable stenoses for PTA are short concentric lesions in large vessels. The balloon is inflated in the lesion under fluoroscopic control when widening of the segment takes place by plaque fracture and intimal disruption/dissection rather than displacement. Although the histopathological appearances can be alarming, PTA has an excellent patency record, especially in larger vessels (Fig. 8.8 A,B). Technical failure to cross the arterial stenosis with a guidewire or to dilate it once crossed affects angioplasty success rates. Patency rates in both iliac and femoropopliteal lesions successfully treated with angioplasty, however, are similar to rates achieved with bypass surgery in the medium term (Wilson et al 1989).

For unfavourable stenoses or occlusions treated by angioplasty, long-term patency can be improved by the percutaneous insertion of metallic stents (Vorverk & Gunther 1992).

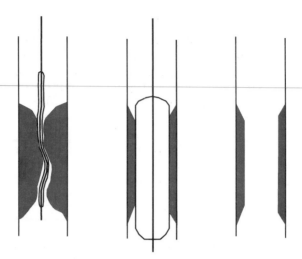

Fig. 8.7 The principle of angioplasty: a balloon catheter is advanced over a guidewire into an arterial stenosis. The balloon is then inflated to dilate the stenosis.

Atherectomy

Where stenoses are eccentric or occlusions cannot be crossed by a guidewire alone, atherectomy may be used to remove atheromatous plaque. A number of appliances are available for this, including side-cutting catheters and rotating drill-like devices. Preliminary treatment with these instruments can be followed by angioplasty with or without stenting. Variable results have been reported but in the femoropopliteal segment atherectomy compares unfavourably with balloon angioplasty alone (Vroegindeweij et al 1992). This topic was reviewed in detail in *Recent Advances in Surgery 16* (O'Malley & Greenhalgh 1993).

Bypass surgery

This remains the mainstay of the treatment of CLI where lesions cannot be treated percutaneously because of their configuration, length, or occurrence at multiple levels. Surgery of the aortoiliac, femoropopliteal and femorocrural segments is well established, but, with increasing availability of specialist vascular expertise, bypass surgery is becoming possible to more distal vessels. Patients with CLI have often had saphenous veins removed for coronary artery bypass or other peripheral reconstructions. In these patients, arm veins can be used for bypass as an alternative to prosthetic materials, and appear to have excellent patency rates (Sesto et al 1992). The construction of long bypasses to the ankle or foot has enabled the treatment of increasing numbers of diabetic patients in whom patent ankle and foot vessels can often be found distal to occluded calf vessels, and aggressive revascularization to small calibre vessels is recognized as worthwhile (Stonebridge et al 1991). Angioscopy has been adopted as an adjunctive technique in some centres. Its use is currently being advocated for 'quality control' of anastomoses, and for valve lysis in in situ femoropopliteal grafts. The expense and limited application of such equipment has contributed to its lack of popularity in the UK and a definite case for its routine use has still to be made.

An essential part of infrainguinal bypass surgery is postoperative surveillance. It has been obvious for some years that autologous vein grafts are prone to develop intrinsic fibrous stenoses within the first year after operation. These strictures progress quickly, and are a major cause of graft failure. Duplex ultrasound examination is a very powerful tool for detection of graft stenoses, and the increasing availability of Duplex ultrasound expertise has made detailed follow-up practical. Stenoses that are detected can be treated by balloon angioplasty (in the case of short discrete stenoses) or by operation. Common follow-up programmes include Duplex examination at 6 weeks, 3, 6 and 12 months after operation, and can be expected to detect approximately 95% of stenoses. Early intervention has been shown to improve long-term patency (Harris 1992)

Prostaglandins

The discovery of prostaglandin E_1 (PGE_1) in 1930 was followed in 1976 by the discovery of a substance with forty times the antiplatelet and vasodilator activity of PGE_1. PGI_1 or prostacyclin as it was subsequently called, is a natural product of endothelial metabolism. Uncontrolled trials of intravenous PGE_1 in critical ischaemia have shown no improvement of PGE_1 over placebo in either ulcer healing or relief of rest pain. Reports of initial studies of prostacyclin in CLI in the early 1980s were encouraging. Administered over several days, intravenous infusion of prostacyclin has been demonstrated in some studies to relieve rest pain for up to a month, but the results of larger studies have not demonstrated such improvements (Belch et al 1983, Norgren 1990). Prostacyclin is expensive and must be given by intravenous infusion daily, requiring inpatient admission. In the light of the equivocal results of even long-term infusion, the treatment of unreconstructable disease in this way cannot be regarded as cost effective.

Evidence is emerging that the once-only or short-term peroperative infusion of prostacyclin may be of value in enhancing distal bypass graft patency rates (Smith et al 1993). There is also experimental evidence to suggest that prostacyclin may modify the reperfusion injury sustained by patients undergoing revascularization procedures for acute CLI (Mohan et al 1992).

If the promise of these initial findings is fulfilled, they are likely to represent a major role for prostacyclin and its analogues.

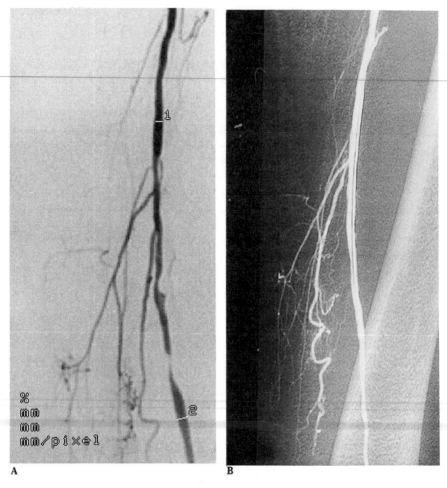

A   B

Fig. 8.8   **A**   This angiogram shows multiple stenoses in a superficial femoral artery between markers 1 and 2.   **B**   Angioplasty has been performed with a good radiological result.

Other drugs

Although many other drugs have been advocated for the treatment of peripheral vascular disease, none is of conclusively proven benefit in limb salvage, and their use cannot be recommended.

Sympathectomy

Performed by either the retroperitoneal approach or, more commonly, by the percutaneous injection of phenol, the aim of lumbar sympathectomy is to destroy vasoconstrictor fibres acting on the leg. There are no controlled studies demonstrating the effect of sympathectomy on CLI, but clinical experience is that it may relieve rest pain in some patients. It is of no benefit once tissue necrosis is established.

FUTURE DEVELOPMENTS IN THE ASSESSMENT AND TREATMENT OF CLI

Prevention

Health education has a major part to play in the prevention of critical peripheral ischaemia. With smoking identified as the major cause in the UK, the expansion of 'no smoking' policies in public places will help; however, significant impact cannot be expected until national policies are formulated and enforced on advertising and the sale of tobacco. Because of the lag time between a reduction in population smoking figures and the expected effect, vascular disease will continue to affect the UK population for some time to come. The impact of treatment of other risk factors such as hypertension, hypercholesterolaemia and diabetes is more difficult to judge, as their role in the development of CLI is less well defined.

Assessment

While clinical assessment will continue to play an important role in the assessment of acute and chronic CLI, vascular surgeons will become increasingly dependent on technology for accurate anatomical localization of disease. The advent of colour Duplex imaging has revolutionized fast, non-invasive assessment of lower limb vessels, and resolution continues to improve. As MRA becomes more available, it is likely that much of our reliance on contrast-based investigations will disappear. MRA not only has the potential to provide anatomical information but haemodynamic data too, and we may eventually be able to interrogate MRA information gained from a single scan session for all that we require.

Treatment

Future improvements in the treatment of acute and chronic CLI will probably focus on adjuvant radiological procedures. Research into the microcirculatory and cellular changes in CLI will hopefully lead to medical therapies designed to modify these effects and increase our 'salvage' rate in acute disease.

Embolectomy and thrombectomy are procedures whose use is rapidly diminishing as the role of thrombolysis is expanding. Rapid thrombolysis with modified delivery techniques and enzyme regimes will extend the use of lytic therapy in acute CLI, and patients currently excluded because of rapidly progressive acute CLI may be treated this way.

Undoubtedly bypass surgery will continue to play a role in the treatment of CLI, and the search will continue for new prosthetic materials and ways of using them. If angioscopy gains more widespread acceptance, the trauma of in situ femorodistal bypass could be reduced by the adoption of semiclosed and even 'closed' minimally invasive techniques.

KEY POINTS FOR CLINICAL PRACTICE

- The treatment of critical limb ischaemia is the most important challenge in vascular practice, and is best managed by a team approach. A judicious combination of imaging, thrombolysis, percutaneous angioplasty and reconstructive surgery can now preserve the great majority of critically ischaemic legs.

- The current definition of CLI is 'persistently recurring ischaemic rest pain requiring regular, adequate analgesia for more than 2 weeks, or ulceration or gangrene of the foot or toes, with an ankle systolic pressure of <50 mmHg or a toe systolic pressure of <30 mmHg'.

- Claudication affects 5% of men over 50 years old and, after the first year, 2–3% per year will progress to CLI. In patients with CLI, there is a 50% 5-year mortality rate, mainly from myocardial infarction. Amputation is necessary in 50% of those surviving 5 years.

- The causes of CLI are diverse, and include abnormalities of cardiac output and rhythm, haemostasis, arteries and veins. In established CLI there are profound changes in the microcirculation, including disturbed vasomotion and maldistribution of blood. Platelets and neutrophils may be activated, and sequestered in the microvessels releasing potent mediators which cause local and distant damage.

- Non-invasive clinical and laboratory assessment of patients with CLI using Doppler and Duplex ultrasound and pulse-generated runoff complements the use of contrast radiology. Indirect assessment of the microcirculation is difficult, unreliable and currently little used in the UK.

- In the treatment of CLI, general measures are necessary to control cardiac and metabolic abnormalities. Patients should be anticoagulated with heparin pending investigation. Rapid assessment allows the rational selection of the many treatments available, including thrombolysis, angioplasty, stenting, bypass surgery and drugs.

REFERENCES

Altman RD 1990 Neutrophil activation: an alternative to prostaglandin inhibition as the mechanism of action of NSAIDS. Semin Arthritis Rheum 19 (Suppl 2): 1–5

Anderson CM, Saloner D, Tsuruda HS et al 1990 Artifacts in maximum intensity projection display of MR angiograms. Am J Roentgenol 154: 623–629

Antiplatelet Trialists Collaboration 1994 Collaborative overview of randomised trials of antiplatelet therapy. 2: Maintenance of vascular graft or arterial patency by antiplatelet therapy. Br Med J 308: 159–168

Beard JD, Nyamekye I, Earnshaw JJ et al 1992 Intraoperative streptokinase removes thrombus the balloon catheter cannot reach. Br J Surg 79: 365

Belch JJF, McArdle B, Pollock JG et al 1983 Epoprostenol (prostacyclin) and severe arterial disease — a double blind trial. Lancet 1: 315–317

Bird D, Leithead CS, Lowe KG 1954 Symmetrical peripheral gangrene in low output heart failure. Lancet 2: 780–782

Bohlin T, Aldman A, Gustavsson PO et al 1988 Hur går det för patienter med viloischemi som ej opereras? Läkartidningen 85: 2398–2399

Bookstein JJ, Valji K 1992 Pulse-spray pharmacomechanical thrombolysis. Cardiovasc Intervent Radiol 15: 228–233

Bylund-Fellenius A-C, Walker P, Elander A et al 1981 Energy metabolism in relation to oxygen partial pressure in human skeletal muscle during exercise. Biochem J 200: 247–255

Caspary L, Creutzig A, Alexander K 1993 Variability of T_cpO_2 measurements at 37°C and 44°C in patients with claudication in consideration of provocation tests. Vasa 22 (2): 129–136

Comerota AJ, Cohen GS 1993 Thrombolytic therapy in peripheral arterial occlusive disease: mechanisms of action and drugs available. Can J Surg 36: 342–348

Conrad MC 1971 Functional anatomy of the circulation to the lower extremities. Year Book Publishers, Chicago

Couch NP 1986 On the arterial consequences of smoking. J Vasc Surg 3: 808–812

Criqui MH, Fronek A, Barrett-Connor E et al 1985 The prevalence of peripheral arterial disease in a defined population. Circulation 71: 510–515

Criqui MH, Langer RD, Fronek A et al 1992 Mortality over a period of 10 years in patients with peripheral arterial disease. N Engl J Med 326: 381–386

Currie I, Wilson YG, Tennant WG et al 1994 Non-invasive aorta-iliac assessment. Br J Surg 1994 (in press)

Dormandy J, Mahir M, Ascady G et al 1989 Fate of the patient with chronic leg ischaemia. J Cardiovasc Surg 30: 50–57

Earnshaw JJ, Scott DJA, Horrocks M et al 1993 Choice of agent for peripheral thrombolysis. Br J Surg 80: 25–27

Ehrly AM, Schroeder W 1978 Oxygen pressure in the ischaemic muscle tissue: a new diagnostic method for evaluating the patients with peripheral arterial occlusion. Vasc Surg 12: 215

Eickhoff JH, Engel HC 1981 Transcutaneous oxygen tension T_cpO_2 measurements on the foot of normal subjects and in patients with peripheral arterial disease admitted for vascular surgery. Scand J Clin Lab Invest 41: 743

European Working Group on Critical Leg Ischaemia 1991 Second European consensus document on chronic critical leg ischaemia. Circulation 84 (Suppl 3)

Fillmore DJ, Yucel EK, Briggs SE et al 1991 MR angiography of vascular grafts in children. Am J Roentgenol 157: 1069–1071

Fitzgerald GA, Smith B, Pederson AK et al 1984 Increased prostacyclin biosynthesis in patients with severe atherosclerosis and platelet activation. N Engl J Med 310: 1065–1068

Fowkes FGR, Housley E, Cawood EHH et al 1991 Edinburgh Artery Study: prevalence of asymptomatic and symptomatic peripheral arterial disease in the general population. Int J Epidemiol 20: 384–392

Franzeck UK, Leibethal R, Diehm C 1987 Mikrovaskulare Flussverteilung und transcutaner Sauerstoffpartialdruck der Hautkapillaren von Patienten mit peripherer arterieller Verschusskrankheit im Stadium 3 und 4. Vasa Suppl 20: 309–310

Gabler WL, Creamer HR 1991 Suppression of human neutrophil functions by tetracyclines. J Periodontol Res 26: 52–58

Gokal R, Dornan TL, Ledingham JGG 1979 Peripheral skin necrosis complicating beta-blockade. Br Med J 1: 721–722

Goldberg M, Serafin D, Klitzman B 1990 Quantification of neutrophil adhesion to skeletal muscle venules following ischaemia-reperfusion. J Reconstr Microsurg 6: 267–270

Harris PL 1992 Vein graft surveillance — all part of the service. Br J Surg 79: 97–98

Hoffman U, Saesseli B, Geiger M et al 1989 Vasomotion in patients with severe ischaemia before and after percutaneous transluminal angioplasty. Int J Microcirc Clin Exp Special Issue, August

Jussila EJ, Niinikoski J 1981 Effect of vascular reconstruction on tissue gas tensions in calf muscles of patients with occlusive arterial disease. Ann Chir Gynaecol 70: 56–60

Kannel WB, D'Agostino RB 1990 Update on fibrinogen as a major cardiovascular risk factor: The Framingham Study. J Am Coll Cardiol 15: 156a

Kannel WB, McGee DL 1985 Update on some epidemiological features of intermittent claudication. J Am Geriatr Soc 33: 13–18

Klausner JM, Paterson IS, Mannick JA et al 1989 Reperfusion pulmonary oedema. JAMA 261: 1030–1035

Kvernebo K, Slagsvold CE, Strandon E 1989 Laser Doppler flowmetry in evaluation of skin post-ischaemic reactive hyperaemia. A study in healthy volunteers and atherosclerotic patients. J Cardiovasc Surg 30: 70–75

Lammer J, Pilger E, Neumayer K et al 1986 Intra-arterial fibrinolysis: long term results. Radiology 161: 159–163

Lantsberg L, Goldman M 1991 Laser Doppler flowmetry, transcutaneous oxygen tension measurements and Doppler pressure compared in patients undergoing amputation. Eur J Vasc Surg 5: 195–197

Lindsberg PJ, Jacobs TP, Frerichs KU et al 1992 Laser Doppler flowmetry in monitoring regulation of microcirculatory changes in spinal cord. Am J Physiol 263: H285–H292

Lowe GDO, Reavey MM, Johnston RV et al 1979a Increased platelet aggregates in vascular and non-vascular illness: correlation with plasma fibrinogen and effect of ancrod. Thromb Res 14: 377–386

Lowe GDO, Morrice JJ, Forbes CD et al 1979b Subcutaneous ancrod therapy in peripheral arterial disease: improvement in blood viscosity and nutritional blood flow. Angiology 30: 594–599

Lowe GDO, Morrice JJ, Forbes CD et al 1982 Double blind controlled clinical trial of ancrod for ischaemic rest pain of the leg. Angiology 33: 46–50

Lowe GDO, Donnan PT, McColl P et al 1991 Blood viscosity, fibrinogen and activation of coagulation and leucocytes in peripheral arterial disease: the Edinburgh Artery Study. Br J Haematol 77 (Suppl 1): 27

McEwan AJ, Ledingham IM 1971 Blood flow characteristics and tissue nutrition in apparently ischaemic feet. Br Med J 3: 220–224

Mahoney JL, Lista FR 1988 Variations in flap blood flow and tissue pO_2: a new technique for monitoring flap viability. Ann Plast Surg 20: 43–47

Matsen FA, Wyss CR, Burgess EM 1980 Transcutaneous oxygen tension in peripheral vascular disease. Surg Gyncol Obstet 150: 525–528

Mohan C, Marini C, Gennaro M et al 1992 the value and limitation of iloprost infusion in decreasing skeletal muscle necrosis. J Vasc Surg 16: 268–273

Mullane KM, Salmon JA, Kraemer R 1987 Leucocyte derived metabolites of arachidonic acid in ischaemia induced myocardial injury. Fed Proc 46: 2422–2433

Mulligan SA, Matsuda T, Langer P et al 1991 Prospective comparison of MR angiography and colour duplex US with conventional angiography. Radiology 178: 695–700

Nash GB, Thomas PRS, Dormandy JA 1988 Abnormal flow properties of white blood cells in patients with severe ischaemia of the leg. Br Med J 296: 1699–1701

Neumann FJ, Waas W, Diehm W et al 1990 Activation and decreased deformability of neutrophils after intermittent claudication. Circulation 82: 922–929

Norgren L 1990 Non-surgical treatment of critical limb ischaemia. Eur J Vasc Surg 4: 449–454

O'Malley MK, Greenhalgh RM 1993 Minimally invasive arterial surgery. In: Taylor I, Johnson CD (eds) Recent advances in surgery 16. Churchill Livingstone, Edinburgh, pp 225–239

O'Riordain DS, O'Donnell JA 1991 Realistic expectations for the patient with intermittent claudication. Br J Surg 78: 861–863

Pellerito JS, Taylor KJ 1992 Doppler color imaging. Peripheral arteries. Clin Diagn Ultrasound 27: 97–112

Potchen EJ 1992 Magnetic resonance angiography. Semin Ultrasound CT MR 13: 225–226

Romanus M, Bagge U, Seifert F et al 1978 Intravital microscopy of the microcirculation in man during and after experimentally controlled ischaemia. Scand J Plast Reconstr Surg 12: 181–187

Ruth B 1993 Skin blood flow evaluated by the laser speckle method and the transcutaneous oxygen tension: interpretation of the dynamics using a simple model. Int J Microcirc Clin Exp 12: 227–254

Scheffler A, Reiger H 1992 Spontaneous oscillations of laser Doppler skin blood flow flux in peripheral arterial occlusive disease. Int J Microcirc Clin Exp 11: 249–261

Scott DJA, Hunt G, Hartnell GG et al 1989 Arteriogram scoring systems and Pulse Generated Runoff in the assessment of patients with critical ischaemia for femorodistal bypass. Br J Surg 76: 1202–1206

Scott DJA, Vowden P, Beard JD et al 1990 Non-invasive estimation of peripheral resistance using pulse generated runoff before femorodistal bypass. Br J Surg 77: 391–395

Seifert H, Jager K, Bollinger A 1988 Analysis of flow motion by the laser Doppler technique in patients with peripheral arterial occlusive disease. Int J Microcirc Clin Exp 7: 223–236

Sesto ME, Sullivan TM, Hertzer NR et al 1992 Cephalic vein grafts for lower extremity revascularisation. J Vasc Surg 15: 543–536

Slagsvold CE, Kvernebo K, Slungaard U et al 1989 Pre- and postischaemic transcutaneous oxygen tension measurements and the determination of amputation level in ischaemic limbs. Acta Chir Scand 155: 527–531

Slagsvold CE, Stranden E, Rosen et al 1992 The role of blood perfusion and tissue oxygenation in the postischaemic transcutaneous pO_2 response. Angiology 43: 155–162

Smith FC, Thomson IA, Hickey NC et al 1993 Adjuvant prostanoid treatment during femorodistal reconstruction. Ann Vasc Surg 7: 88–94

Soini HO, Takala J, Nordin AJ et al 1992 Peripheral and liver tissue oxygen tensions in hemorrhagic shock. Crit Care Med 20: 1330–1334

Stonebridge PA, Tsoukas AI, Pomposelli FB et al 1991 Popliteal to distal bypass grafts for limb salvage in diabetics. Eur J Vasc Surg 5: 265–269

Svedman P, Holmberg J, Jacobsson S et al 1982 On the relation between transcutaneous oxygen tension and skin blood flow. Scand J Plast Reconstr Surg 16: 133

Vorverk D, Gunther RW 1992 Stent placement in iliac arterial lesions: three years of clinical experience with the Wallstent. Cardiovasc Intervent Radiol 15: 285–290

Vroegindeweij D, Kemper FJM, Tielbeek AV et al 1992 Recurrence of stenoses following balloon angioplasty and Simpson atherectomy or the femoropopliteal segment: a randomised comparative 1 year follow-up study using colour flow duplex. Eur J Vasc Surg 6: 164–171

Welbourn CRB, Goldman G, Paterson IS et al 1991 Pathophysiology of ischaemia reperfusion injury: central role of the neutrophil. Br J Surg 78: 651–655

Werns SW, Luccesi BR 1989 Myocardial ischaemia and reperfusion: the role of oxygen radicals in tissue injury. Cardiovasc Drugs Ther 2: 761–769

Widmer LK, Biland L, DaSilva A 1985 Risk profile and occlusive peripheral artery disease. Proceedings of the 13th international congress on angiology Athens

Wilson SE, Wolf GE, Cross AP et al 1989 Percutaneous transluminal angioplasty versus operation for peripheral arteriosclerosis. J Vasc Surg 9: 1–8

Wiseman S, Kenchington G, Dain R et al 1989 Influence of smoking and plasma factors on patency of femoropopliteal vein grafts. Br Med J 299: 643–646

Zahavi J, Zahavi M 1985 Enhanced platelet release reaction, shortened platelet survival time and increased platelet aggregation and plasma thromboxane B_2 in chronic obstructive arterial disease. Thromb Haemost 53: 105–109

9

Surgical aspects of urinary incontinence

A. R. Mundy

Urinary incontinence is extremely common. We all start off our lives incontinent and many of us end up that way as well. Between the two extremes of life it is estimated that incontinence affects 10–25% of adolescents and adults (Cardozo 1991). It is so common in fact that most women expect to get it after childbirth; most men expect to get it with advancing years in association with 'prostate problems'; and jokes about 'weak bladders' and incontinence are the stuff of everyday humour. To those who suffer urinary incontinence it can be an extremely debilitating symptom, both socially and professionally.

In some instances, namely those patients with neurological disease, incontinence may be associated with impaired renal function, but in most patients urinary incontinence exists in isolation.

THE AETIOLOGY OF INCONTINENCE

There are many different causes of incontinence as listed in Table 9.1 Such a list by being comprehensive fails to give attention to frequency. Detrusor instability and stress incontinence are very much commoner than any of the neuropathic causes or extrasphincteric causes of incontinence. Patients with those two problems are the commonest to present for investigation and treatment and most commonly require surgery. Equally, senility affects most people who live long enough and bed-wetting affects the whole of mankind initially, but in neither of these instances is surgical treatment indicated. When reading such a list one therefore needs a degree of perspective.

On the subject of causes of incontinence it is perhaps worth pointing out that incontinence has knock-on effects which are not always immediately apparent. Incontinence is the commonest reason why a patient with neurological disease is admitted to hospital and one of the commonest reasons why the elderly are admitted to hospital as well. There are therefore considerable implications in funding and provision of health services which may not be immediately apparent.

Table 9.1 Causes of urinary incontinence

Transsphincteric
A. Non-neuropathic
    a. Detrusor instability
    b. Sphincter weakness incontinence (stress incontinence)
    c. Overflow incontinence
    d. Postmicturition dribbling
    e. Incontinence due to loss of awareness
        i. By night: simple bed-wetting
        ii. All the time: in association with senility
    f. Iatrogenic incontinence
        i. Due to drugs (especially diuretics, hypnotics)
        ii. Due to surgery (especially prostatectomy)

B. Neuropathic
    In association with spina bifida and other congenital cord lesions, spinal cord injury,
    Parkinson's disease, cerebrovascular accidents, disseminated sclerosis and other acquired
    non-traumatic spastic paraplegias

Extrasphincteric
Ectopia vesicae (exstrophy of the bladder)
Vesicovaginal, ureterovaginal and other urinary fistulae
Congenital ectopic ureter

THE INITIAL APPROACH TO THE PROBLEM

All patients should have a detailed history and physical examination and on the basis of this most can be allocated to a provisional diagnosis. When the symptoms are not entirely clear from the history, patients can be given a chart to complete on which they note the timing and volume of urine voided and whether or not they are dry or wet at that time. The timing and volume of intake is also useful information. In the absence of neurological disease, or one of the unusual extrasphincteric causes, treatment can usually be empirical on the basis of the history and the frequency/volume chart. First-line treatment of detrusor instability will be with bladder training and anticholinergic drugs. The first-line treatment of presumed simple stress incontinence is with the use of pelvic floor exercises or, in some postmenopausal patients, topical oestrogens.

Patients with chronic retention due to benign prostatic hyperplasia will usually have a transurethral resection in the first instance but sometimes the chronically distended bladder will never contract again and clean intermittent self-catheterization may be necessary to give complete bladder emptying.

Postmicturition dribbling is diagnosed from the history and does not require any form of investigation or treatment let alone surgical treatment, just explanation. Incontinence due to loss of awareness requires containment and attention to circumstances rather than treatment. Patients with iatrogenic incontinence need an assessment and possibly a change of their drug regimen if this is at fault. Patients with postsurgical iatrogenic incontinence usuallyrequire surgical intervention; this essentially refers to patients with postprostatectomy incontinence.

Patients with ectopia vesicae (exstrophy) or epispadias need the attention of a paediatric urologist as do those with ectopic ureters which may be either reimplanted, or removed by nephroureterectomy if there is no useful remaining renal function. Patients with fistulae should have them repaired if catheterization of the bladder fails to give prompt improvement.

Those patients with detrusor instability or stress incontinence that fails to respond to simple measures, those with postprostatectomy incontinence and all patients with neuropathic incontinence require urodynamic investigation to define exactly the cause and nature of their problem so that treatment can be planned. Other types of patients, as indicated above, will either require more appropriate investigation or no investigation at all.

This is not the place to describe or discuss the techniques and interpretation of urodynamic investigation, but the reader is unlikely to understand the subject of incontinence and its treatment without at least a rudimentary grasp of the principles of urodynamics, so should consult references such as those given at the end of this chapter.

GENERAL TREATMENT

The first and most important step before proceeding to surgery is to make an accurate urodynamic diagnosis. The second and almost equally important question is to make sure that the patient understands the advantages and disadvantages of surgery and to satisfy the surgeon that he/she is properly motivated. It is important to realize that nobody ever died of wetting themselves but they do occasionally die as a result of surgical intervention, however well intentioned that surgery may have been. It is important therefore to have a properly informed and well-motivated patient who understands what surgery can offer and also what it can not. A particular point worth mentioning at this stage is that surgery does not always cure a patient, it simply converts symptoms from a socially unacceptable level to a socially acceptable level and often produces a degree of voiding difficulty. This voiding difficulty may be to such a degree that clean intermittent self-catheterization is required to empty the bladder if the bladder is no longer able to empty itself adequately. This is not common in patients undergoing surgery for stress incontinence but is common in patients undergoing surgery for detrusor instability and all patients should be warned of the possibility of requiring clean intermittent self-catheterization and those who find such a prospect unacceptable should not be submitted to surgery. The same applies to surgical treatment of neuropathic bladder dysfunction.

It goes without saying that surgical treatment of urinary incontinence is only used when non-surgical methods have failed or are inappropriate. This particularly applies to the surgical treatment of stress incontinence, detrusor instability and neuropathic bladder problems. Most ladies with significant stress incontinence will require surgery, but surgery is rarely required in detrusor instability which usually responds to a combination of bladder retraining and anticholinergic drugs. In neuropathic bladder conditions there are likewise many patients who respond to non-surgical treatment and many others for whom surgical treatment is unrealistic because of their associated neurological problems. This point will not be repeated but it should be born in mind throughout this chapter that surgery is only indicated when non-surgical methods have failed or are inappropriate.

DETRUSOR INSTABILITY

Detrusor instability is the term given to the occurrence of involuntary bladder contractions when the patient is trying to hold urine in the bladder (Abrams et al 1988). These contractions may occur spontaneously or on provocation by factors such as coughing or a change of posture. The contractions cause an urgent desire to void (urgency), frequency because they generally occur at a low bladder capacity, and urge incontinence if the contraction cannot be contained by voluntary contraction of the urethral sphincter mechanism.

The cause of this is not known but appears to be due to 'instability' — hypopolarization — of the smooth muscle cell membrane, perhaps as a result of partial cholinergic denervation of the detrusor but this is, to say the least, arguable (Broding & Tuner 1994). Detrusor instability may be secondary to bladder outflow obstruction in males but does not appear to be so related in females, although outflow obstruction in females (using the same terms of reference) is rare. Detrusor instability is similar to detrusor hyper-reflexia seen in patients with neurological disease and may have a similar aetiological basis, but, until that is proven, the two separate terms are given to an identical urodynamic pattern.

The strong association of anxiety states with overaction bladder states has been recognized for years (Frewen 1980) and a failure of maturity has been cited by many as a cause of the unstable bladder but this is a hypothesis that remains unproven.

Surgery for detrusor instability

Such surgery is relatively recent when compared with surgery for stress in-continence. None the less, it is well established. Techniques such as bladder transection, transvesical injection of pelvic plexus with phenol, endoscopic bladder transection and neurosurgical procedures on the sacral nerve roots have had a vogue (Mundy 1988) and the occasional patient may be considered for ileal conduit urinary diversion but in general the surgical procedure for detrusor instability is the so-called 'clam' ileocystoplasty which is a form of augmentation cystoplasty (Mundy & Stephenson 1985). The bladder is subtotally bisected (Fig. 9.1) and a section of gut equal in length to the circum-ference of the bisected bladder is isolated on its vascular pedicle (Fig. 9.2)

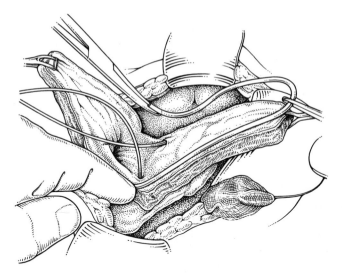

Fig. 9.1 Ileocytoplasty. The bladder has been subtotally bisected in the coronal plane and the circumference of the bladder is being measured with a length of plastic tubing.

and opened to form a patch (Fig. 9.3) and sewn into the bladder to close it (Fig. 9.4). This works very well but, as mentioned above, is commonly associated with voiding difficulty thereafterwards — a symptom that patients are usually happy to exchange for their previous frequency, urgency and urge

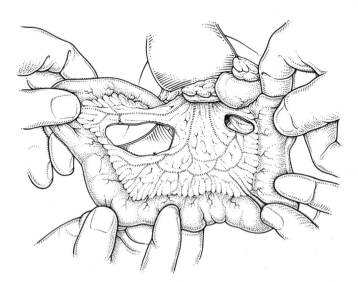

Fig. 9.2 A section of ileum, equal in length to the circumference of the bisected bladder, is being mobilised on its vascular pedicle.

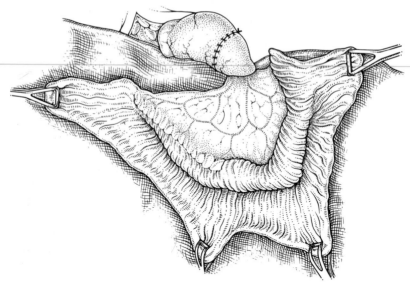

Fig. 9.3 The ileal segment has been opened along its antimesenteric border to form a patch.

incontinence but one which may occasionally require clean intermittent self-catheterization to provide emptying thereafterwards.

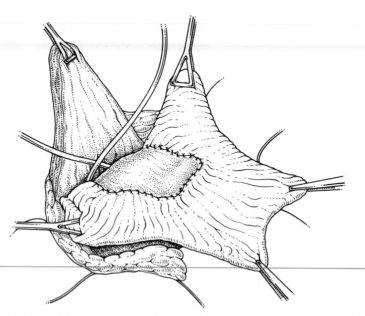

Fig. 9.4 Partly completed ileocytoplasty. The patch has been sewn to the posterior bladder wall and is about to be sewn to the anterior bladder wall. A catheter has been passed up each ureter for orientation.

SPHINCTER WEAKNESS INCONTINENCE
(STRESS INCONTINENCE)

This refers to incontinence on coughing, laughing, sneezing, lifting or any other form of activity causing a rise in intra-abdominal pressure. It occurs most commonly in women after pregnancy and childbirth but there are other causes. For example, bilateral single ectopic ureters are associated with a malfunctioning of the bladder neck and sphincter mechanism and there are other congenital types of sphincter weakness, most notably epispadias, but these are all rare. More commonly sphincter weakness may be secondary to direct trauma or scarring from urethral or periurethral surgery and may be secondary also to radiotherapy for reasons that are not entirely clear. Such conditions should be looked for in the history and on physical examination but further discussion of such problems is beyond the scope of this chapter.

After pregnancy and childbirth sphincter weakness incontinence is thought to be due to a combination of loss of support to the bladder outflow as a result of relaxation of the ligamentous structures of the pelvic floor during pregnancy and overstretching during delivery, and denervation of the urethral sphincter mechanism as a result of overstretching of the nerves of the pelvic plexuses during delivery (Snooks & Swash 1984). In most patients loss of support seems to predominate.

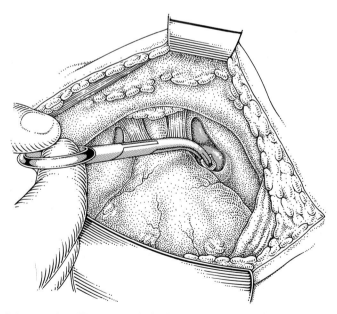

Fig. 9.5 Colosuspension. The endopelvic fascia on the right side of the bladder neck has been incised and the plane between the bladder base and the anterior vaginal wall is being developed with a 'peanut'.

Surgery for stress incontinence

This is the most well-established form of surgery for incontinence and generally takes the form of one of two types of bladder neck suspension: open retropubic bladder neck suspension or transvaginal so-called 'endoscopic' bladder neck suspension. Both seek to provide support for the bladder neck so that the urethral sphincter mechanism can work to its best advantage. Open bladder neck suspension may be achieved by any one of the numerous very similar techniques which have been described of which the best known are the colposuspension described by Birch and the Marshall–Marchetti–Kranz procedure. The Birch colposuspension (Stanton 1986) is the better procedure in which, through a Pfannenstiel incision, the endopelvic fascia is disrupted on either side of the bladder neck (Fig. 9.5) so that the anterolateral vaginal wall can prolapse through (Fig. 9.6). This is then stitched to the side wall of the pelvis, usually the pectineal ligament, on each side (Figs. 9.7, 9.8) to elevate and support the bladder neck and urethra.

The same procedure (more or less) can be performed transvaginally using techniques such as those described by Raz (1981), Stamey (1973), Peyrera and many others. Bladder neck suspension is now also being performed laparoscopically. Whichever technique is used is usually a reflection of personal bias, although other factors such as vaginal prolapse and how it may be simultaneously treated may influence the decision.

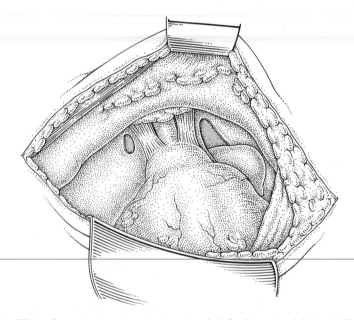

Fig. 9.6 With a finger in the vagina, the lateral vaginal fornix on the right-hand side is being 'tented' up towards the pectineal ligament.

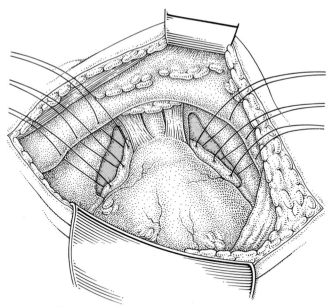

Fig. 9.7   Having mobilised the vaginal fornix on each side, sutures have been placed to hitch the vaginal wall up to the pectineal ligament.

For those with more severe and intractable forms of stress incontinence which have failed to respond to standard techniques, procedures such as sling

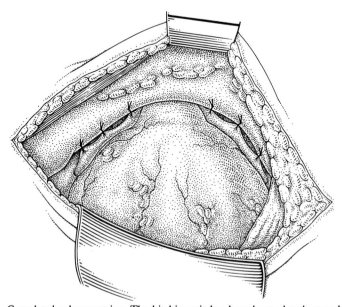

Fig. 9.8   Completed colosuspension. The hitching stitches have been placed on each side.

suspension of the bladder neck or implantation of an artificial sphincter may be contemplated (for review see Raz 1985). Slings are generally most useful when the bladder neck and urethra cannot be stabilized in any other way when it is loss of support that is the problem. When the urethral sphincter mechanism is intrinsically too weak so that even a well-suspended bladder outflow cannot function adequately then an artificial sphincter is the only reliable way of treating the incontinence.

OVERFLOW INCONTINENCE

This is generally the result of chronic retention of urine secondary to benign prostatic hyperplasia but may be associated with other conditions such as diabetic autonomic neuropathy, dyssynergic bladder neck obstruction in males and occasionally other forms of outflow obstruction in either sex. It is generally diagnosed with ease on clinical examination by the ready palpation of a grossly distended bladder. The treatment is to either use clean intermittent self-catheterization or alternatively, in males with bladder outflow obstruction, to relieve the obstruction. Although relieving the obstruction seems the obvious approach, this often fails to give symptomatic relief because the acontractile bladder state that results from chronic distension persists. Clean intermittent self-catheterization then becomes necessary despite relief of the obstruction (Lapides et al 1972). This will also not be considered further.

POSTMICTURITION DRIBBLE

This can occur in females but generally occurs in male of middle age and onwards when the bulbocavernosus muscle fails to empty the urethra at the end of voiding. The characteristic story is that the individual finishes voiding, dresses himself and then, as he turns and walks away, leaks a few drops of urine; that is the one and only symptom. It should be identified in the history, does not require further investigation but simply requires strong reassurance and advice on the merits of patience.

BED-WETTING

This is an extremely common problem and when it occurs in the absence of daytime symptoms is rarely associated with any urodynamic abnormality but is due to a failure of the brain to afferent impulses indicating a full bladder. It occasionally responds to alarms or the use of imipramine but generally gets better spontaneously in its own good time, although it may be difficult to persuade the patient and particularly the parents to accept this.

SENILITY

With advancing years or disease the individual may fail to recognize the desirability of going to empty the bladder in a particular place put aside for that purpose. In addition the aged patient may also suffer from stress incontinence if they are female, or urge incontinence in either sex, and the male patient may be subject to prostatic problems as well. All of these may cause or predispose to or worsen urinary incontinence and it can be a very difficult and sometime depressing problem to treat. The first thing to do is to see if the patient is taking any drugs (see below) that might make matters worse and look for any other treatable cause, i.e. to assess mobility and see if simple modification of everyday life — including paying attention to the ease with which the patient can get to the toilet might give an easy solution. If not, there is generally little that one can offer other than containment. Indwelling catheters should be resisted as they can be pulled out with even a fully inflated balloon with remarkable ease — and considerable bleeding. Appropriately designed undergarments with protective pads are far more suitable.

IATROGENIC INCONTINENCE DUE TO DRUGS

Individuals with borderline control, particularly after the menopause in females and with advancing years in both sexes, particularly when mobility is restricted, may find that the overenthusiastic use of diuretics or hypnotics turns them from borderline continence to borderline incontinence. In any patient the drug regimen should be the first line of questioning before proceeding to any detailed investigation.

IATROGENIC INCONTINENCE DUE TO SURGERY

This most commonly follows transurethral resection of the prostate which necessarily destroys the bladder neck sphincter mechanism and, if performed incompetently or sometimes for no apparent reason, may destroy or otherwise interfere with the urethral sphincter mechanism as well. Over enthusiastic use of blind internal urethrotomy in female patients is another occasional cause.

Surgery for postprostatectomy incontinence

Surgery for postprostatectomy incontinence, if sufficiently severe to warrant surgery in a patient fit enough to undergo it, means implantation of an artificial urinary sphincter (Mundy 1991). The Brantley Scott artificial sphincter in its AS800 model (Fig. 9.9) is the only device in regular clinical use. It is a hydraulic device with a cuff around a selected point of the bladder outflow — usually the bulbar urethra in post-prostatectomy incontinence (Fig. 9.10) — a pressure-regulating balloon that produces the occlusive force, and a control pump. The occlusive force is constantly maintained by the direction

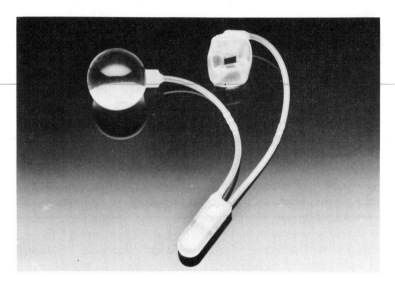

Fig. 9.9   The AS800 'Brantley Scott' artificial urinary sphincter.

of fluid flow from balloon to cuff (Fig. 9.11A) except when the pump is squeezed when fluid flow is reversed (Fig. 9.11B) to empty the cuff into the balloon thereby allowing voiding to occur.

The results are particularly good with the artificial sphincter in such patients (as they are in those women with refractory simple stress incontinence) but occasional problems from mechanical failure of the device, or, more importantly, from infection and consequent erosion, are a serious, albeit infrequent, nuisance.

The important point is to be sure by video-urodynamic evaluation that the incontinence is due to sphincter weakness/damage as incontinence in many of these patients is actually due to coincidental detrusor instability rather than a consequence of the prostatectomy (Fitzpatrick et al 1979).

NEUROPATHIC INCONTINENCE

This is much less common than non-neuropathic incontinence but is generally more severe and associated with disturbances of bowel function, sexual function and of lower limb function as well, all of which serve to make matters worse. A specific feature of neuropathic incontinence is the common association of detrusor dysfunction with sphincteric obstruction leading to high-pressure bladder outflow obstruction which may cause impairment of renal function and eventually renal failure. All such patients require careful investigation of both the upper and lower urinary tract.

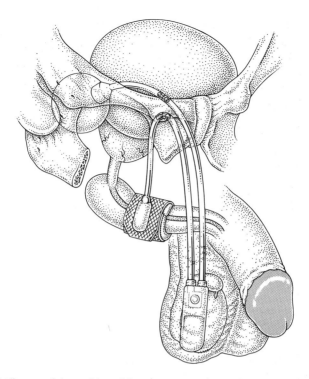

Fig. 9.10 A diagram of the position of the components of the AS800 artificial sphincter in a patient with post prostatectomy incontinence in whom the cuff has been implanted around the bulbar urethra.

Surgery for neuropathic bladder dysfunction

This is more complicated because the urodynamic problem is more compli-cated as there is usually a combination of both bladder and sphincter dysfunction. The bladder or the sphincter may be overactive or underactive in any combination (Rickwood et al 1982). Bladder underactivity and sphincteric obstruction (overactivity), particularly in combination, are usually amenable to treatment by clean intermittent self-catheterization (Lapides et al 1972) to ensure adequate bladder emptying if it cannot be achieved otherwise. Bladder overactivity and sphincter weakness usually in combination and most commonly in association with a variable degree of sphincteric obstruction are unfortunately much more common, the former — detrusor hyperreflexia — requring an augmentation cystoplasty if anticholinergic drugs cannot make the bladder docile and sphincter weakness requiring implantation of an artificial urinary sphincter unless attention to bladder overactivity allows the system to be sufficiently docile for the individual to attain reasonable continence even with a relatively weak sphincter (Parry et al 1992).

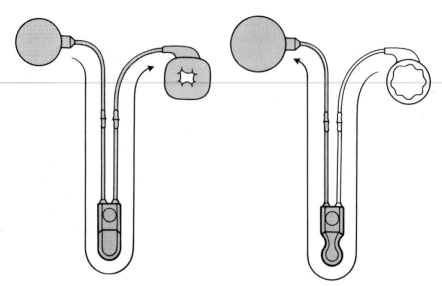

Fig. 9.11 Under 'resting' circumstances fluid flow in the AS800 is from the balloon through the control mechanism of the control pump to the cuff providing an occlusive force.

Fig. 9.12 When the pump is squeezed the cuff is emptied through the valve mechanism of the control pump into the balloon temporarily to allow voiding to occur.

A combination of clam ileocystoplasty and implantation of an artificial urinary sphincter may be a daunting procedure in some patients with neuropathic bladder dysfunction, particularly those who are confined to a wheelchair, and in such patients a urinary diversion may be a more realistic alternative.

In recent years, techniques of continent urinary diversion have been developed in which a catheterizable stoma runs from a selected point on the anterior abdominal wall through a valve mechanism into a substitute bladder, the valve mechanism serving to provide continence (Duckett & Snyder 1986, Woodhouse & Pope 1993). The individual therefore has a stoma, but a very much smaller stoma than that associated with an ileal conduit, and does not have to wear a bag because of the continence mechanism between the stoma and substitute bladder. This procedure, in its various different forms, has been a godsend for those patients who warrant surgical intervention but lack the mobility that makes orthotopic reconstruction by cystoplasty and an artificial sphincter realistic. The first technique of continent diversion available was the so-called Kock pouch (Kock et al 1978) but this proved unreliable sufficiently often that most people have now gone over to the so-called Mitrofanoff procedure (Mitrofanoff 1980) where the continence mechanism is a flap valve usually using the appendix as the continent catheterizable channel when available (Fig. 9.13) or the ureter when it is not (Fig. 9.14) rather than the nipple valve system used in the Kock pouch technique.

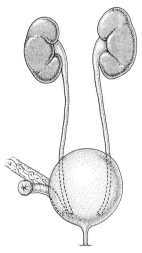

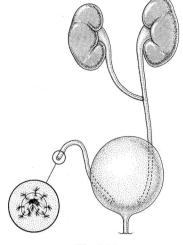

Fig. 9.13   Fig. 9.14

Another recent development is the sacral anterior root stimulator developed by Brindley (Brindley et al 1986) for use in spinal injured patients. It can
only be used in patients with a complete cord transection and viable nerve
roots and sacral spinal cord below. In such patients the device can be used to
stimulate bladder emptying, usually in conjunction with a posterior rhizotomy
to abolish involuntary detrusor contractility and poor bladder compliance. It
can also be used for bowel emptying and erection as well although it is less
successful in these two areas.

Unfortunately in many patients with neuropathic bladder, particularly those
congenital types with associated problems such as hydrocephalus or those
with progressive disease such as Parkinson's disease, the associated disabilities
make any form of treatment difficult and complex surgery in particular
unrealistic. In such patients with particularly intractable incontinence an ileal
conduit urinary diversion may be the best way of securing dryness if
conservative methods fail.

EXTRASPHINCTERIC CAUSES OF INCONTINENCE

Ectopia vesicae (bladder exstrophy) and epispadias are usually obvious that
epispadias in females may be overlooked. Gynaecologica fistulae are usually
obvious or can be deduced from the history. It is easy, however, to overlook
an ectopic ureter into the vagina in a young or adolescent girl as a cause of
incontinence but persistent intractable incontinence not associated with stress
or urgency between otherwise normal voiding episodes does not occur in any
other situation, so should be picked up in the history and the finding of a pool
of urine on examination of the vagina should strengthen the suspicion.

KEY POINTS FOR CLINICAL PRACTICE

It is generally possible to make anybody who is incontinent continent with the range of surgical procedures now available. It is not therefore so much a question of which operation is appropriate for which patient but in determining in the first place which patient is suitable for operation at all. When surgery for incontinence fails, particularly in more complex cases, it is usually as a result of poor selection and performing surgery on inappropriate patients rather than performing it inadequately.

ACKNOWLEDGEMENTS

Figures 9.1–9.14 are reproduced from Mundy A R 1993 Urodynamic and reconstructive surgery of the lower urinary tract. Churchill Livingstone, Edinburgh.

REFERENCES

Abrams P, Blaivas JG, Stanton SG et al 1988 The standardisation of terminology of lower urinary tract function. ICS Committee on Standardisation of Terminology. Scand J Urol Nephrol Suppl 114: 5–19

Brading AF, Turner WH 1994 The unstable bladder: towards a common mechanism. Br J Urol 73: 3–8

Brindley GS, Polkey CE, Rushton DN et al 1986 Sacral anterior root stimulators for bladder control in paraplegia: the first 50 cases. J Neurol Neurosurg Psychiatry 49: 1104–1114

Cardozo L 1991 Urinary incontinence in women: have we anything new to offer? Br Med Bull 303: 1453–1456

Duckett JW, Snyder HM 1986 Continent urinary diversion: variations on the Mitrofanoff principle. J Urol 135: 58–62

Fitzpatrick JM, Gardiner RA, Worth PHL 1979 The evaluation of 68 patients with post-prostatectomy incontinence. Br J Urol 51: 552–555

Frewer WK 1980 The management of urgency and frequency of micturition. Br J Urol 52: 367–369

Kock NG, Nilson AF, Norlen L et al 1978 Urinary diversion via a continent ileum reservoir: clinical experience. Scand J Urol Nephrol Suppl 49: 23–31

Lapides J, Diokuo AL, Silber SJ et al 1972 Clean intermittent self-catheterisation in the treatment of urinary tract disease. J Urol 107: 458–461

Mitrofanoff P 1980 Cystotomie continente trans-appendiculaire dans le traitement des vessies neurologiques. Chir Pediatr 21: 297–305

Mundy AR 1988 Detrusor instability. Br J Urol 62: 393–397

Mundy AR 1991 Artificial sphincters. Br J Urol 67: 225–229

Mundy AR, Stephenson TP 1985 'Clam' ileocystoplasty for the treatment of refractory urge incontinence. Br J Urol 57: 641–646

Parry JRW, Nurse DE, Boucaut HAP et al 1990 Surgical management of the congenital neuropathic bladder. Br J Urol 65: 164–167

Raz S 1981 Modified bladder neck suspension for female stress incontinence. Urology 18: 82

Raz S 1985 Symposium on female urology. Urol Clin North Am 12 (2)

Rickwood AMK, Thomas DG, Phip NH et al 1982 Assessment of the congenital neuropathic bladder by combined urodynamic and radiological studies. Br J Urol 54: 507–511

Snooks S, Swash M 1984 Abnormalities of the innervation of the urethral situated sphincter musculature in incontinence. Br J Urol 56: 401–405

Stamey TA 1973 Cystoscopic suspension of the vesical neck for urinary incontinence. Surg Gynecol Obstet 136: 547 1993

Woodhouse CRJ, Pope AJ 1993 Alternatives to urinary diversion with a bag: results in 100 patients. Br J Urol 72: 580–585

GENERAL REFERENCES

Mundy AR, Stephenson TP, Wein AJ Urodynamics: principles, practice and application. Churchill Livingstone, Edinburgh
Mundy AR 1993 Urodynamic and reconstructive surgery of the lower urinary tract. Churchill Livingstone, Edinburgh

10

Modern hernia management

A. N. Kingsnorth

In the UK, approximately 80 000 hernia repairs are performed per year; in males this is the commonest operation and overall it is the third commonest operation performed. By the age of 65 years, 3% of men will have had a groin hernia repair. Hernia surgery rates in the UK are low. The age-standardized hernia surgery rate of 100 per 100 000 population per annum compares with figures of 180 and 280 respectively for Australia and the USA. The age-specific rates have a peak in infancy and a peak in the 55–85-year age group (Fig. 10.1).

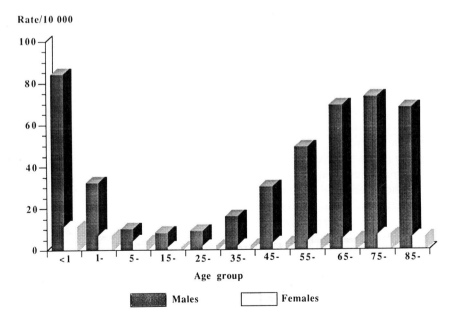

Fig. 10.1 Age-specific surgery rates for inguinal hernia per 10 000 for males and females, England 1989–1990

159

HERNIA CHARACTERISTICS

Ninety per cent of inguinal hernia operations are on males. In adult European males, 65% of inguinal hernias are indirect and 55% are right-sided. Bilateral hernias are four times more commonly direct than indirect. Many hernias exist in the community undiagnosed, undetected and unreported. The results of insurance examination surveys show that only 20–50% of men with inguinal hernia report the condition at medical interviews. Femoral hernia is three times more common in females than males, although females themselves undergo three times as many inguinal hernia repairs as femoral hernia repairs. Femoral hernia, which is very rare under the age of 35 years, is most common in multiparous women and is as prevalent in men as in nulliparous women.

PATHOGENESIS

An indirect inguinal hernia is not simply a congenital defect represented by a persistent patent processus vaginalis. Autopsies reveal that 10–20% of men have indirect sacs and no hernia during life, indicating that a processus vaginalis can remain patent throughout life without the development of a hernia. A proportion of patent processus vaginales apparently obliterate while others persist. For instance at presentation for repair of an infantile inguinal hernia the clinical incidence of contralateral hernia is 20% and the operative incidence of patent processus vaginalis is 50%. During 20 years of follow-up after infant hernia repair, 22% of men will develop a contralateral inguinal hernia (Given & Rubin 1989).

In males beyond adolescence, simple removal of an indirect hernia sac results in an unacceptably high recurrence rate indicating that other factors are involved in the pathogenesis. Moreover, the high frequency of indirect hernias in middle-aged and older people suggests a pathological change in the connective tissue of the posterior inguinal wall. Thus, the susceptibility to inguinal hernia is based both on the presence of a congenital sac and on failure of the transversalis fascia. These facts should guide the surgeon when managing indirect hernias in adult males.

Pathogenesis of direct inguinal hernia is more complex. In the majority of patients there is no peritoneal sac and the occurrence parallels ageing and other factors such as smoking. Thus the incidence would appear to be more directly related to a failure of the posterior inguinal wall or transversalis fascia. Additional factors include anatomical abnormalities such as a deficient medial half of the transversalis fascia and failure of the insertion of the internal oblique aponeurosis onto the superior pubic ramus. Metabolic abnormalities have been identified including a generalized deficiency in collagen, particularly in smokers and patients with abdominal aortic aneurysms (Lehnert & Wadouh 1992). A high incidence of hernia in Eskimos in the West Arctic of Greenland, where there is a high frequency of the HLA-B27 allele resulting in instability of mesenchymal tissues, points to a more specific genetic and collagen metabolic abnormality (Harvald 1989).

NATURAL HISTORY

The incidence of strangulated hernias in the UK is 13 per 100 000 per annum with a peak in the 80-year age group. Strangulation occurs in 10% of patients with no previous history of groin hernia. Because of an ageing population the mortality following strangulation has remained between 10% and 15% over the last 30–40 years. Mortality is highest when bowel resection is necessary.

The risk of strangulation is low. Neuheuser studied a population in Columbia where hernia repair was virtually unobtainable and found a strangulation rate of 0.29% per annum (Neuhauser 1977). However, in the USA in 1964, 2070 patients died from intestinal obstruction secondary to hernia and in 1967 this was one of the ten leading causes of death.

The different types of groin hernia carry different risks of strangulation. By far the greatest risk is associated with femoral hernia, with 40% of patients admitted as emergency cases with strangulation or incarceration. By contrast, direct inguinal hernia represents only 3% of hernias which strangulate. This clearly indicates that differing priorities must be given to the elective management of femoral and direct inguinal hernia. Asymptomatic direct inguinal hernias have been observed for up to 10 years without enlargement even in labourers (Berliner 1990). Because of the low risk of strangulation counterbalanced by the slight but low risk of morbidity or mortality for elective repair, inguinal hernioplasty in a 65-year-old man does not increase life expectancy.

The relative risk of strangulation of groin hernia is not constant from year to year (Gallegos et al 1991). The cumulative probability of strangulation is greater in the first 3 months for both inguinal and femoral hernias. After 3 months, the cumulative probability of strangulation for inguinal hernia is 2.8% rising to 4.5% after 2 years (Fig. 10.2). For femoral hernia, it is 22% at 3 months, rising to 45% at 21 months (Fig. 10.3). In a patient over the age of 60 years with a complicated hernia there is a 20-fold increased risk of dying from attempted repair compared with patients who undergo elective hernioplasty.

Based on the above observations the following recommendations can be made. High-risk groups can be identified such as patients having had previous infantile hernia repair, smokers, the elderly and patients with abdominal aortic aneurysms. The public, especially the elderly, should be warned of the potential dangers of a lump in the groin and general practitioners should be encouraged to refer such patients promptly, i.e. in the first 3 months of the existence of a hernia. A recent survey indicates that this is not current practice. Not only general practitioners but also geriatricians and surgeons are exercising a selective policy in the elderly for groin hernioplasty. For example, only 21% of general practitioners would refer a 79-year-old male with a small

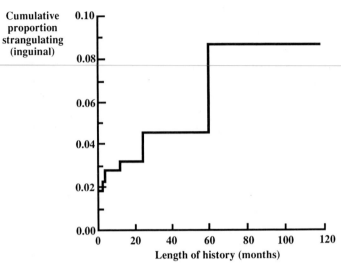

Fig. 10.2 Plot of the cumulative proportion of inguinal hernias strangulating versus length of history. (Reproduced with permission from Gallegos et al 1991.)

painless reducible inguinal hernia to a surgeon for a further opinion and only 61% of geriatricians would refer a frail 80-year-old female for elective surgery on account of an asymptomatic femoral hernia (Allen et al 1987).

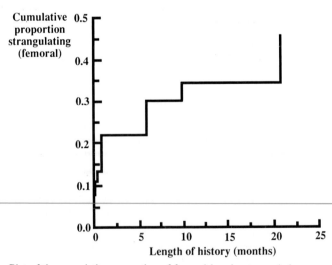

Fig. 10.3 Plot of the cumulative proportion of femoral hernias strangulating versus length of history. (Reproduced with permission from Gallegos et al 1991.)

CLASSIFICATION AND DIAGNOSIS

Although specialized units have attempted to promulgate one specific type of hernioplasty for all groin hernias, this may not be appropriate. Recently, attempts have been made to classify hernias and match the type of hernia with specific operations. The classifications of Gilbert (Table 10.1) and Nyhus (Table 10.2) have been popularized in the USA and have been used as a means of limiting the indications for the use of prosthetic material and the indications for laparoscopic hernia repair. For instance, prosthetic mesh may only be indicated where the posterior inguinal wall is significantly weak and laparoscopic repair may only be indicated in the smaller types of hernia such as indirect inguinal with no fascial defect or indirect inguinal with minor dilatation of the internal ring or femoral hernia. No consensus, however, has been reached concerning the individualization of hernia repair. Herniography is a useful adjunct particularly in patients with obscure groin pain with a normal or inconclusive physical examination (Gullmo 1989). Complication rates are low and the false-positive rate is negligible. This approach should be considered mandatory in the professional sportsman with chronic groin pain before hernioplasty is considered because of the long list of differential diagnoses (Malycha & Lovell 1992).

Table 10.1   The five types of inguinal hernia (after Gilbert)

Indirect	Type I	Snug internal ring, intact canal floor	
	Type II	One finger breadth internal ring, intact canal floor	
	Type III	Two finger breadth internal ring, defective canal floor (scrotal and sliding hernias)	
Direct	Type IV	Entire canal floor defective, no peritoneal sac anterior to canal floor, intact internal ring	
	Type V	Diverticular defect admitting no more than one finger, internal ring intact	

Table 10.2   Classification of groin hernias (after Nyhus)

Type I	Indirect inguinal hernia: internal inguinal ring normal (e.g. child's hernia)
Type II	Indirect inguinal hernia: internal ring dilated but posterior inguinal wall intact, inferior deep epigastric vessels not displaced
Type III	Posterior wall defects
	A. Direct inguinal hernia
	B. Indirect inguinal hernia: internal ring dilated, medially encroaching or destroying the transversalis fascia of the Hesselbach triangle (e.g. massive scrotal, sliding or pantaloon hernias)
	C. Femoral hernia
Type IV	Recurrent hernias

MANAGEMENT POLICY

The truss

The majority of patients treated with a truss grain poor hernia control with considerable discomfort (Law & Trapnell 1992). The reasons for this may be related to the fact that 21% of patients are prescribed a truss before referral to a surgeon, 44% receive no instructions concerning the fitting of the truss and as a consequence 77% fitted the truss whilst standing. A poorly fitted truss can increase the complications of hernia and result in atrophy of the spermatic cord and the fascial margins of the inguinal region. These problems may contribute significantly to morbidity as 40 000 trusses are sold annually, mostly through retail outlets in the UK.

Day care surgery

Although enthusiasts, such as James Nicoll from Glasgow and Eric Farquaharson from Edinburgh, have actively encouraged day care for inguinal hernioplasty for at least 40 or 50 years, such enthusiasm remained isolated until the last decade. Currently in the USA 70% of inguinal hernioplasty is performed on a day case basis and the majority of patients are discharged within 4 h of surgery. A recent survey in the UK indicated that only 11% of the surgeons were regularly undertaking day case inguinal hernioplasty (Morgan et al 1992). Medical fitness may not be the most important criterion governing early discharge and in the elderly social support becomes the overriding factor (Millat et al 1993). A recent study from the French Association of Surgical Research found that only 10% of patients received 1-day surgery for inguinal hernioplasty and 60% were discharged within 48 h. The figures quoted above from the USA come from free-standing specialist facilities and are not representative of the entirety of hernia surgery practice. For instance, the length of stay for inguinal hernioplasty in the US Army is 4.6 days and Metropolitan Life Insurance Company statistics indicate that length of stay for their clients averaged 2.9 days. The Royal College of Surgeons of England (1993) estimates that 50% of groin hernia surgery can be performed on a day case basis.

Local anaesthesia

Local anaesthesia is a valuable option. However, it is not suitable for anxious, obese or uncooperative patients or those with complex hernias. Safety standards in the operating theatre should be rigorously enforced and include knowledge of the safe dose of local anaesthesia administered on a mg/kg body weight basis. Intraoperative monitoring, intravenous access and pulse oximetry are essential, especially if intravenous sedation is being administered.

Local anaesthetic hernia repair should not be undertaken by junior surgeons until they are adept at surgical technique and achieving good results from surgery performed under general anaesthesia. Junior surgeons will slip back down the learning curve when adopting local anaesthesia for hernioplasty and should be given close supervision whilst learning the local anaesthetic technique (Kingsnorth et al 1981). Bupivacaine blockade of the inguinal field is just as effective when given before wound incision as after wound closure. The duration of anaesthesia when no oral or parenteral analgesia is required lasts for between 10 and 12 h (Kingsnorth et al 1979).

TECHNIQUE OF REPAIR

The 1880–1890 period in the last century could justifiably be termed 'the decade of the inguinal hernia'. Significant contributors included Lucas-Champonnière (incision and opening of the external oblique fascia). Banks (high ligation of peritoneal sac), Marcy (closure of the transversalis fascia/iliopubic tract) and Bassini (complete division of the fascial floor of the inguinal canal from the internal ring to the pubis and closure with a layer of non-absorbable sutures). The decade of the 1990s may have equivalent significance in the 20th century due to the enthusiastic uptake of prosthetic mesh and laparoscopic techniques for hernioplasty.

The darn

In this operation, the transversalis fascia is not incised but is imbricated with a continuous suture, which almost certainly results in local ischaemia and subsequent healing with disorganized collagen resulting in areas of weakness of the posterior wall which inevitably enlarge and allow further herniation of the posterior inguinal wall. The latest (and perhaps best) report of the imbrication–darn technique, which incorporates the Kinmonth modification of the Maloney darn, results in recurrence rates at 5 years of 3.5% for primary hernias and 8.3% for recurrent hernias (Lifschultz & Juler 1986). Notwithstanding these poor results, 35% of consultant surgeons use the Maloney darn as their sole method of inguinal hernioplasty (Morgan et al 1991).

Shouldice operation (Figs 10.4, 10.5)

In spite of a Hunterian Lecture to the Royal College of Surgeons of England by Dr Frank Glassow given more than 10 years ago, describing a less than 1% recurrence rate in over 100 000 hernioplasties, this technique generally has not been adopted by UK surgeons. The Shouldice operation alone or in combination is used in less than 20% of inguinal hernioplasties in England (Morgan et al 1991). Good results with the Shouldice operation have been reproduced by specialists both in the UK and elsewhere (Table 10.3) but have only recently been put to the test of the randomized prospective controlled

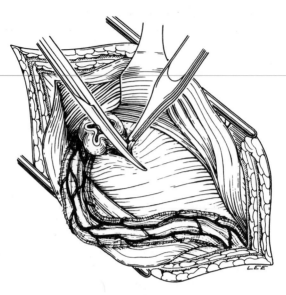

Fig. 10.4   Dissection of the transversalis fascia in the Shouldice repair. (Reproduced with permission from Devlin 1988.)

trial in the hands of trainee surgeons. A higher failure rate from trainees has been apparent from Barwell's figures for some years and the randomized trials

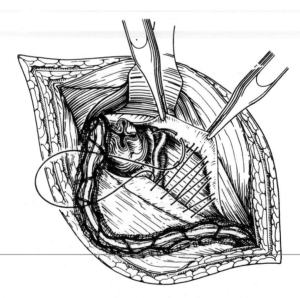

Fig. 10.5   Suturing the lower lateral flap of fascia transversalis to the undersurface of the medial flap along the 'white line' or 'arch' in the Shouldice repair. (Reproduced with permission from Devlin 1988.)

Table 10.3 Results of the Shouldice repair (percentage recurrence)

	Indirect		Direct	Recurrent	Total
Glasgow 1954–1986	0.9		1.1	3.5	20 485
Devlin 1970–1982		0.8			718
Barwell 1974–1991	0.8		2.6	3.0	2512
Berliner 1972–1983		1.6		5.9	2513
1980–1983		1.1			1017
Barwell trainees 1974–1991	4.9		4.9	3.0	1196
Shouldice Hospital 1945–1990		0.5		1.5	200 271
Wantz		0.9			2470

reported in 1992 indicate a recurrence rate for trainees of between 4% and 10% (Kingsnorth et al 1992, Panos et al 1992, Tran et al 1992, Fingerhut & Hay 1993). The enthusiasts of the Shouldice hernioplasty are unwittingly performing the operation of Bassini as illustrated by Attilio Catterina (Wantz 1989). It is salutary to reflect that, within 30 years of Bassini's report of 2.7% recurrence rate for his new technique, surgeons in general were reporting recurrence rates of approximately 10–12%. Approximately the same attrition rate may now be applying to the Shouldice operation in the hands of trainee surgeons who perform the bulk of this type of operation in the UK.

For the present, however, the current world literature supports the Shouldice operation as providing the best results for inguinal hernioplasty, and junior surgeons should be trained to adopt this technique until the new approaches to groin hernioplasty have been field-tested not only in specialist units but also in randomized prospective controlled trials in the 'real world' of general hospitals and trainee surgeons.

Tension-free hernioplasty (Lichtenstein technique) (Figs 10.6, 10.7)

Usher was the first to suggest prosthetic mesh to be a useful adjunct in inguinal hernioplasty. The polyethylene material used in this era, however, was not biocompatible and caused significant problems in terms of local rejection and held back the development of mesh in inguinal hernioplasty for several decades. It is largely the efforts of Lichtenstein which have popularized the use of prosthetic mesh. Controversy still surrounds the ideal material, polypropylene, Dacron, Prolene and expanded polytetrafluoroethylene being some of the products currently in use. Excellent results of several thousand operations performed by the Lichtenstein technique using polypropylene mesh have been reported (Lichtenstein 1987). The problem with mesh rejection has been solved and wound infection rates are insignificant. In this specialist unit, the recurrence rate is less than 1% and patients recover rapidly

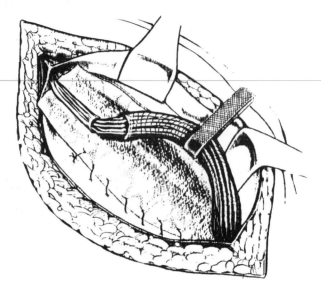

Fig. 10.6   A 6-inch by 3-inch patch slit to accommodate the spermatic cord is fixed to cover the posterior inguinal wall with overlap. (Reproduced with permission from Shulman 1993).

with a minimum of postoperative pain. Once again, the testing ground for this operation should be in the hands of trainee surgeons and in other non-specialist centres. Preliminary results from two European centres reporting on small numbers of patients are encouraging (Rutten et al 1992, Davies et al 1994).

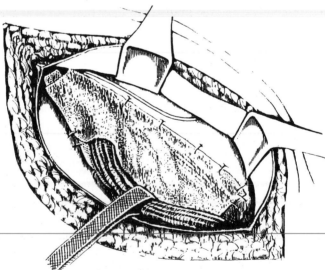

Fig. 10.7   Final position of the mesh with 'tails' closed around lateral margin of the deep ring. (Reproduced with permission from Shulman 1993).

Table 10.4 The history of external mesh and hernia repair

1958	Usher	Mesh prosthesis to buttress and reinforce a previously sutured repair
1974	Lichtenstein	'Plug' repair for femoral and recurrent inguinal hernia
1984	Martin & Max	Reinforcement of repair with mesh
1986	Lichtenstein	'Onlay' mesh patch as primary hernia repair
1988	Capozzi & Berkenfeld	Sutured onlay mesh ($n = 745$)
1991	Gilbert	'Sutureless' repair of small to moderate-sized by inguinal hernia cones and swatches ($n = 412$)
1992	Celdran	Mesh and triangular extension anchored to Cooper's liagment ($n = 43$)
1992	Bellis	Mesh with rectus abdominus tendon transfer ($n = 27\,267$)
1993	Robbins & Rutkow	Mesh-plug hernioplasty for all inguinal hernia and femoral hernias ($n = 1563$)
1993	Horton & Florence	Preperitoneal patch through the anterior route ($n = 100$)

Other external mesh repairs (Table 10.4)

A variety of mesh designs and mesh placements have flourished since Lichtenstein showed that mesh could be used successfully for hernioplasty. French surgeons favour Dacron mesh placed in the preperitoneal space over a large area (Stoppa 1984). Recovery from this type of extensive surgery is more prolonged and it may be better reserved for complex or recurrent hernias. Prolene mesh can be utilized in a similar technique as the Lichtenstein repair while polypropylene with a triangular extension to cover the femoral canal but is otherwise similar to the Lichtenstein technique and has been successfully employed in specialist units (Capozzi et al 1988, Barnes 1987, Celdran et al 1992).

Expanded polytetrafluoroethylene has been adopted for both the external approach and preperitoneal approach with good results. However, the limitations of this material include expense and its lack of incorporation into the tissues by fibroblast and collagen proliferation. It is for these reasons that it is perhaps an ideal material for large abdominal incisional hernias.

A more controversial use of prosthetic materials concerns its use configured as a swatch, bung, plug, or sutureless patch. In this context a roll or dart of material is placed in a hernial orifice with or without suture to obstruct the passage of the hernia to the exterior. A sutureless patch may then be placed over the whole of the posterior inguinal wall to reinforce this 'swatch' (Gilbert 1992; Rutkow & Robbins 1993). The specialist units reporting these techniques indicate a low recurrence rate, early return to work and minimal complications. Extreme caution, however, should be observed in generally recommending these techniques which have been adopted in subclassifications of hernia, subdivided by strict criteria and definitions indicating the size of the internal ring and the extent of the defect in the posterior inguinal wall. It is doubtful whether junior surgical trainees could practise this type of hernia surgery successfully.

Laparoscopic repair

Since the pioneering work of Ger (Ger et al 1990) there has been an explosion in interest in laparoscopic hernia repair following closely on the heels of successful adoption of the laparoscope for cholecystectomy. The specific goals of the laparoscopic hernia surgeon are to improve on the external approaches by decreasing postoperative morbidity, in particular the amount of subjective operative pain, and to reduce postoperative disability and allow an early return to work. These two objectives must be achieved in the context of low recurrence rates. Currently three techniques are being evaluated, viz. the intraperitoneal onlay mesh, the transabdominal pre-peritoneal repair (requiring laparoscopy and then a second incision in the peritoneum to enter the preperitoneal space) and the extraperitoneal hernioplasty (Filipe et al 1992). The transabdominal preperitoneal repair may be suitable for direct, femoral and combined direct and femoral hernias whereas the intraperitoneal onlay mesh has been recommended for indirect and large direct hernias. It is likely that there will not be one laparoscopic technique applicable to all types of inguinal hernia. The laparoscopic surgeon is faced with many of the problems of surgeons using mesh in the preperitoneal space where it has been found that a large area of mesh is required to cover all the myoperitoneal orifices; the deep internal ring should be adequately closed with sutures and hernial sacs sufficiently resected.

The literature abounds with reports of series containing less than 100 patients which convey useful hints to the laparoscopic learner surgeon enabling him to eliminate obvious mistakes on his early learning curve. Nevertheless, significant complications have been encountered including severe thigh pain due to stapling of the lateral cutaneous nerve of thigh, scrotal hydrocele and injury of intra-abdominal organs such as the bladder. A recent analysis of the cost of laparoscopic hernioplasty showed that the per hour cost in the operating theatre was 37% greater than that of open repair as a consequence of the more complex technology and the mean operating time was 90 min against 55 min for an open repair. This resulted in the actual cost for laparoscopic repair being 50% higher than for open repair (Wexner 1993). At this point in time, the laparoscopic operation is rapidly evolving and will require further study and better understanding of the anatomy. As techniques and technology improve this operation may find its way into the general armamentarium of the hernia surgeon. Nevertheless, surgeons should not be pushed prematurely into mass utilization of this as yet unproven technique.

Preperitoneal repair for primary and recurrent hernia

There is no standard technique for the repair of a recurrent hernia; more than 100 articles have been written on the subject in the world literature over the last 20 years attesting to the fact that no single approach is universally successful. Small, apparently direct recurrences can be repaired successfully by the Shouldice technique or a mesh plug. However, this is at the risk of further disturbance of the vasculature of the spermatic cord and testis with the risk of ischaemic orchitis and possible testicular infarction. Complex recurrent hernias are more amendable to repair by the preperitoneal technique using large pieces of prosthetic material. The hernia defect is best closed with interrupted non-absorbed sutures and the repair reinforced by prosthetic mesh anchored to Cooper's ligament, tacking sutures placed above the repair of the transversalis fascia and folded cephalad to fit beneath the wound entry (Nyhus 1993). In this way, the mesh covers all peritoneal orifices including the potential hernial spaces, i.e. direct, indirect and femoral canal. This type of surgery cannot be performed on an ambulatory basis. The morbidity is higher than for primary hernia surgery but recurrence rates in the hands of experts or experienced hernia surgeons are less than 5%.

STRATEGY FOR ADDITIONAL PROBLEMS

Bilateral hernias

The dilemma of how to deal with patients with simultaneous bilateral inguinal hernia repair is not inconsequential as 12% of patients present in this way. Patients should be selected for simultaneous or sequential repair. Because simultaneous bilateral repair carries a much higher risk of urinary retention with urinary tract infection and prolonged hospital stay (15% of patients versus 6% of those having unilateral repair), the elderly and particularly those with symptoms of bladder outflow obstruction should have their operations performed sequentially or preferably under local anaesthesia (Miller et al 1991). The short-term recovery including wound complications, postoperative respiratory complications and ability to return to normal activity is not impaired by simultaneous operation nor are recurrence rates. The advantage in young patients is that operating time and hospital stay are both reduced, resulting in a saving in costs and inconvenience for both patient and hospital.

Comorbidity

Colorectal disease

Several studies have evaluated the diagnostic role of flexible sigmoidoscopy as a means of screening for asymptomatic colorectal disease in patients with groin hernia. All have shown a 16–28% incidence of neoplastic (malignant or premalignant) lesions. This has led to the assumption that inguinal hernia justifies sigmoidoscopy. These claims, however, have been refuted by a study in which a control group of patients without groin hernia, having no gastrointestinal symptoms or family history of gastrointestinal malignancy and having negative faecal occult blood examination, were compared with 100 groin hernia patients also negative for faecal occult blood (Wheeler et al 1991). No differences were found between the two groups in terms of the incidence of neoplastic colorectal lesions.

Urinary retention

Because urinary retention is the single most common cause of unplanned hospital admission following inguinal hernia repair, the preferential order for inguinal hernia repair and prostatectomy has been questioned. Benign prostatic hypertrophy and inguinal hernia are both common: 3% of men over the age of 65 years will have, or have had, an inguinal hernia, more than 50% of men over the age of 65 years will have symptoms of urinary obstruction and inguinal hernia is found in 25% of prostatectomy patients. In a study comparing two groups of patients, one having prostatectomy prior to having a hernia repair and the other having inguinal hernia repair prior to prostatectomy, the incidence of urinary tract infection was 31% in those having the inguinal hernia repair as the initial operation. The incidence of urinary tract infection correlated with the duration of bladder catheterization following postoperative retention (Cramer et al 1983). These results suggest that, in patients having inguinal hernia and symptomatic prostatic obstruction, prostatectomy should be performed first, thus reducing urinary tract infections with no additional risk related to the hernia.

Advanced age

Elective surgery can be undertaken with zero mortality even in octogenarians of ASA (American Society of Anesthetists) grade 3 (severe systemic disease that limits activity but is not incapacitating) provided that there is accurate preoperative diagnosis and treatment of systemic disease and there is a judicious choice of anaesthesia. In the elderly, mortality for emergency surgery with bowel resection and groin hernia repair remains at 10–60%.

Peritoneal dialysis

Inguinal hernias are found in approximately 6% of patients on chronic ambulatory peritoneal dialysis. The factors involved in this high incidence include anatomical (patent processus), hydrostatic (continuous presence of dialysate), and metabolic (uraemia, muscle wasting). The mode of presentation is scrotal swelling but, at this stage, the differential diagnosis between peritonitis and obstruction or strangulation of the hernia is difficult (Engeset & Youngson 1984). In patients on chronic ambulatory peritoneal dialysis it is recommended that they are examined regularly for hernia, they are warned of the potential dangers of the development of a reducible groin swelling and, once detected, prompt repair of any clinical defect should be carried out.

RECOVERY AND RETURN TO ACTIVITY

In spite of decades of information indicating that patients may return to work within 2–4 weeks of inguinal hernia surgery, long periods of time off work and convalescence are commonplace. Patients actually take a mean of 7 weeks off work (those in sedentary occupations take more time off work) whilst surgeons advise a mean of 4.4 weeks off work and general practitioners 6.2 weeks (Robertson et al 1993). The only significant factors accounting for time a patient takes off work after hernia surgery relate to social security benefits, occupation and personal sickness insurance. Age, social class, previous medical history, respiratory disease, grade of surgeon performing the operation and postoperative complications do not significantly alter the variation in time off work after hernia surgery. In a recent survey, most patients based the expected time they took off work on information gained from colleagues: their general practitioner was seen as the most important factor in delayed return to work (Rider et al 1993). Well-motivated, fit and younger patients travelling some distance to attend specialist centres will return to work earlier than the bulk of patients in the 55–85-year-old age group having hernia surgery under a centralized system of health care.

Strangulated hernia

The National Confidential Enquiry into Perioperative Deaths, 1991–1992 investigated 210 deaths following inguinal hernia repair and 120 deaths following femoral hernia repair (Campling et al 1993). Although many of the patients were elderly (45 were aged between 80 and 89 years) and unfit (24 were ASA grade 3 and 21 were ASA grade 4), only 19% of the patients were operated on by consultants and a further 25% by senior registrars. Complications were related to pre-existing cardiorespiratory problems rather than to the hernia surgery. Analysis by experts of the events leading to death suggested that the outcome could have been improved if the experience of the surgeon had been matched with the ASA grade of the patient, adequate resuscitation had been performed preoperatively and postoperative care had taken place in a high dependency unit or intensive care unit. In moribund patients, interventional surgery could have been withdrawn. The high risk of mortality in these patients demands a high quality of surgical and postoperative care.

COMPLICATIONS OF SURGERY

Less than one-quarter of complications after hernia surgery will be detected in hospital. Wound complications should not exceed 5% and this incidence is not increased with the use of prosthetic materials. Scrotal complications are of equal importance and include haematoma, hydrocele, genital oedema and damage to the vas or testicular vessels. The problem of nerve injury and persistent postoperative pain and that of ischaemic orchitis and testicular atrophy warrant special comment.

The incidence of groin pain after hernia surgery is surprisingly common in hernia centres which carry out regular annual review and clinical examination of all their patients. Approximately one-quarter of patients have some degree of residual dysesthesia (Gilbert 1993). Amongst this large group of patients there are a small number with a well-defined postoperative neuralgia affecting the ilioinguinal, iliohypogastric or genitofemoral nerves. The term 'nerve entrapment' is best avoided in this situation as it aggravates both the patients and their desire for litigation. The neuralgias are best tackled with a judicious nerve block or surgical division of the sensory nerve at a higher level.

The occurrence of ischaemic orchitis and testicular atrophy is likely to bring the surgeon into confrontation with his patient in the law courts. The cause is not related to tight closure of the internal ring at hernia repair (Fong & Wantz 1992). The testis has a rich collateral supply from the inferior epigastric vesicle, prostatic and scrotal vessels, and interference at one level is unlikely to induce ischaemia. Ischaemic orchitis will only occur when extensive dissection along the entire length of the spermatic cord down to the testis has been performed with damage to the collateral arterial supply at several levels and interruption of the venous pampiniform plexus. On this basis it is recommended that distal indirect sacs should never be dissected beyond the pubic tubercle nor should the spermatic cord be mobilized beyond the pubic tubercle. Observing these two simple rules, the incidence of ischaemic orchitis can be reduced below 1%. The clinical manifestations of ischaemic orchitis occur between 2 and 5 days after hernia surgery, with pain, tenderness and swelling with induration lasting for up to 4–5 months. Subsequent testicular atrophy occurs in approximately one-quarter of patients. Testicular atrophy related to previous inguinal hernioplasty is a significant cause of infertility in men attending fertility clinics, with up to 11% giving a history of previous unilateral hernioplasty. In this group of men, semen quality (sperm concentrations, motility and morphology) are markedly reduced in comparison to that of fertile men (Yavetz et al 1991).

OTHER HERNIA TYPES

Femoral hernia

The high approach is recommended for the majority of primary hernias with the exception of thin female patients in whom the crural or low operation may be performed. The femoral ring is narrowed by a darn between Cooper's ligament and the inguinal ligament. The plug repair is an alternative in which a strip of mesh 20 cm long and 3 cm wide is rolled up to create a firm plug which is anchored in the femoral canal with four or five sutures after reduction of the hernial sac and its contents (Shulman et al 1992). The preperitoneal approach should be used when the patient has undergone previous groin surgery or when obstruction or strangulation is present.

Incisional hernia

A symptomatic bulge will develop in up to 10% of abdominal incisions and require surgical intervention. In complex hernias, the risk of strangulation can be high and operative intervention is indicated. Wound failure is common in obese patients, particularly those suffering postoperative wound infection; the type of wound most at risk is the lower midline. These factors tend to produce a group of patients who are elderly, unfit, often with diabetes mellitus in whom the musculotendinous elements that insert onto the pubis have become totally disrupted (Hesselink et al 1993, Bendavid 1990).

The patients can be divided essentially into two groups. First, those in whom there is no tissue defect and repair of the incisional hernia can be effected by reconstituting the normal anatomy with a non-absorbable monofilament suture material taking large bites of tendon/aponeurosis/fascial layers to achieve a suture length to wound length of 4:1. Secondly, a variety of prosthetic materials can be used when a tissue defect exists (Molloy et al 1991, Van der Lei et al 1989, Wantz 1991). If peritoneal closure can be achieved then extraperitoneal Dacron or Marlex mesh is appropriate, placed superficial or deep to the rectus abdominus muscles. If peritoneal closure cannot be achieved, or is doubtful, then the preferable material is expanded polytetrafluoroethylene because the risk of adhesion by loops of bowel to this material is minimal. The defect must be covered widely with at least a 5 cm rim of mesh extending in all directions beyond the limits of the hernia defect. The mesh must be fixed to the margins of the defect and also at its periphery.

Umbilical hernia

In adults, one operation that has stood the test of time for nearly a century for the correction of this defect is the Mayo repair (Devlin 1988). Intertrigo and inflammation of the skin around an umbilical hernia is common and antibiotic prophylaxis is recommended. Although many of these patients are elderly and obese, operation is strongly recommended because of the high risk of strangulation. A better result can be obtained by removing the umbilical cicatrix, but the patient must be warned beforehand than an effective repair will remove this feature of their anatomy. A first-time repair which uses the strong fascial layers of the linea alba will rarely require prosthetic mesh for reinforcement although this may become necessary for the repair of recurrent umbilical hernia.

CONCLUSIONS

Inguinal hernia is a common condition and there are unexplained variations in clinical practice resulting in variations in use of resources and outcome. Although there are insufficient research data on which to recommend best practice, the 'Clinical guidelines on the management of groin hernia in adults' published by the Royal College of Surgeons of England are a valuable base from which to start. These guidelines are helpful for training junior surgeons, can provide patients with some certainty about outcome and provide a standard against which practice can be audited. In addition, the possibility of 'outside agencies' imposing standards of hernia surgery is eliminated.

Levels of training should be defined for junior surgeons undertaking primary inguinal hernioplasty, complex recurrent hernioplasty, incisional hernioplasty or surgery for strangulated hernia, especially in the elderly or unfit. New techniques must be field-tested in the 'real world' where junior trainees undertake the bulk of this type of surgery, with personal follow-up. Once defined, guidelines should be regularly updated and incentives given for adherence. Finally, every surgeon should be aware of his own results.

KEY POINTS FOR CLINICAL PRACTICE

- Femoral hernias should be repaired as soon as possible after presentation.
- Asymptomatic direct inguinal hernias in the elderly (where the diagnosis is confident) do not require operation.
- Day case surgery and local anaesthesia should be offered to mobile patients with adequate social support.
- The available literature supports the Shouldice inguinal hernioplasty as giving the best results.
- Prosthetic mesh and laparoscopic repair should be carefully and prospectively evaluated and used only after discussion with the patient.
- Immediate mobilization and return to work should be advised within 2 (sedentary workers) to 4 (labourers) weeks.
- In laparoscopic surgery the presence of an apparent patent processus vaginalis in the absence of a clinical hernia is not an indication for surgical intervention.

REFERENCES

Allen PIM, Zager M, Goldman M 1987 Elective repair of groin hernias in the elderly. Br J Surg 74: 987
Barnes JP 1987 Inguinal hernia repair with routine use of Marlex Mesh. Surg Gynecol Obstet. 165: 33–37
Bendavid R 1990 Incisional parapubic hernias. Surgery 108: 898–901
Berliner SD 1990 When is surgery necessary for a groin hernia? Postgrad Med 87: 149–152
Campling EA, Devlin HB, Hoile RW et al (eds) 1993 The Report of the National Confidential Enquiry into Perioperative Deaths 1991–1992, NCEPOD, London
Capozzi JA, Berkenfeld JA, Cherry JK 1988 Repair of inguinal hernia in the adult with prolene mesh. Surg Gynecol Obstet 167: 124–128
Celdran A, Vorwald P, Merono E 1992 A single technique for polypropylene mesh

hernioplasty of inguinal and femoral hernias. Surg Gynecol Obstet 175: 359–361

Cramer SO, Malangoni MA, Schulte WJ et al 1983 Inguinal hernia repair before and after prostatic resection. Surgery 94: 627–630

Davies N, Thomas M, McIlroy B et al 1994 The Lichtenstein tension-free hernia repair: early results from the UK. Br J Surg 1994 (in press)

Devlin HB 1998 Umbilical hernia in adults. In: Management of abdominal hernias. Butterworth, London, pp 111, 140–145

Engeset J, Youngson GG 1984 Ambulatory peritoneal dialysis in hernial complications. Surg Clin North Am 64: 385–392

Filipe CJ, Fitzgibbons, RJ, Salerno GM et al 1992 Laparoscopic herniorrhaphy. Surg Clin North Am 72: 1109–1124

Fingerhut A, Hay JM 1993 Seventh annual meeting of the French Association for Surgical Research (ARC) and the First French–Germany Joint Meeting with the Permanent Working Party on Clinical Studies (CAS) of the German Surgical Society, 27 March 1993, Paris, France. Theor Surg 8: 163–167

Fong Y, Wantz GE, 1992 Prevention of ischaemic orchitis during inguinal hernioplasty. Surg Gynecol Obstet 174: 399–402

Gallegos NC, Dawson J, Jarvis M et al 1991 Risk of strangulation in groin hernias. Br J Surg 78: 1171–1173

Ger R, Monroe K, Duvivier R et al 1990 Management of indirect inguinal hernias by laparoscopic closure of the neck of the sac. Am J Surg 159: 370–373

Gilbert AI 1992 Sutureless repair of inguinal hernia. Am J Surg 163: 331–335

Gilbert AI 1993 Medical legal aspects of hernia surgery: personal risk management. Surg Clin North Am 73: 583–593

Given JP, Rubin SZ 1989 Occurrence of contralateral inguinal hernia following unilateral repair in a pediatric hospital. J Pediatr Surg 24: 963–965

Gullmo A 1989 Herniography. World J Surg 13: 560–568

Harvald B 1989 Genetic epidemiology of Greenland. Clin Genet 36: 364–367

Hesselink VJ, Luijendijk RW, de Wilt JHW et al 1993 An evaluation of risk factors in incisional hernia recurrence. Surg Gynecol Obstet 176: 228–234

Kingsnorth AN, Wijesinha SS, Grixti CJ, 1979 Evaluation of dextran with local anaesthesia for short stay inguinal herniorrhaphy, Ann R Coll Surg Engl 61: 456–458

Kingsnorth AN, Britton BJ, Morris PJ 1981 Recurrent inguinal hernia after local anaesthesia repair. Br J Surg 68: 273–275

Kingsnorth AN, Gray MR, Nott DM 1992 Prospective randomised trial comparing the Shouldice technique and plication darn for inguinal hernia. Br J Surg 79: 1068–1070

Law NW, Trapnell JE 1992 Does a truss benefit a patient with inguinal hernia? Br Med J 304: 1092

Lehnert B, Wadouh F 1992 High incidence of inguinal hernias and abdomial aortic aneurysms. Ann Vase Surg 6: 134–137

Lichtenstein IL 1987 Herniorrhaphy: a personal experience with 6321 cases. Am J Surg 153: 553–559

Lifschultz H, Juler GL 1986 The inguinal darn. Arch Surg 121: 717–719

Malycha P, Lovell G 1992 Inguinal surgery in athletes with chronic groin pain: the Sportman's hernia. Aust NZ J Surg 62: 123–125

Millat B, Fingerhut A, Gignoux M et al and the French Associations for Surgical Research 1993 Factors associated with early discharge after inguinal hernia repair in 500 consecutive unselected patients. Br J Surg 80: 1058–1060

Miller AR, van Heerden JA, Naessens JM et al 1991 Simultaneous bilateral hernia repair: a case against conventional wisdom. Ann Surg 213: 272–276

Molloy RG, Moran KT, Waldron RP et al 1991 Massive incisional hernia: abdominal wall replacement with marlex mesh. Br J Surg 78: 242–244

Morgan M, Reynolds A, Swan AB et al 1991 Are current techniques of inguinal hernia repair optimal? A survey in the United Kingdom. Ann R Coll Surg Engl 73: 341–345

Morgan M, Beech R, Reynolds A et al 1992 Surgeons: view of day surgery: is there a consensus among providers. J Public Health Med 14: 192–198

Neuhauser D 1977 Elective inguinal herniorrhaphy versus a truss in the elderly. In: Bunker JP, Barnes BA, Mostella FA (eds) Costs, risks and benefits of surgery. Oxford University Press, New York.

Nyhus LM 1993 Iliopubic tract repair of inguinal and femoral hernia: the posterior (pre-peritoneal) approach. Surg Clin North Am 73: 487–499

Panos RG, Beck DE, Maresh JE et al 1992 Preliminary results of prospective randomised study of Cooper's ligament versus Shouldice herniorrhaphy technique. Surg Gynecol Obstet 175: 315–319

Rider MA, Baker DM, Locker A et al 1993 Return to work after inguinal hernia repair. Br J Surg 80: 745–746

Robertson GSM, Haynes IG, Burton PR 1993 How long to patients convalesce about inguinal herniorrhaphy? Current principles and practice. Ann R Coll Surg Engl 75: 30–33

Royal College of Surgeons of England 1993 Report of a Working Party. Clinical guidelines for the management of adult groin hernia

Rutkow IM, Robbins AW 1993 Tension-free inguinal herniorrhaphy. A preliminary report on the 'mesh plug' technique. Surgery 114: 3–8

Rutten P, Ledecq M, Hoebeke Y et al 1992 Hernial inguinal primaire: hernioplastie ambulatoire selon Lichtenstein. Premiers resultants cliniques et implications économiques étude des 130 premiers cas opères. Acta Chir Belg 92: 168–171

Shulman AG, Amid PK, Lichtenstein IL 1992 Prosthetic mesh plug repair of femoral and recurrent inguinal hernias: the American experience. Ann R Coll Surg Engl 74: 97–99

Stoppa RE 1984 The use of Dacron in the repair of hernias of the groin. Surg Clin North Am 64: 269–285

Stoppa RE 1989 Treatment of complicated groin and incisional hernias. World J Surg 13: 545–554

Tran VK, Putz T, Rohde H 1992 A randomized controlled trial of inguinal hernia repair to compare the Shouldice and the Bassini–Kirschner operation. Int Surg 77: 235–237

Van der Lei B, Bleichrodt RP, Summermacher RKJ et al 1989 Expanded PTFE patch for the repair of large abdominal wall defects. Br J Surg 76: 803–805

Wantz GE 1989 The operation of Bassini as described by Attillio Catterina. Surg Gynecol Obstet 168: 67–68

Wantz GE 1991 Incisional herniplasty with mersilene. Surg Gynecol Obstet 172: 129–137

Wexner SD 1993 Laparoscopic hernia repair: a plea for science and statistics. Surg Endosc 7: 150–151

Wheeler WE, Wilson SL, Kurncz J et al 1991 Flexible sigmoidoscopy screening for asymptomatic colorectal disease in patients with and without inguinal hernia. South Med J 84: 876–878

Yavetz H, Harash B, Yogev L et al 1991 Fertility of men following inguinal hernia repair. Andrologia 23: 443–446

11

Oncology for surgeons: monoclonal antibodies

C. Y. Yiu

The hybridoma technique (Kohler & Milstein 1975) enables the production of monoclonal antibodies with desired specificities, in pure form, and indefinitely, in contrast to polyclonal antisera which may vary from batch to batch, contaminated with undesirable proteins, immunoglobulins or other substances. Monoclonal antibodies have superseded polyclonal antibodies in many immunological reactions, and have found widespread applications in oncology. This chapter concentrates mainly on the experience of the clinical applications of monoclonal antibodies in the diagnosis and therapies of common malignancies, the problems encountered in immunolocalization, and recent advances in the generation of antibodies; many laboratory-based experimental studies such as clearing bone marrow of malignant cells, antibody directed enzyme prodrug therapy, endothelium targeting by antibodies, and active specific immunotherapy using antigens identified by monoclonal antibodies are not included.

STRUCTURE OF ANTIBODY

An antibody consists of a pair of identical heavy and light chains. Each of these consists of a constant region and a variable region made up of different domains or folds joined together by intrachain and interchain disulphide bonds. The variable regions contain the antigen binding sites. The different domains forming an antibody can be separated. Enzyme cleavage divides an antibody into the bivalent $F(ab')_2$, or monovalent Fab antigen binding fragments. Smaller antibody fragments with antigen binding activities can be constructed by genetic engineering techniques. Fv fragments are formed by the variable region heavy (V_H) and light (V_L) chain domains. These fragments are unstable but stability can be improved by a peptide linker joining the V_H and V_L domains to form single chain Fv fragments (scFv). The binding unit consisting of the V_H domain alone is called a single domain antibody (dAb) fragment (Winter & Milstein 1991). The domain for effector functions is the Fc fragment. Fig. 11.1 illustrates how an antibody can be divided into various fragments which can be conjugated to different chemicals or genetically engineered for diagnostic or therapeutic purposes.

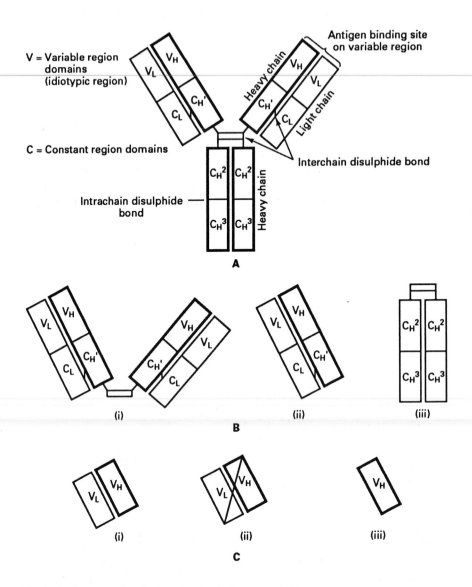

Fig. 11.1 Structure of antibody and antibody fragments. **A** Whole antibody (150 kDa) formed by two heavy and two light chains. **B** Proteolytic enzyme cleavage results in: (i) bivalent F(ab')₂ fragment (100 kDa); (ii) monovalent Fab fragment (50 kDa); (iii) Fc fragment (effector functions). **C** Genetic engineering construction of antibody fragments: (i) variable region fragments (Fv) (25 kDa); (ii) variable region fragments with peptide linker forming single chain Fv (scFv) which is more stable than Fv (27 kDa); (iii) single domain antibody fragment (dAb) consisting of heavy chain variable domain.
V_H = heavy chain variable domain; V_L = light chain variable domain. C_H^1, C_H^2, C_H^3 = heavy chain constant domains; C_L = light chain constant domain (adapted from Hawkins et al 1993).

APPLICATION OF MONOCLONAL ANTIBODIES IN ONCOLOGY

Diagnosis

Histopathology

Monoclonal antibodies have revolutionized diagnostic histopathology. Their significance is comparable to what CT (computed tomography) or MRI (magnetic resonance imaging) scans are to radiology or endoscopy is to gastroenterology (Gatter 1989). By using a panel of monoclonal antibodies, each recognizing an antigen characteristic of a particular tumour, an anaplastic tumour can be typed into lymphoma, carcinoma or other tumours. Fig. 11.2 shows the application of monoclonal antibodies in diagnosing anaplastic tumours.

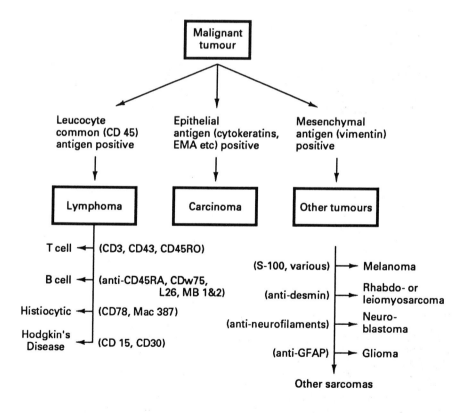

Fig. 11.2   Immunohistochemical diagnosis of malignant tumours. (Reproduced by permission of John Wiley & Sons Ltd from Gatter 1989.)

Radioimmunoscintigraphy (RIS)

Mach et al (1981) were the first to use radiolabelled monoclonal antibodies against carcinoembryonic antigen (CEA) for cancer detection. Many other anti-mucin monoclonal antibodies have been used for RIS; for example, epithelial membrane antigen (EMA) (Yiu et al 1991a,b), and tumour associated glycoprotein 72 (TAG-72) (Doerr et al 1993). By 1992 RIS had been performed in 110 clinical studies (Larson 1991), including more than 20 different cancers, such as colorectal, breast, ovarian, lung, melanoma, and T-cell lymphoma, pancreatic cancer, neuroblastoma, glioma, cervical carcinoma, hepatocellular carcinoma, sarcoma, prostatic carcinoma, trophoblast and germ cell tumours, thyroid carcinoma, insulinoma, seminoma (Goldenberg & Larson 1992), using over 52 different monoclonal antibodies and five different radionuclides (Larson 1990). Colorectal cancer is the most extensively investigated with RIS, followed by ovarian and breast cancer (Goldenberg & Larson 1992).

In RIS, radiolabelled antibodies, typically between 500 µg to 1 mg with an activity of 120 MBq (Yiu et al 1991a,b), are injected intravenously. Short-lived high-signal radioisotopes such as iodine-125 or technetium-99 give better images than long-lived low-activity radioisotopes such as iodine-131 (Britton & Granowska 1991). Imaging of high-signal radionuclides occurs within a few hours of antibody injection, whereas with low-energy radionuclides optimal imaging takes place a few days later. Indium-111 has the disadvantage of high uptake by the spleen, the bone marrow and the liver (Yiu et al 1991a,b).

The radiolabelled uptake by the tumour is less than 1% of the injected dose. Using planar imaging the smallest size of tumour detected was about 2.5 cm and weighing about 2–3 g; many tumours detected are greater than 4 cm in diameter (Larson 1990). However, lesions as small as 0.5–1 cm can be detected by single-photon emission tomography (SPECT). A combination of SPECT and technetium-99m labelled antibodies achieved the best results (Goldenberg & Larson 1992). In colorectal cancer RIS detects between 46% and 95% of tumours. False positive results can be obtained in areas of inflammation such as diverticular abscess or bone abscess (Yiu et al 1991b), degenerative joint disease, abdominal aneurysms, postoperative bowel adhesions. These conditions can account for up to 13% of positive scans (Goldenberg & Larson 1992).

The most successful radiolabelled antibody localization results obtained to date are with anti-T-cell, anti-neuroblastoma and anti-CEA monoclonal antibodies (Larson 1990). Indium-111 labelled T101 monoclonal antibody has a high detection rate of occult T-cell malignancies in lymph nodes; iodine-131 labelled monoclonal antibody F8 localized to over 90% of neuroblastoma with a concentration of 0.04% injected dose/g tumour; several anti-CEA monoclonal antibodies give good localization to colorectal cancers.

So far very few toxic side-effects have been reported. The general adverse reaction rate to mouse monoclonal antibodies is estimated to be 1 per 1100

(Goldenberg & Larson 1992). An indium-111 labelled monoclonal antibody against the TAG-72 antigen, called 'Oncoscint', has been approved recently by the Food and Drug Administration in the USA for clinical imaging (Larson et al 1994).

Colorectal cancer

Serum marker

CEA is the most well-known serum marker for colorectal cancer. Other markers reactive with monoclonal antibodies include: CA 19-9, which is a circulating epitope of the Lewis blood group antigen, sialylated lacto-N-fucopentose II (sialyl-Le^a); TAA CA 50 which consists of two carbohydrate structures, sialyl-Le^a and sialosyl-lactotetraose; and TAA 195 (CA 195), which contains epitopes of Le^a and sialyl-Le^a. There is strong overlap for these markers in benign colorectal conditions and cancers, indicating a lack of specificity (Van der Schouw et al 1992). Two other mucin markers CA 242 (Ward et al 1993) and CA M43 (Van Kamp et al 1993) are no better than CEA as indicators of colorectal cancer status.

Micrometastases/malignant cells in bone marrow or lymph nodes

Bone marrow micrometastases provide independent prognostic information. In 88 colorectal cancer patients a monoclonal antibody reactive with cytokeratin 18 detected micrometastases in 32% of patients. These patients had significantly reduced disease-free survival compared to those without metastases (Lindemann et al 1992).

A retrospective study of the lymph nodes of 50 patients diagnosed as having Dukes' B colorectal cancer were examined with monoclonals against cytokeratin (AE1/AE3) and TAG-72 antigen (CC49). Micrometastases were found in 14 patients. These had poorer prognosis and six died within 66 months (Greenson et al 1994).

Radioimmunoscintigraphy

Radiolabelled mouse monoclonal antibodies. Iodine-125 labelled anti-CEA monoclonal antibody F(ab')$_2$ or Fab fragments and SPECT detected correctly between 71% and 93% of patients with clinically confirmed or suspected colorectal cancers (Bischof-Delaloye et al 1989). Some recurrent tumours, particularly those in the pelvis and inside the abdomen, were diagnosed only by RIS using the monoclonal indium-111 CYT-103 (Doerr et al 1993). RIS also detected some cases of liver metastases a month ahead of CT or ultrasound scanning (Bischof-Delaloye et al 1989).

RIS has been used to assess the effectiveness of radiotherapy or chemo-therapy, and to differentiate between postoperative fibrous tissue and tumour deposits indistinguishable by other imaging techniques (Britton & Granowska 1991). Iodine-125 labelled anti-CEA antibody A5B7 (Blair et al 1990) and monoclonal CC49 (Triozzi et al 1994) have also been used to detect tumours at operation by means of a hand-held gamma counting probe.

Radiolabelled human monoclonal antibodies. Administration of human monoclonal antibodies has the advantage of avoiding the human anti-mouse antibody response (HAMA). In RIS, iodine-131 labelled human monoclonal 28A32, 16–88, reactive with cytokeratins, detected between 55% and 75% of metastatic colorectal tumours (Steis et al 1990, Boven et al 1991). Another iodine-131 labelled human monoclonal, COU-1, also reactive with cytokeratin, detected colorectal cancers in seven out of nine patients. The tenth patient who had no tumour had a negative scan (Ditzel et al 1993).

Breast cancer

Serum marker

CA 15.3 is a high molecular weight glycoprotein identified by two monoclonal antibodies: monoclonal 115D8, generated against milk fat globule membrane, and monoclonal DF3, raised against breast carcinoma subcellular membranes (Dixon et al 1993a). In advanced breast cancer, a combination of CEA, CA 15.3 and ESR is effective in assessing response and in guiding treatment to endocrine therapy (Robertson et al 1991) or chemotherapy (Dixon et al 1993a,b). Patients with metastatic breast cancer in the bone, lung, and viscera, and who had negative test for serum CA 15.3 might have a positive test for epithelial mucin core antigen (EMCA) (Dixon et al 1993a). Serum level of EMCA showed significant correlation with UICC assessment of response at 2, 4 and 6 months. The EMCA assay is easier to perform than that for CA 15.3 may be potentially more useful than CA 15.3 (Dixon et al 1993a).

Histological markers

Oestrogen receptor immunocytochemical assay (ERICA). Oestrogen receptor (ER) is a nuclear protein involved in the regulation of transcription with specific sequence. It is a marker for responsiveness of invasive breast cancer to hormonal therapy and less aggressive tumour behaviour, and even better survival (Poller et al 1993). Previously ER in breast cancer was measured by a radioligand binding technique. ER can now be detected on histological sections, for example, by using monoclonal antibody H 222 (Poller et al 1993). ER is found in about 60% of invasive breast carcinomas. In ductal carcinoma in situ (DCIS) ER was present in 31.8% of cases and was associated with non-comedo appearance, small cell size, higher S-phase fraction and lack of c-*erbB*-2 protein overexpression. ER status guides endocrine therapy of invasive breast carcinoma and DCIS (Poller et al 1993).

c-erbB-*2*.   The oncogene c-*erbB*-2, also known as *neu* or *HER-2* or *HER-2/neu*, codes for a growth factor receptor related to tyrosine kinase. Expression of this oncogene correlates with poorly differentiated and advanced tumours, although confirmation is required (Perren 1991). c-*erbB*-2 is present in 61% of DCIS. It is always associated with large-cell comedo type and never in small-cell cribriform/micropapillary type of DCIS (Bartkova et al 1990). It is uncertain if c-*erbB*-2 expression is related to invasiveness of DCIS.

pS2 protein.   pS2 protein is expressed by many epithelial cancers but few normal tissues. It has a similar sequence to that of pancreatic spasmolytic polypeptide (hSP) (Luqmani et al 1993). Immunohistochemical demonstration of pS2 protein in breast cancer was consistent with a better survival and response to endocrine therapy. In DCIS pS2 was present in 63–67% of cases with comedo, solid, cribriform and micropapillary types. There is a good correlation with progesterone receptor status but not with oestrogen receptor status (Luqmani et al 1993).

Ovarian cancer

Patients with advanced ovarian carcinoma have a 5-year survival varying from 7% to 62%. CA 125, a tumour-associated antigen secreted by ovarian cancer, measured in the serum, is effective in predicting the prognosis of these patients following treatment with chemotherapy. Those with a level of 450 U/ml have a poor survival of 7 months. Those with a level of less than 55 U/ml have a median survival of 23 months, 58–221 U/ml a survival of 16 months, and 228–434 U/ml of 15 months (Fisken et al 1993).

Pancreatic cancer

CA 242, CA 50 and CEA have been compared as serum marker for pancreatic cancer. It was found that CA 242 has a higher specificity for pancreatic cancer than the other two (Pasanen et al 1993).

Monoclonal antibodies in the therapy of cancer

Monoclonal antibodies may be used as carriers for cytotoxic agents, such as radioisotopes or toxins in cancer therapy. It can be used in unmodified form by acting as a vaccine through the generation of anti-idiotypic (anti-binding site) antibodies by patients. Administration of a monoclonal antibody (MAb1) may induce the production of an antibody (MAb2, an anti-idiotypic antibody) to the binding site of MAb1. The structure of the binding region of MAb2 mimics the tumour antigen identified by MAb1. MAb2 can in turn stimulate production of an anti-idiotypic MAb3 which has binding features similar to those of MAb1, and reacts against the tumour (Herlyn et al 1991).

Toxins from plant (e.g. ricin, abrin) and bacteria (e.g. diphtheria toxin, *Pseudomonas* exotoxin) have been conjugated to monoclonals. Immunotoxins kill both resting and dividing cells by their actions on the Golgi apparatus (Vitetta et al 1993). Many immunotoxin trials are at phase I and II stages where assessments are made on their toxicities and maximum tolerated doses. Immunotoxins may have hepatotoxicity, may cause myalgias, and may cause vascular leak syndrome and pulmonary oedema, possibly due to reaction with endothelial cells (Vitetta et al 1993).

Clinical studies of monoclonal antibody therapies

Colorectal cancer

Radioimmunotherapy. Radioimmunotherapy in colorectal cancer is still in its infancy with studies being confined to dosimetry calculation for different antibodies and radioisotope preparations. For example, a phase I trial of chimaeric iodine-131 labelled B72.3 monoclonal showed that therapeutic doses caused significant bone marrow suppression. The maximum tolerated dose was 36 mCi/m^2 (Meredith et al 1992). A phase II trial of iodine-131 labelled monoclonal CC49, showed no significant effect at a dose of 75 mCi/m^2 (Murray et al 1994). Rhenium-186 labelled anti-CEA antibody Fab'_2 fragment NR-CO-O2 achieved a maximal tolerated dose of 200 mCi/m^2 which is higher than intact antibody (Breitz et al 1992).

Therapy with MAb1. In colorectal cancer monoclonal antibody therapy compares favourably with other forms of adjuvant therapies, and is free from side-effects. In a randomized control trial involving 189 patients with Dukes' C colorectal cancer, the treatment group received 500 mg of monoclonal 17-1A (MAb1) within 2 weeks of surgery and a further four injections of 100 mg of antibody at monthly intervals. At a median follow-up of 5 years, the death rate in the treatment group was 30% lower. The distant but not local recurrence rate had fallen by 27%, possibly reflecting a difference in tumour loads at these sites (Riethmuller et al 1994). Monoclonal antibodies may exert their effects on cell receptors, resulting in: activation or inactivation of cells; the destruction of cells by activating complement, opsonization, antibody-dependent cellular cytotoxicity systems, or induction of apoptosis via anti-Fas (Apo-I) antibodies; induction of cytotoxic T-cells; and induction of anti-idiotypic antibodies with anti-cellular activity (Riethmuller et al 1994).

Therapy with MAb2. An anti-idiotypic human monoclonal antibody 105AD7 (human MAb2) has also been used for immunization against colorectal cancer (Durrant et al 1993). This antibody was isolated from a patient administered with a mouse monoclonal antibody 791T/36 for imaging. In a phase I clinical trial of patients with advanced colorectal cancer, 13 patients received up to seven immunizations each. Lymphocytes were available from 11 patients, seven of whom showed anti-tumour T-cell responses. Interleukin-2 was also detected in eight out of 13 patients. Six patients had positive responses to both T-lymphocytes and interleukin-2. The median survival for the immunized patients was 12 months compared with 3 months for the control group (Durrant et al 1993).

Granulocyte-macrophage colony-stimulating factor (GM/CSF). Antibody-dependent cellular cytotoxicity can be enhanced by pretreatment of effector cells with granulocyte-macrophage colony-stimulating factor (GM/CSF). Twenty patients with advanced metastatic colorectal cancer were given human recombinant GM/CSF before treatment with monoclonal 17-1A. Two patients achieved complete remission: one with disappearance of para-aortic nodes; the other had resolution of retroperitoneal lymph nodes and a lung metastasis. One patient had reduction of tumour bulk by up to 50%, three patients had disease stabilized for greater than 3 months (Ragnhammar et al 1993).

Immunotoxins. A phase I study involving 17 patients with colorectal metastases with the monoclonal antibody 791T/36 conjugated to ricin toxin A chain, showed reversible side-effects related to the toxin, consisting of low serum albumin, flu-like symptoms with fever, proteinuria and mental state changes. Human antibody response developed to both the antibody and the toxin within 3 weeks. Mixed tumour regression occurred in five patients (Byers et al 1989).

Ovarian cancer

Radioimmunotherapy. In an extended phase I–II trial 52 patients with epithelial ovarian cancer were given intraperitoneal yttrium-90 labelled monoclonal HMFG1 following surgery and chemotherapy (Hird et al 1993). The only adverse reaction was reversible myelosuppression. The median follow-up was 35 months. Twenty-one out of the 52 patients had no residual disease, two patients died. Radioimmunotherapy reduced tumour recurrence rate and improved long-term survival, and should be considered as adjuvant therapy in ovarian cancer (Hird et el 1993).

Idiotypic therapy. In advanced ovarian cancer, patients who underwent RIS and who developed anti-idiotypic response to the anti-CA 125 monoclonal, had longer than expected survival for their disease stages. This was probably due to the therapeutic effect of the anti-idiotypic antibodies (Baum et al 1994).

Gliomas

Radioimmunotherapy. Monoclonal antibody BC-2 recognizes the glycoprotein tenascin, expressed by the stroma of malignant gliomas but not by normal cerebral tissue (Riva et al 1992). BC-2 labelled with iodine-131 was injected directly into recurrent glioblastoma in ten patients who had not responded to surgery, chemotherapy or radiotherapy. Many patients had multiple injections with a total radiation dose delivered to the tumours of between 7000 and 41 000 cGy. CT and NMR (nuclear magnetic resonance) scans revealed that two patients had partial remissions with a reduction of >50% of tumour volume, one had complete remission, three patients had stabilization of the disease, while four patients did not respond. The patients who responded remained in remission for at least 11–17 months (Riva et al 1992).

Monoclonal antibody with LAK cells.   Lymphokine-activated killer (LAK) cells have been used to treat malignant glioma. LAK cells were pre-treated with a bispecific antibody prepared by the chemical conjugation of an anti-CD3 monoclonal (reactive with LAK cells) and a glioma reactive monoclonal, NE150. The antibody pretreated cells were more effective in the therapy of grade III and IV glioma than LAK cells alone. Of the ten patients thus treated, two did not respond, four showed regression of tumour, four had eradication of tumour cells left after surgery. No recurrence was detected 10–18 months after treatment, compared with a historical control group of ten patients treated with LAK cells alone, nine of whom developed recurrence within a year (Nitta et al 1990).

Malignant melanoma

Direct effect of monoclonal antibody.   Gangliosides, which are cell matrix interacting molecules, are produced by melanomas. These include GD2, GM2, 9-O-acetylated GD3 and GD3. Human monoclonal antibodies have been generated against gangliosides GD2 (L72) and GM2 (L55). Intralesional injection of these antibodies resulted in tumour regression by 50% in some patients (Irie et al 1989).

Idiotypic therapy.   Twenty-five patients with stage IV melanoma were immunized with a mouse anti-idiotypic monoclonal antibody MK2-23 (MAb2). Fourteen patients responded to immunization and had significantly longer survival than the nine who did not. Three patients showed partial response with reduction in size of metastatic lesions in one lasting for 52 weeks, and in the other two lasting for 93 weeks (Mittelman et al 1992).

Non-Hodgkin's lymphoma

Direct effect of monoclonal antibody.   Two patients with non-Hodgkin's lymphoma were treated with a re-shaped human monoclonal antibody (CAMPATH-1H) which reacts with the CAMPATH-1 antigen expressed on nearly all lymphoid cells and monocytes but not by other cells (Hale et al 1988). Antibody (1–20 mg) was injected daily intravenously for up to 43 days. Lymphoma cells were cleared from the circulation and the bone marrow, and splenomegaly and lymphadenopathy were resolved. Haemopoeisis returned to normal in one patient and partially in another (Hale et al 1988).

Idiotypic therapy.   B-cell lymphomas have on their cell surface immunoglobulins or idiotypes which act as distinct markers for monoclonal antibody therapy. After failure of conventional treatment, 14 patients were treated with anti-idiotypic monoclonal antibodies. Eight patients had complete or partial responses for over 6 months; one patient had complete remission lasting 6 years (Brown et al 1989). Another 11 patients were given interferon additionally. Ten patients showed objective evidence of tumour regression at 2 weeks. There were two complete responses, seven partial and two minor responses. The duration of response varied from 2 months to more than 24 months (Brown et al 1989).

Immunotoxins.   In eight different phase I trials where immunotoxins were given to patients with high tumour load, partial or complete remissions were obtained in between 12% and 75% of patients. Under similar circumstances chemotherapeutic agents can only expect a 5% response rate (Vitetta et al 1993). Immunotoxin (anti-B-blocked ricin) was administered to 12 patients in complete remission following autologous bone marrow transplant for relapse of B-cell non-Hodgkin's lymphoma. Eleven patients remain in complete remission at 13–36 months post-treatment (Grossbard et al 1993).

PROBLEMS WITH MONOCLONAL ANTIBODY LOCALIZATION

Experience with radioimmunoscintigraphy has revealed a number of problems associated with antibody localization to tumours. Solutions to these difficulties are discussed below.

Human anti-mouse antibody response (HAMA)

Mouse monoclonal antibodies induce a HAMA in up to 50% of patients after first administration and up to 90% after two to three administrations (Hand et al 1994). This reaction may be directed at the immunoglobulins in general or at the idiotypic regions. HAMA may be suppressed or prevented by cyclosporin A therapy (Ledermann et al 1988, Weiden et al 1994). However, this response can be best avoided by the administration of human monoclonal antibodies or 'humanized' mouse antibodies, described below.

Low concentration of antibody localization to tumours

There are three physiological barriers affecting localization of macromolecules such as antibodies to tumours. These are (1) variable blood supply, (2) raised interstitial pressure, (3) significant distance between stroma and tumour cells (Jain 1990). Other barriers include basement membrane and junctions between cells (Dvorak et al 1991). Antibodies which react with tumour antigens expressed on the stroma side may achieve greater localization to tumours (Boxer et al 1994). Improved antibody localization to tumours can be achieved by the following methods.

Enzyme cleavage of antibodies – fragments F(ab')₂, Fab

The smaller $F(ab')_2$ fragments produced by enzyme cleavage of antibodies (Fig. 11.1) can penetrate tissue spaces and tumours more readily. Excretion of free circulating antibody fragments is faster, thus reducing the background activity during RIS. There is no binding by Fc receptor to cells in liver, lung and spleen. Improved imaging results have been reported by Mariani et al (1991) using technetium-99m labelled $(F(ab')_2$ fragments of anti-CEA monoclonal antibody F023C5. Smaller antibody fragments such as single chain antibody fragments (scFv) (Fig. 11.1) can now be produced by molecular techniques described below. These have the advantages of better tumour penetration and being less immunogenic in human.

Regional delivery of antibodies

Regional administration of antibodies may overcome low antibody concentration or high systemic radiation dose and destruction of antibodies by liver and other normal organs associated with intravenous administration of antibodies (Rowlinson-Busza et al 1991). For example, intravesical administration of monoclonal AUA1 is taken up selectively by bladder tumours but not by normal urothelium (Bamias et al 1993). Iodine-131 labelled monoclonals, reactive against CD10 and CD19 antigens, were administered intrathecally to seven children with central nervous system relapse of acute lymphoblastic leukaemia. Six patients showed demonstrable responses (Pizer et al 1993). Intraperitoneal administration of iodine-131 radiolabelled antibodies is effective in the therapy of ovarian carcinoma (Hird et al 1993).

Intratumour delivery of antibodies

Monoclonal antibodies, reactive with N-CAM (neural cell adhesion molecules), were administered directly to the tumours in patients with recurrent or cystic malignant gliomas of grade III–IV (Papanastassiou et al 1993). The antibodies were retained longer in tumours than when given intrathecally. Radiation doses to the whole body were reduced. There was no bone marrow toxicity which occurred with intrathecal administration of antibodies (Papanastassiou et al 1993).

Enhanced antigen expression by tumours

Interferon treatment significantly increased tumour CEA expression in a xenograft from 809 ng CEA per g tumour to 5598 ng CEA per g tumour. It doubled the radiation dose of yttrium-90 radiolabelled anti-CEA monoclonal antibody ZCE025 delivered to the tumours and significantly improved the results of radioimmunotherapy (Kuhn et al 1991).

Tumour heterogeneity

Immunohistochemical staining shows that different antigens may be expressed by cells within a tumour, or tumours from different patients. To overcome tumour heterogeneity in antibody localization, a cocktail of monoclonal antibodies, each recognizing different antigenic epitopes, can be used. In a clinical study, a mixture of $F(ab')_2$ fragments of monoclonal antibodies achieved better tumour detection rate than a single antibody (Chatal et al 1984).

RECENT ADVANCES IN ANTIBODY PRODUCTION

Bispecific antibodies

A bispecific antibody with one arm binding to a tumour and another to an effector agent is produced by fusion of two different hybridomas. A bispecific monoclonal antibody reactive with methotrexate and a tumour associated antigen (gp72) (Pimm et al 1990), a monoclonal with specificity for cytotoxic T-cells and ovarian cancer (Garrido et al 1990), and a humanized antibody reactive with CEA and radiolabelled chelate diethylenetriaminepentaacetic acid (DTPA-^{90}Y) for radioimmunotherapy (Bruynck et al 1993), have been produced.

In clinical applications the bispecific antibody is localized to the tumour first. After clearance of unbound antibody, the effector agent is administered. This antibody-targeting approach reduces background activity, with maximal cytotoxic effects being exerted to the tumour and minimal side-effects to normal tissues.

Human monoclonal antibodies

Unlike the production of mouse monoclonal antibodies, the generation of human monoclonal antibodies has been fraught with difficulties. The frequency of cell fusion is low, the hybridomas are unstable and secrete few antibodies, but ultimately they are dependent on a natural process of immunization in the patients. Thus only a few human monoclonal antibodies to cancer have been reported. Anti-cancer humoral responses in humans appear to be directed at intracellular antigens such as cytokeratins (O'Hare & Yiu 1987).

Colorectal cancer

Peripheral blood lymphocytes from autologous tumour immunized patients were used to generate human monoclonal antibodies, two of which have been used in RIS. 16–88 reacts with cytokeratins 8, 18 and 19 expressed to a greater extent in colorectal cancer than normal colon, while 28A32 reacts with both cytoplasmic and surface determinants (Steis et al 1990).

Human colorectal monoclonal antibodies derived from draining lymph node lymphocytes include COU-1 (Erb et al 1992) and SK1 (Chang et al 1993a), both are IgM. COU-1 reacts with a cytokeratin-like cytoplasmic protein with a molecular weight of 43 000 and is probably a modified cytokeratin 18 (Erb et al 1992). SK1 reacts with cells from the gastrointestinal tract, but otherwise shows a restricted tissue distribution and lyses cells in the presence of complements (Chang et al 1993b). The reactive antigen is a sialoglycoprotein of molecular weight 42 000 (Chang et al 1993a). Other human antibodies reactive with live colonic cell line LS174T but few other epithelial cells on fluorescence-activated cell scan have been reported (Yiu et al 1992). Some of these antibodies reacted with colorectal cancer xenografts on immunocytochemistry.

Breast cancer

Human monoclonal antibody reactive against the mouse mammary tumour virus (MuMTV) polypeptides was generated from a breast cancer patient (Shoenfeld et al 1987). Other breast monoclonals (YBB-190, YBM-209, YBY-088) react with cytokeratin (Ryan et al 1988). Monoclonal F86 reacts with surface antigens of five different breast cancer cell lines and several malignant myelomonocytic cell lines but not normal mononucleocytes (Posner et al 1991).

Malignant melanoma

A human monoclonal recognizing the ganglioside GD2, secreted by Epstein–Barr virus transformed cell L72, reacts with malignant cells of neuroectoderm origin, including melanoma, glioma and neuroblastoma but not other cell or tumour types (Katano et al 1984).

Lung cancer

A human IgM monoclonal antibody NCC-1004, produced from a papillary adenocarcinoma of lung, reacts with blood group i antigen. It reacts with squamous carcinomas of lung and oesophagus, carcinoma of thyroid, red blood cells, B-lymphocytes, basal cells of bronchial epithelium, stratified squamous epithelium, endothelium and alveolar epithelium (Hirohashi et al 1986).

Ovarian cancer

In vitro immunization of lymphoid cells with OCCSA, a 200-kDa ovarian cell surface antigen, produced a human antibody, TC5. It is specific for ovarian cancer and early stage breast cancer. There was no reaction with normal ovary, uterus, cervix, endocervix, fallopian tubes, lung, heart, pancreas, liver or breast (Chaudhuri et al 1994).

Rapid cloning of variable (V) genes

Antibody specificities are determined by the variable regions. Specificity is achieved by rearrangement of the heavy and light chain V genes. The rearranged or functional V genes are similar at either end, and can be cloned by means of polymerase chain reaction (PCR). Antibody genes can be cloned from any antibody secreting cells, for example B-lymphocytes or hybridoma cells. The starting materials can be RNA or DNA; cDNA can be generated from RNA. The cloned genes are available for genetic engineering and can be inserted into plasmid vectors and transfected into mammalian cells, bacteria or other cell types for antibody fragment expressions. The fragments produced will have antigen binding property of the intact immunoglobulin (Hawkins et al 1993).

Antibody fragments and antibody fusion proteins

Antibody fragments consisting of only the variable heavy (VH) and light (VL) chain domains can be constructed by genetic engineering. In this system plasmids are used as vectors to insert cDNA of VH and VL, joined together by a polypeptide linker, into *Escherichia coli* which express the antibody fragments. These are called single chain variable fragments (scFv) (Fig. 11.1). scFv have been constructed from the mouse anti-placental alkaline phosphatase monoclonal H17E2 (Savage et al 1993a). Genetic engineering also enables antibody fragments to be linked to unrelated protein. Thus in a feasibility study, an anti-lysozyme scFv was joined to interleukin-2, a cytokine produced by T helper cells, to form an anti-tumour fusion protein (Savage et al 1993b).

Humanized mouse monoclonal antibodies

To reduce the immunogenicity of the mouse antibody in human, two approaches have been used.

1. *Chimaeric antibodies*

In this process cDNA coding for the mouse immunoglobulin variable region is cloned from the mouse hybridoma and joined to human constant region genes, such as human genomic gamma 4 and kappa constant region genes. The chimaeric immunoglobulin genes are transfected by virus into COS-1 cells which express the chimaeric antibody. Several chimaeric antibodies have been constructed, for example B6.2 (Sahagan et al 1986), anti-colorectal cancer antibodies 17-1A (Sun et al 1986) and B72.3 (Whittle et al 1987), anti-breast cancer antibody MBr1 (Orlandi et al 1991). The binding reactivity and specificity of chimaeric antibodies are similar to those of the original mouse antibodies.

2. *Reshaped or CDR grafted human antibodies*

The antigen binding surface of an antibody is composed of six hypervariable loops of amino acids, known as complementarity determining regions (CDRs), which are mounted on relatively constant framework of the variable regions. Genetic manipulations enable grafting of CDRs from mouse antibody to human framework of the variable regions, producing humanized or reshaped human antibody, so that the major part of the immunoglobulin is of human origin (Hawkins et al 1993). A reshaped human antibody directed to human ovarian and testicular tumours has been constructed from the mouse monoclonal antibody H17E2 (Verhoeyen et al 1991).

Phage display antibodies

Antibody genes can be cloned into filamentous bacteriophages (phages) instead of bacteria. Phages are viruses with a single-stranded DNA genome that infect bacteria. They have on their surface a protein (gene III protein) used for attachment to bacteria. An antibody gene may be inserted onto one end of gene III which will express the encoded antibody fragment on the phage surface (Fig. 11.3). The antibody on the phage surface is immunoreactive and the phage remains infective. Thus phages behave like functional B-lymphocytes, with antibodies displayed on the surfaces, and the genes encoding the antibodies contained within. Screening of genetically modified phages selects not only the reactive antibodies but also the relevant antibody genes, which may be used to produce large amounts of antibodies in *E. coli* or stored (Hawkins et al 1993).

Bypassing hybridoma to produce antibodies

Phage-antibody technique has been used to generate antibodies, for example chimaeric antibodies to epidermal growth factor receptor (EGFR). Phage-antibody libraries were prepared from RNA of the immunized mouse B-cells to construct cDNA coding for the variable heavy and light chains. The PCR-amplified genes were cloned into phagemid vector and the ligation mixtures were electroporated into *E. coli*. The library stock thus generated was screened for reactivity to EGFR. Two reactive scFv expressed on phages were converted into whole immunoglobulin molecules (Kettleborough et al 1994). Phage antibodies with better affinity to CEA than mouse monoclonal antibodies have also been produced (Chester et al 1994).

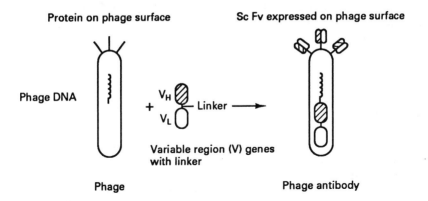

Fig. 11.3 Production of phage antibody. cDNA of V genes, prepared from mRNA of B-lymphocytes, is amplified by PCR. The linked V_H and V_L genes are cloned into the phage producing a phage antibody.
V_H = heavy chain variable domain; V_L = light chain variable domain; scFv = single chain variable fragments.

Bypassing immunization to produce human antibodies

It is theoretically possible to generate human antibody without immunization by mimicking the antigen-driven response of B-lymphocytes in vitro. A 'naive' phage library of rearranged V genes was created from the peripheral blood lymphocytes of two healthy volunteers. The phage library bound with 15 antigens which included CEA, MUCI mucin, tumour necrosis factor-alpha, turkey egg white lysosome, bovine serum albumin and bovine thyroglobulin (Marks et al 1991). These bindings were generally of low intensity. However, increased affinity of antibody fragments to antigens can be manipulated in vitro by molecular techniques (Winter & Milstein 1991).

SCID mice for production of human monoclonal antibodies

Human monoclonal antibodies may be generated in mice with severe combined immunodeficiency (SCID) which lack both functional T- and B-cells. The immune responses generated in these mice are similar to those in normal animals following transplantation of human fetal or mature immune cells (Borrebaeck et al 1993).

CONCLUSION

Monoclonal antibodies have found many applications in oncology, the most significant of which has been in diagnostic histopathology. Their potential to detect markers of tumour progression or prognosis is promising but requires further confirmation. Radioimmunoscintigraphy using technetium-99m la-belled antibodies and single-photon emission computed tomography can often detect occult metastatic colorectal cancers not revealed by conventional imaging techniques, and could play a more active role in the management of this disease. Immunotherapy is most successful in haematological malignan-cies where there is better access of antibodies to target cells. In solid tumours the absolute amount of antibodies localized remains low. Recent development in the humanization of mouse antibodies, the progress being made in genetically engineered antibodies with desirable binding properties and smaller fragments, increasing understanding of the biology of tumour circulation and stromal environment, novel methods of antibody delivery and discovery of new tumour markers such as oncogene protein products or cell surface receptors, all act to increase the chances of success of antibody targeted therapy. The use of monoclonal antibodies, or molecules identified by antibodies, as vaccines is an exciting prospect. Thus the multidisciplinary approach that has been adopted should ensure that monoclonal antibodies make a significant contribution to the management and therapy of cancer.

KEY POINTS FOR CLINICAL PRACTICE

- Monoclonal antibodies play an important role in the histological diagnosis of undifferentiated tumours.
- ERICA (oestrogen receptor immunocytochemical assay) has simplified the assessment of oestrogen receptor status in breast cancer.
- In colorectal cancer radioimmunoscintigraphy may detect tumours not revealed by other imaging techniques.
- Unmodified antibody and anti-idiotypic antibody therapies have shown encouraging results in colorectal cancer and other tumours.
- Human anti-mouse antibody response is diminished by the construction of humanized mouse antibodies and antibody fragments using genetic engineering techniques.
- Genetic engineering techniques can be used to produce antibodies or antibody fusion protein better suited than mouse monoclonals for clinical application.

REFERENCES

Bamias A, Ogden C, Krausz T et al 1993 Intravesical administration of HMFG2 monoclonal antibody in superficial bladder carcinomas. In: Epenetos AA (ed) Monoclonal antibodies 2. Applications in clinical oncology. Chapman and Hall, London, pp 97–101
Bartkova J, Barnes DM, Millis RR et al 1990 Immunohistochemical demonstration of c-erbB-2 protein in mammary ductal carcinoma in situ. Hum Pathol 21: 1164–1167
Baum RP, Niesen A, Hertel A et al 1994 Activating anti-idiotypic human anti-mouse antibodies for immunotherapy of ovarian carcinoma. Cancer 73: 1121–1125
Bischof-Delaloye A, Delaloye B, Buchegger F et al 1989 Clinical value of immunoscintigraphy in colorectal carcinoma patients: a prospective study. J Nucl Med 30: 1646–1656

Blair SD, Theodorou NA, Begent RHJ et al 1990 Comparison of anti-fetal colonic microvillus and anti-CEA antibodies in peroperative radioimmunolocalisation of colorectal cancer: Br J Cancer 61: 891–894

Borrebaeck CAK, Martensson C, Ifversen P et al 1993 Evaluation of the scid-hu mouse as a model to generate human monoclonal antibodies. In: Epenetos AA (ed). Monoclonal antibodies 2. Applications in clinical oncology. Chapman and Hall, London, pp 481–491

Boven E, Haisma HJ, Bril H 1991 Tumor localisation with 131I-labelled human IgM monoclonal antibody 16.88 in advanced colorectal cancer patients. Eur J Cancer 27: 1430–1436

Boxer GM, Abassi AM, Pedley RB et al 1994 Localisation of monoclonal antibodies reacting with different epitopes on carcinoembryonic antigen (CEA) — implications for targeted therapy. Br J Cancer 69: 307–314

Breitz HB, Weiden PL, Vanderheyden JL 1992 Clinical experience with rhenium-186-labeled monoclonal antibodies for radioimmunotherapy: results of phase I trials. J Nucl Med 30: 1646–1656

Britton KE, Granowska M 1991 The role of radiolabelled antibodies in cancer diagnosis. In: Epenetos AA (ed) Monoclonal antibodies. Applications in clinical oncology. Chapman and Hall, London, pp 223–236

Brown SL, Miller RA, Horning SJ et al 1989 Treatment of B cell lymphomas with anti-idiotype antibodies alone and in combination with alpha interferon. Blood 73: 651–661

Bruynck A, Seemann G, Bosslet K 1993 Characterisation of a humanised bispecific monoclonal antibody for cancer therapy. Br J Cancer 67: 436–440

Byers VS, Rodvien R, Grant K et al 1989 Phase I study of monoclonal antibody-ricin A chain immunotoxin XomaZyme-791 in patients with metastatic colon cancer. Cancer Res 49: 6153–6160

Chang HR, Koda K, Chang S et al 1993a AgSK1, a novel carcinoma associated antigen. Cancer Res 53: 1122–1127

Chang HR, Chavoshan B, Park H 1993b Human monoclonal antibody SK1-mediated cytotoxicity against colon cancer cells. Dis Colon Rectum 36: 1152–1157

Chatal JF, Saccavini JC, Fumoleau P 1984 Immunoscintigraphy of colon carcinoma. J Nucl Med 25: 307–314

Chaudhuri TR, Zinn KR, Morris JS et al 1994 Human monoclonal antibody developed against ovarian cancer cell surface antigen. Cancer 73: 1098–1104

Chester K, Begent RHJ, Robson L et al 1994 Phage libraries for generation of clinically useful antibodies. Lancet 343: 455–456

Ditzel H, Rasmussen JW, Erb K et al 1993 Tumor detection with 131I-labeled human monoclonal antibody COU-1 in patients with suspected colorectal carcinoma. Cancer Res 53: 5920–5928

Dixon AR, Price MR, Hand CW et al 1993a Epithelial mucin core antigen (EMCA) in assessing therapeutic response in advanced breast cancer — a comparison with CA15.3. Br J Cancer 68: 947–949

Dixon AR, Jackson L, Chan SY et al 1993b Continuous chemotherapy in responsive metastatic breast cancer: a role for tumour markers? Br J Cancer 68: 181–185

Doerr RJ, Herrera L, Abdel-Nabi H 1993 In-111 CYT-103 monoclonal antibody imaging in patients with suspected recurrent colorectal cancer. Cancer 71: 4241–4247

Durrant LG, Denton GW, Robins RA 1993 Immunization with human monoclonal antiidiotypic antibody in colorectal cancer. Ann NY Acad Sci 690: 334–336

Dvorak HF, Nagy JA, Dvorak AM 1991 Structure of solid tumours and their vasculature: implications for therapy with monoclonal antibodies. Cancer Cells 3: 77–85

Erb K, Borup-Christensen P, Ditzel H et al 1992 Characterization of a human-human hybridoma antibody, C-OU1 directed against a colon tumor-associated antigen. Hybridoma 11: 121–134

Fisken J, Leonard RCF, Stewart M et al 1993 The prognostic value of early CA125 serum assay in epithelial ovarian carcinoma. Br J Cancer 68: 140–145

Garrido MA, Valdayo MJ, Winkler DF 1990 Targeting human T-lymphocytes with bispecific antibodies to react against human ovarian carcinoma cells growing in *nu/nu* mice. Cancer Res 50: 4227–4232

Gatter KC 1989 CL Oakley Lecture (1989). Diagnostic immunocytochemistry: achievements and challenges. J Pathol 159: 183–190

Goldenberg DM, Larson SM 1992 Radioimmunodetection in cancer identification. J Nucl Med 33: 803–814

Greenson JK, Isenhart CE, Rice R et al 1994 Identification of occult micrometastases in pericolic lymph nodes of Dukes' B colorectal cancer patients using monoclonal antibodies against cytokeratin and CC49. Cancer 73: 563–569

Grossbard ML, Gribben JG, Freedman AS et al 1993 Adjuvant immunotoxin therapy with anti-B4-blocked ricin after autologous bone marrow transplantation for patients with B-cells non-Hodgkin's lymphoma. Blood 81: 2263–2271

Hale G, Dyer MJS, Clark MR et al 1988 Remission induction in non-Hodgkin lymphoma with reshaped human monoclonal antibody, CAMPATH-1H. Lancet 2: 1395–1401

Hand PH, Kashmiri SVS, Schlom J 1994 Potential for recombinant immunoglobulin constructs in the management of carcinoma. Cancer 73 (suppl 3): 1105–1113

Hawkins RE, Llewelyn MB, Russell SJ 1993 Monoclonal antibodies in medicine. In: Basic molecular and cell biology, 2nd edn. BMJ Publishing Group, London, pp. 111–131

Herlyn D, Caton A, Koprowski H 1991 Anti-idiotypes in cancer immunotherapy. In: Epenetos AA (ed) Monoclonal antibodies. Applications in clinical oncology. Chapman and Hall, London, pp 283–290

Hird V, Maraveyas A, Snook D et al 1993 Adjuvant therapy of ovarian cancer with radioactive monoclonal antibody. Br J Cancer 68: 403–406

Hirohashi S, Clausen H, Nudelman E et al 1986 A human monoclonal antibody directed to blood group i antigen: heterohybridoma between human lymphocytes from regional lymph nodes of a lung cancer patient and mouse myeloma. J Immunol 136: 4163–4168

Irie RF, Matsuki T, Morton DL 1989 Human monoclonal antibody to ganglioside GM2 for melanoma treatment. Lancet 1: 786–787

Jain RK 1990 Physiological barriers to delivery of monoclonal antibodies and other macromolecules in tumors. Cancer Res 50 (Suppl 3): 814S–819S

Katano M, Jien M, Irie RF 1984 Human monoclonal antibody to ganglioside GD2-inhibited human melanoma xenograft. Eur J Cancer Clin Oncol 20: 1053–1059

Kettleborough CA, Ansell KH, Allen RW et al 1994 Isolation of tumor cell-specific single-chain Fvs from immunized mice using phage-antibody libraries and the reconstruction of whole antibodies from these antibody fragments. Eur J Immunol 24: 952–958

Kohler G, Milstein C 1975 Continuous cultures of fused cells secreting antibody of predefined specificity. Nature 256: 495–497

Kuhn JA, Beatty BG, Wong JYC et al 1991 Interferon enhancement of radioimmunotherapy for colon carcinoma. Cancer Res 51: 2335–2339

Larson SM 1990 Clinical radioimmunodetection, 1978–1988: overview and suggestions for standardisation of clinical trials. Cancer Res (Suppl) 50: 892S–898S

Larson SM 1991 Radioimmunology. Imaging and therapy. Cancer 67: 1253–1260

Larson SM, Chaitanya RD, Scott AM 1994 Overview of clinical radioimmunodetection of human tumors. Cancer 73: 832–835

Ledermann JA, Begent RHJ, Bagshawe KD et al 1988 Repeated antitumour antibody therapy in man with suppression of the host response by cyclosporin A. Br J Cancer 58: 654–657

Lindemann F, Schlimok G, Dirschedl P et al 1992 Prognostic significance of micrometastatic tumour cells in bone marrow of colorectal cancer patients. Lancet 340: 685–689

Luqmani YA, Campbell T, Soomro S et al 1993 Immunohistochemical localisation of pS2 protein in ductal carcimona in situ and benign lesions of the breast. Br J Cancer 67: 749–753

Mach J-P, Buchegger F, Forni M et al 1981 Use of radiolabelled monoclonal anti-CEA antibodies for the detection of human carcinomas by external photoscanning and tomoscintigraphy. Immunol Today 2: 239–249

Mariani M, Bonino C, Tarditi M et al 1991 Early clinical results with Tc-99m-labelled F(ab′)₂. In: Epenetos AA (ed) Monoclonal antibodies. Applications in clinical oncology. Chapman and Hall, London, pp 297–307

Marks JD, Hoogenboom HR, Bonnett TP et al 1991 By-passing immunization: human antibodies from V-gene libraries displayed on bacteriophage. J Mol Biol 222: 581–597

Meredith RF, Khazaeli MB, Plot WE et al 1992 Phase I trial of iodine-131-chimeric B72.3 (human IgG4) in metastatic colorectal cancer. J Nucl Med 33: 23–29

Mittelman A, Chen ZJ, Yang H et al 1992 Human high molecular weight-melanoma associated antigen (HMW-MAA) mimicry by mouse anti-idiotypic monoclonal antibody MK-23: induction of humoral anti-HMW-MAA immunity and prolongation of survival in patients with stage IV melanoma. Proc Natl Acad Sci USA 89: 466–470

Murray JL, Macey DJ, Kasi LP et al 1994 Phase II radioimmunotherapy trial with ^{131}I-CC49 in colorectal cancer. Cancer 73: 1057–1066

Nitta T, Sato K, Yagita H et al 1990 Preliminary trial of specific targeting therapy against malignant glioma. Lancet 335: 368–371

O'Hare MJ, Yiu CY 1987 Human monoclonal antibodies as cellular and molecular probes: a review. Mol Cell Probes 1: 33–54

Orlandi R, Figini M, Tomassetti A et al 1991 Biochemical and biological characterization of the chimeric MBr1 antibody. In: Epenetos AA (ed) Monoclonal antibodies. Applications in clinical oncology. Chapman and Hall, London, pp 31–36

Papanastassiou V, Pizer B, Tzanis S et al 1993 Use of radioimmuno-conjugates in the treatment of malignant glioma. In: Epenetos AA (ed) Monoclonal antibodies 2. Applications in clinical oncology. Chapman and Hall, London, pp 179–185

Pasanen PA, Eskelinen M, Partanen K et al 1993 Receiver operating characteristic (ROC) curve analysis of the tumour markers CEA, CA 50 and CA 242 in pancreatic cancer; results from a prospective study. Br J Cancer 67: 852–855

Perren TJ 1991 CerbB2 oncogene as a prognostic marker in breast cancer. Br J Cancer 63: 328–332

Pimm MV, Robins RA, Embleton MJ et al 1990 A bispecific monoclonal antibody against methotrexate and a human tumour associated antigen augments cytotoxicity of methotrexate–carrier conjugate. Br J Cancer 61: 508–513

Pizer BL, Papanastassiou V, Hancock J et al 1993 Intrathecal radioimmunotherapy for central nervous system acute lymphoblastic leukaemia in childhood. In: Epenetos AA (ed) Monoclonal antibodies 2. Applications in clinical oncology. Chapman and Hall, London, pp 255–262

Poller DN, Snead DRJ, Roberts EC et al 1993 Oestrogen receptor expression in ductal carcinoma in situ of the breast: relationship to flow cytometric analysis of DNA and expression of the c-erbB-2 oncoprotein. Br J Cancer 68: 156–161

Posner MR, Elboim HS, Tumber MB et al 1991 An IgG human monoclonal antibody reactive with a surface membrane antigen expressed on malignant breast cancer cells. Hum Antibodies Hybridomas 2: 74–83

Ragnhammar P, Fagerberg J, Frodin JE et al 1993 Effect of monoclonal antibody 17-1A and GM-CSF in patients with advanced colorectal carcinoma — long lasting, complete remissions can be induced. Int J Cancer 53: 751–758

Riethmuller G, Schneider-Gadicke E, Schlimok G et al 1994 Randomised trial of monoclonal antibody for adjuvant therapy of resected Dukes' C colorectal carcinoma. Lancet 343: 1177–1183

Riva P, Arista A, Sturiale C et al 1992 Treatment of intracranial human glioblastoma by direct intra-tumoral administration of ^{131}I-labelled anti-tenascin monoclonal antibody BC-2. Int J Cancer 51: 7–13

Robertson JFR, Pearson D, Price MR et al 1991 Objective measurement of therapeutic response in breast cancer using tumour markers. Br J Cancer 64: 757–763

Rowlinson-Busza G, Bamias A, Krausz T et al 1991 Monoclonal antibody uptake and distribution following intra-tumour injection. In: Epenetos AA (ed) Monoclonal antibodies. Applications in clinical oncology. Chapman and Hall, London, pp 149–156

Ryan KP, Dillman RO, DeNardo SJ et al 1988 Breast cancer imaging with In-111 human IgM monoclonal antibodies: preliminary studies. Radiology 167: 71–75

Sahagan BG, Doral H, Saltzgaber-Muller J et al 1986 A genetically engineered murine/human chimeric antibody retains specificity for human tumor-associated antigen. J Immunol 137: 1066–1074

Savage P, Rowlinson-Busza G, Verhoeyen M et al 1993a Construction, characterisation and kinetics of a single chain antibody recognising the tumour associated antigen placental alkaline phosphatase. Br J Cancer 68: 738–742

Savage P, So A, Spooner RA, Epenetos AA 1993b A recombinant single chain antibody interleukin-2 fusion protein. Br J Cancer 67: 304–310

Shoenfeld Y, Hizi A, Tal R et al 1987 Human monoclonal antibodies derived from lymph nodes of a patient with breast carcinoma react with MuMTV polypeptides. Cancer 59:

43–50

Steis RG, Carrasqillo JA, McCabe R et al 1990 Toxicity, immunogenicity, and tumor radioimmunodetecting ability of two human monoclonal antibodies in patients with metastatic colorectal carcinoma. J. Clin Oncol 8: 476–490

Sun LK, Curtis P, Rakowicz-Szulczynska E et al 1986 Chimeric antibodies with 17-1A-derived variable and human constant regions. Hybridoma 5: S17

Triozzi PL, Kim JA, Aldrich W et al 1994 Localization of tumor-reactive lymph node lymphocytes in vivo using radiolabeled monoclonal antibody. Cancer 73: 580–589

Van der Schouw YT, Verbeek ALM, Wobbes Th et al 1992 Comparison of four serum tumours markers in the diagnosis of colorectal carcinoma. Br J Cancer 66: 148–154

Van Kamp GJ, von Mensdorff-Pouilly S, Kenemans P et al 1993 Evaluation of colorectal cancer-associated mucin CA M43 assay in serum. Clin Chem 39: 1029–1032

Verhoeyen M, Broderick L, Eida S et al 1991 Re-shaped human anti-PLAP antibodies. In: Epenetos AA (ed) Monoclonal antibodies. Applications in clinical oncology. Chapman and Hall, London, pp 34–44

Vitetta ES, Thorpe PE, Uhr JW 1993 Immunotoxins: magic bullets or misguided missiles. Immunol Today 14: 252–259

Ward U, Primrose JN, Finan PJ et al 1993 The use of tumour markers CEA, CA-195 and CA-242 in evaluating the response to chemotherapy in patients with advanced colorectal cancer. Br J Cancer 67: 1132–1135

Weiden PL, Wolf SB, Breitz HB et al 1994 Human anti-mouse antibody suppression with cyclosporin A. Cancer 73: 1093–1097

Whittle N, Adair J, Lloyd C et al 1987 Expression in COS cells of a mouse-human chimaeric B72.3 antibody. Protein Eng 1: 499

Winter G, Milstein C 1991 Man-made antibodies. Nature 349: 293–299

Yiu CY, Baker L, Boulos PB 1991a Anti-epithelial membrane antigen monoclonal antibodies and radioimmunolocalization of colorectal cancer. Br J Surg 78: 1212–1215

Yiu CY, Baker L, Davidson BR et al 1991b Immunoscintigraphy of colorectal cancer using a monoclonal antibody 77–1. Eur J Surg Oncol 17: 495–501

Yiu CY, Baker L, Olabiran Y et al 1992 Generation of human monoclonal antibodies from colorectal diseases. Br J Surg 79: S36

12

Surgical lasers and photodynamic technology

S. Evrard   J. Marescaux

Since 1967 and the introduction of the first CO_2 laser, many applications have been proposed for laser technology in general surgery, always with abundant optimism but often with poor success. Obviously, lasers are infrequently employed by the general surgeon, a fact mainly due to the cost of these devices and the satisfactory performance of electrocautery. In other specialities such as ophthalmology and dermatology, lasers have gained large acceptance. They were not merely substituted for electrocautery but used for new applications. A similar approach might be appropriate in general surgery. At least two original applications will be discussed for laser technology: (1) telesurgery whose future development will require special tools not only for coagulation, section, and welding, but also robotic guiding; (2) photodynamic technology including therapy and fluorescence imaging. Indeed, the latest research in lasers was directed towards tissue targeting and to achieving specific biological effects. In the past, industrial demands led to the development of lasers which physicians adapted for their use in the best possible way. Now, recent understanding of laser–tissue interactions favours the development of new systems designed for specific medical applications (Parrish & Wilson 1991). In return, the surgeon must have a competent knowledge of photobiology.

BASIC PRINCIPLES

Scientific background

Laser is the acronym of Light Amplifier Stimulated Emission of Radiation. It has two fundamental characteristics: (1) production of identical photons by a stimulated emission process; (2) amplification of this stimulated emission. The first characteristic originated in the quantum theory proposed by Einstein in 1917. Atoms excited by energy rise to higher metastable states for a very short period of time. The restitution of energy implies a photonic emission by three different mechanisms: spontaneous emission, absorption and stimulated emission. Only the latter type of emission allows recruitment of identical photons, i.e. coherent across time and space. As a direct consequence, the laser beam is monochromatic: all the photons have the same wavelength and

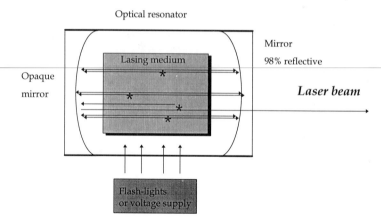

Optical resonator

Fig. 12.1   Outline of laser system.

the same energy. The second characteristic of laser is amplification of the beam based on the optical resonator theory proposed by Bohr. Schematically, an optical resonator consists of two mirrors facing each other, one of them being only 98% reflective. The small number of photons passing through this mirror is the collimated laser beam (Fig. 12.1).

The first laser by Maiman in 1960 used ruby as a medium. Now a wide range of solids, gas, liquids or vapours are available as lasing media. Fig. 12.2 summarizes most of the available medical lasers and their wavelengths of emission. The latest laser technology developed is the diode laser. Diode lasers are electronic semiconductor devices that emit laser light as electrical current passes through them. Their high electrical-to-optical efficiency permits the design of high-power air-cooled lasers that are lightweight and compact (Manni 1992). Semiconductor diode lasers are the future of medical laser applications. Finally, it should be observed that laser output can be of two different modes: the continuous mode, in which a continuous level of energy is produced, and the pulsed mode, in which high energy bursts are obtained.

From a practical point of view, a laser (i.e. a lasing medium) is well defined by its wavelength which will determine the interaction between laser beam tissue and its output.

WAVELENGTH

The wavelength directly influences the depth of penetration of tissue. For wavelength of the visible spectrum and the near infrared, the longer the wavelength, the deeper the tissue distribution. In the bands of the far infrared, light transmission into the tissues decreases rapidly. Tissue penetration can be estimated at about 1 mm for ultraviolet, 2–4 mm for green light, 5–10 mm for red light, 10–30 mm for near infrared light and only 0.05–0.1 mm for far infrared. Laser light with low transmission and high absorption rates

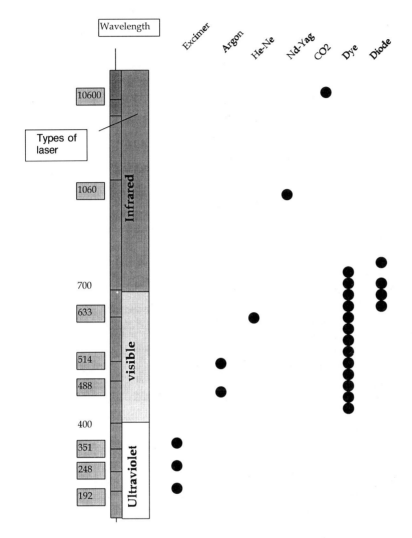

Fig. 12.2   Wavelengths of medical lasers.

dissipates its energy in a small volume inducing vaporization. At the opposite, laser light with a high transmission rate dissipates its energy in a larger volume with less thermal effect.

Medical laser wavelengths range from the ultraviolet to the near infrared with many useful bands in the visible part of the spectrum (Fig. 12.2). Some wavelengths can be transmitted along flexible quartz fibres; others have to be transmitted by articulated mirrors (far infrared of CO_2 laser and excimer lasers) or multifibre catheters (ultraviolet of 351 nm excimer laser). It should be noted that wavelengths of some lasing media are tunable.

Laser output

The output is determined by the lasing medium and its possibilities of pumping by voltage supply or light flashes. It may be expressed by the power which is the time rate of energy flux (in watts) and the energy which is the power per unit time (in joules). In clinical practice, power and energy must be plotted to the light area where they are delivered. An exact dosimetry of laser output is often difficult to determine because of the frequent heterogeneity of the biological targets.

Laser–tissue interaction

Interaction of light with tissue is very complex (Svaasand & Doiron 1983). Biological tissues are characterized by their heterogeneity (cells, vessels, fat, water, etc.), their different rates of blood flow and the concentration of pigments or chromophores. All these parameters may markedly affect the tissue/light behaviour. Incident light upon tissue may be reflected, scattered, transmitted or absorbed. Biological activity of light is due to the sole absorption phenomenon by chromophores. Natural biological chromophores are water, haemoglobin and melanin; photodynamic therapy uses artificial chromophores named photosensitizers. Laser light which is absorbed by chromophores is converted to kinetic energy: heat for power densities, photooxidation for non-thermal power densities. In general, less than $50\ J\ cm^{-2}$ produces a non-thermal effect, $50–400\ J\ cm^{-2}$ produce a gradual dehydration and coagulation of the tissues, more than $400\ J\ cm^{-2}$ vaporizes the tissues.

THERMAL APPLICATIONS

Applications are the same as for electrocautery except that the delivery devices of laser energy by flexible quartz fibres will be more appropriate for telesurgery.

Laser type

Non-tunable lasers

Excimer lasers. Excimer (EXCIted diMER) lasers are ultraviolet sources producing very short energy pulses (Linsker et al 1984) at a wavelength of 193, 248 or 351 nm. All excimer lasers use a gas mixture of about 0.1% of xenon chloride or argon fluoride, 1% rare gas and the remainder a buffer gas, either helium or neon or both. A photoablative effect by disruption of intermolecular bonds can be obtained with excimer laser. At present, ophthalmology is the main field of application but tissue welding could prove to be interesting especially for telesurgery. Mechanically assisted sutureless anastomosis of gut, vessels or bile duct could be possible in the future.

Argon laser.   Argon laser produces two wavelengths at 488 and 514 nm. Tissue depth penetration is only 1 mm because of absorption of haemoglobin. Cutting with argon laser light induces adjacent tissue coagulation and controls haemostasis from vessels of 1 mm in diameter (Fuller 1983) with a low rate of smoke production. Argon light transmission by quartz fibres is available but argon technology is more expensive than CO_2.

Nd-YAG and KTP lasers.   The lasing medium is a crystal of yttrium-aluminium-garnet (YAG) doped with a small quantity of the rare-earth metal neodynium (Nd). It produces a 1060 nm invisible infrared light easily transmitted by optical fibres. Targeting of the invisible Nd-YAG laser beam is obtained by coupling with an helium–neon pilot laser (red beam). Nd-YAG energy has less specific absorption by haemoglobin and water than CO_2 or argon lasers (Dixon et al 1979), so only 60% of it will be absorbed. Tissue penetration is about 10–20 mm and vessels of 3 mm in diameter are coagulated (Fuller 1983). The KTP laser is a Nd-YAG doubled in frequency (wavelength 532 nm). The KTP beam is visible (green) but induces an obliteration of the television image.

CO_2 laser.   The lasing medium is CO_2 and N_2 gas. The CO_2 near infrared laser beam is also invisible with a wavelength at 10 600 nm. CO_2 energy is strongly absorbed by water but not air. Tissues are vaporized but only for 0.1 mm, and coagulation is obtained for vessels of only 0.5 mm in diameter. Because there is no adjacent tissue coagulation, a small spot of 600 μm is ideal for cutting (Bruhat & Mage 1979). Laparoscopic CO_2 laser use is advocated by gynaecologists even though it has three drawbacks: (1) CO_2 pneumoperitoneum partly absorbs the laser beam energy; (2) vaporization of the tissue induces smoke which requires ventilation of pneumoperitoneum; and (3) transmission of the CO_2 laser beam requires a series of mirrors and an articulating arm, but flexible fibres will be available in the future (Bouquet de la Jolinière et al 1989).

Tunable lasers

Dye lasers.   Lasing media are dyes in a liquid state energized by different lasers such as argon laser, metal-vapour laser, diode laser, etc., or by flash-lights. The more frequently used dyes are Kiton red, DCM and rhodamine. They are employed in photodynamic therapy between 630 and 750 nm and as lithotriptors (Chang et al 1987). Stone destruction involves the generation of plasma upon application of the laser light. The laser light is absorbed in the generated plasma causing plasma electrons to equilibrate with plasma ions; the hot plasma then produces a thermal wave which propagates through the stone, causing a reactionary shock wave which fractures the stone (Gitomer & Jones 1987, Dayton et al 1988). The possibility of thermal injury to the common bile duct wall requires an energy threshold compatible with safe surgical conditions.

Diode laser.   Semiconductor technology has brought a new concept: the diode lasers. These small diode lasers (size of a box of matches!) are tunable with a high electrical-to-optical efficiency. Currently, there are two basic types of high-power diode lasers suitable for surgical applications. Aluminium gallium arsenide (AIGaAs) diode lasers emit at a nominal laser wavelength of 800 nm, which can be transmitted efficiently through quartz fibres, with an output of 25 W. Equipped with a hot-tip fibre, a thermal tissue necrosis of about 0.5 mm can be achieved (Manni 1992). In the near future, another diode (AlGaInP) lasing in the 640–700 nm range will be available for photodynamic therapy.

Diode lasers may find a use in tissue welding. Laser function is obtained in a non-contact mode with low energy power. Another technique often referred to as 'laser soldering' uses 800 nm diodes and a solution of indocyanine green and fibrinogen applied to the junction to be sealed. The dye enhances the absorption of the diode energy, and the fibrinogen improves the mechanical strength of the tissue junction (Manni 1992).

Delivery devices

The optimal delivery system of laser energy for minimal access surgery is by flexible quartz fibres for both non-contact and contact applications. A quartz lens is usually coupled with the laser beam and the fibre. The fibre has a central core of high-quality glass coated with a thin layer of glass at a slightly lower refractive index (Murray et al 1992). Light is transmitted along the fibre by total internal reflection. Fibres range approximately from 0.1 to 1 mm. Bare fibres can be used in a non-contact (coagulation), near-contact (vaporization) or contact (purely thermal) mode (Hunter 1991).

Recently a variety of industrial sapphire and ceramic contact tips for handheld or endoscopic use have been introduced. They allow cutting with the side of the fibre and provide a tactile feedback to the surgeon (Hunter 1991). Contact fibres have two disadvantages: they are slightly more expensive and they stay hot for 10 s after use, risking contact burn to adjacent organs.

Clinical applications

Liver

Experimental studies indicate the possibility of liver resection with CO_2 or Nd-YAG lasers or the two combined. Tranberg et al (1986) compared the Nd-YAG laser and the ultrasonic dissector with the routine blunt dissection for liver resection. They observed that non-contact Nd-YAG laser use resulted in a significant reduction in operating time compared with the other two methods, a decreased perioperative blood loss but caused more extensive tissue necrosis. Joffe et al (1985) have demonstrated the superiority of the contact

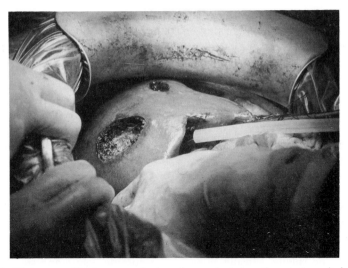

Fig. 12.3 High-power CO_2 laser vaporization of two colonic hepatic metastases during a Pringle manoeuvre. (Courtesy of R. Sultan.)

artificial sapphire technique over the non-contact approach in the rat as did Schroder et al (1987) in a canine model.

Recently Katkhouda et al (1992) reported the first case of laparoscopic liver hydatid cyst laser resection. The authors suggested that this technique using a Nd-YAG laser was probably also indicated for small liver metastases or benign tumours. Palliative vaporization of scattered hepatic metastases (Fig. 12.3), especially in tumours of endocrine origin, is advocated (Dixon 1988).

Biliary

Laparoscopic laser cholecystectomy has been proposed as an alternative to electrocautery (Hunter 1991; Reddick & Olsen 1990). It should be observed that no prospective data are yet available on this subject. Electrosurgical dissection may be faster and is less costly, whereas laser dissection may be more precise (Hunter 1991). Other authors deny any place for laser in laparoscopic cholecystectomy (Voyles et al 1990).

Common bile duct stones may be fragmented using the photoacoustic effect of laser beam. In this contact technique, the laser light induces a plasma which, when hot, produces a shock wave which fractures the stone (Gitomer & Jones 1987). The most appropriate type of laser seems to be the pulsed dye laser. This high energy pulsed device allows reduction in the size of the stone with minimal thermal effect. In the same way, common bile duct stones can be treated at the time of laparoscopic cholecystectomy in one procedure avoiding the need for conversion to an open common bile duct exploration or the need for subsequent endoscopic retrograde cholangiography, papillotomy and stone extraction. A flexible laparoscopic choledocoscope driving the quartz fibre may be introduced either into the cystic duct or by choledocotomy. Rapid saline flow irrigates the stone fragments through the sphincter of Oddi into the duodenum.

Pancreas

Joffe et al (1985) have performed both experimental and clinical pancreatic resections with Nd-YAG laser. Total pancreatectomies were also performed with CO_2 laser in dogs (Donna 1981). A significant reduction in operating time and blood loss was reported.

Spleen

Dixon et al (1980) have described an open technique for segmental or partial splenectomy involving ligature of selected hilar vessels and Nd-YAG vaporization of the splenic capsule, superficial sinusoidal tissue and smaller peripheral vessels. The coagulated material was aspirated. As the hilum was approached, larger vessels were divided and clipped. Laparoscopic splenectomies have already been performed and laser may find a role in such a procedure.

Head and neck

CO_2 laser excision of head and neck tumours induces less blood loss and decreased operating times (Aronoff 1981). Polyps of the larynx and tracheal region have been treated successful (Shapsay & Simpson 1983) as have lymphangiomas of the head and neck in children (White & Adkins 1986).

Oesophagogastrointestinal

Contact Nd-YAG laser has been advocated as a useful instrument for visceral dissection (especially stomach and intestine) during open procedures (Hira & Moore 1987, Skobelkin et al 1987). Laparoscopic surgery may also benefit by this laser scalpel.

Hunter et al (1984) have reported a laser version of the Taylor procedure in dogs. Following posterior vagotomy an argon laser myotomy was used for the lesser curvature. Serosa and muscularis were coagulated but mucosa was preserved. Secretory studies were shown to be satisfactory.

Endoscopic laser surgery has been widely used as palliative therapy of gastrointestinal malignancy. Cancers of the oesophagus, stomach, colon and rectum have been managed in order to relieve dysphagia, obstruction or to control bleeding (Fig. 12.4). Laser treatment can be carried out under light sedation on an outpatient basis. Relief of obstruction requires between one and five sessions.

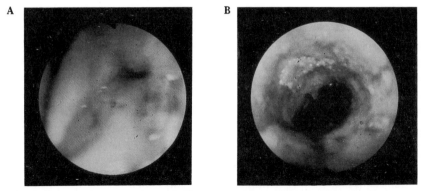

Fig. 12.4   Endoscopic laser palliation. **A** Malignant and postradiotherapy stenosis of the upper oesophagus. **B** Nd-YAG laser palliative recanalization of the oesophagus. (Courtesy of D. Coumaros.)

Fleischer & Sivak (1985) obtained a 92% rate of dysphagia relief, in 68 patients with oesophageal cancer but perforation occurred in 12%. Using the laser alone, Barr et al (1990) observed a lower complication rate than using the laser followed by endoscopic intubation. Perforations occur in about 5% of cases and must be treated by intubation, although it is often fatal (Murray et al 1992). Fleischer & Sivak (1984) have also reported temporary control of bleeding and restoration of transit in a small series of gastric carcinomas.

Inoperable bleeding and obstructing colorectal carcinomas may also be treated by Nd-YAG laser. Brunetaud et al (1990) experienced good palliative results by treating their patients every 6 weeks without waiting for symptoms to recur. Loizou et al (1990) have reported that eradication of small tumour (less than 3 cm diameter) is possible in 100%. Extensive tumour treatment may be complicated by bowel perforation leading to colostomy formation.

Miniaturized robotic guiding

Instrumentation for laparoscopic surgery is in its infancy and no doubt much progress is likely in the near future, especially in the development of three-dimensional imaging and microinstrumentation. The concept of miniaturized robots assisted by computers to cut with precision, to perform endocorporeal knots, etc., seems futuristic but not impossible. Research in this field is in progress. Lasers would be useful to pilot these microdevices as they do in military technologies.

PHOTODYNAMIC TECHNOLOGY

Basic principles

Photodynamic therapy (PDT) is a new anticancer treatment attracting considerable interest because of its selectivity. The preferential uptake and retention of intravenously administered photosensitizers in malignant tissue in relation to the surrounding normal tissues sets up a relative therapeutic ratio. Thereafter activation at an appropriate light wavelength produces singlet oxygen and other free radicals (Foote 1982) which are cytotoxic and induce the selective destruction of the cancer. These transitory radicals are thought to damage blood vessel endothelium and cause destruction of the tumour microcirculation (Star et al 1986). Direct disruption of cell membrane (Valenzeno 1987) as well as of subcellular organelles (Gibson & Hilf 1983) has been described.

Furthermore, the excitation of the photosensitizer by the incident photon produces re-emission of a fluorescent photon which can be used to localize the reaction. Detection of this fluorescence might be useful to demonstrate small tumour deposits.

Although haematoporphyrin derivatives remain the most widely used photosensitizers, they offer poor chemical homogeneity and relatively weak absorption in the clinically useful red part of the spectrum where light penetration of tissues is strong. Much research is now in progress to develop second generation photosensitizers.

PDT may be applied to destroy the tumour within its organ of origin (Patrice et al 1989, McCaughan et al 1989a) or to destroy tumour cells dispersed in different peripheral tissues, such as cellular fat or lymph, as intraoperative adjunctive treatment.

Photodynamic therapy

Endoscopic applications of PDT have been reported for the treatment of head and neck (Grossweiner et al 1987), lung (Balchum & Doiron 1985), bladder (Shumaker & Hetzel 1987) and gastrointestinal tumours (Patrice et al 1989). Oesophageal tumours may be treated either by cylinder diffuser tipped fibres (Fujimaki & Nakayama 1986) or by interstitial illumination (McCaughan et al 1989b). Complications are local oedema and fibrosis. PDT appears to be an effective method of palliation of the malignant dysphagia caused by oesophageal cancer, and phase III clinical trials are now ongoing to compare this method with other established methods of palliation (Marcus 1990). Advanced colorectal tumours have also been treated endoscopically by PDT with similar results (Jin et al 1989, Patrice et al 1989).

Gastrointestinal surgeons are becoming more interested in photodynamic therapy (Amato 1993) and the basis of such an intra-abdominal application has been extensively reviewed (Evrard et al 1993).

PDT was used as adjuvant treatment following curative resection as well as in palliative treatment of surgically unresectable colorectal cancer recurrence in 14 patients from the Roswell Park Memorial Institute (Herrera-Ornelas et al 1986). Irradiation was by a Kiton red laser pumped by an argon laser. The photosensitizer used was Photofrin®. Laser illumination was 100–400 J/cm². Tumour residues more than 1 cm deep were irradiated interstitially. No local or systemic complications were observed after intravenous administration of the sensitizer. Fluorescence with a Wood's light was closely related to positive biopsies and tumour sampling after PDT showed haemorrhagic necrosis. The results in terms of survival were poor, as expected in view of patient selection, but PDT was able to sterilize areas of microscopic tumour recurrence. Furthermore, many patients experienced considerable relief of pelvic pain.

Another feasibility study was performed by a second surgical team at Roswell Park Memorial Institute (Nambisan et al 1988). This was a second-look study in ten patients with recurrence of sarcoma. Photofrin II® was used at a dose of 2.5–5 mg/kg; illumination was by a Kiton red laser emitting at 630 nm, and a total light dose of 30–288 J/cm² was delivered. Two late serious skin photosensitization accidents occurred. Two patients had a complete surgical resection followed by irradiation of the tumour bed, and were in total remission at 24 and 28 months respectively. Three patients had a further recurrence at the margins of the treated zone. All other patients developed distant metastases but no local recurrence. This study suggested excellent tolerance of PDT and the benefit of tumour fluorescence in achieving a total en bloc resection.

A third study is a case report from Colombus, Ohio (USA) (McCaughan et al 1991). A 57-year-old woman underwent cholecystectomy in 1985 and a common bile duct adenocarcinoma was noted. A T-tube was first inserted followed by a U-tube coursing through the skin. Intraluminal PDT was performed seven times during 4 years using a cylinder diffuser tip at the end of a quartz fibre. Dihaematoporphyrin ether was used at a dose of 2 mg/kg, 48–96 h before illumination. The laser was a Kiton red dye laser pumped by an argon laser. Between 200 to 400 J were delivered per cm of diffusing tip. The biological tolerance of both dihaematoporphyrin ether and PDT was excellent. The patient survived for more than 4 years when metastases appeared in the pleura.

The last report is from the National Cancer Institute at Bethesda (USA) and was devoted to treatment of peritoneal carcinomatosis (Sindelar et al 1991) in 23 patients. They underwent surgical debulking of as much tumour as possible leaving behind no neoplastic nodules greater than 5 mm. Two dye lasers emitting at 630 nm were used in tandem delivering 1.5–7.5 W. Maximum delivered light dose was 3 J cm^{-2} with a total energy delivered to each patient ranging from 2997 to 56 460 J. Dihaematoporphyrin ether was used as photosensitizer. A dilute lipid emulsion was used to cover peritoneal surfaces and to improve homogeneity of dose delivery. The mean duration of the procedure was 8.5 h. Five complications occurred following therapy: one haemoperitoneum, one necrotizing pancreatitis, two intestinal fistulas and one urinoma. There was no postoperative mortality. It is difficult to determine the relative contribution of these complications to aggressive surgical debulking or photodynamic therapy. Among the 13 patients treated for ovarian cancer, 11 demonstrated progressive disease while two have remained free of recurrence (8–14 months). Among the eight patients treated for widespread sarcoma, two had no evidence of disease progression (8–9 months). Two patients treated for pseudomyxoma peritoneii remained free of progressive disease for 9–18 months.

Photodynamic imaging

The use of optical spectroscopy for tissue diagnosis is a new approach in medical diagnostics. Biological chromophores such as tryptophan, elastin, collagen, melanin, flavins, etc., and endogenous porphyrin, may fluoresce under ultraviolet illumination. Furthermore, a non-fluorescent chromophore like haemoglobin may absorb fluorescence (Anderson-Engels et al 1991). Based on differences in laser-induced fluorescence spectra, it has been possible to discriminate normal and benign pathology such as atherosclerosis or carious teeth and non-tumoral and cancerous tissues (Fig. 12.5) (Andersson et al 1987a, Kapadia et al 1990). Another approach requires the prior administration of a photosensitizer to the patient, which preferentially localizes to the tumoral tissue. Using a Wood's light, Herrera-Ornelas et al (1986) found an excellent correlation between observed sites of fluorescence and the presence of tumour in biopsies of the same sites. Nevertheless, the fluorescence detection signal is limited by tissue autofluorescence (Baumgartner et al 1987, Balchum et al 1987). Andersson et al (1987b) have demonstrated that the ratio between autofluorescence and photosensitizer fluorescence may allow a dimensionless monitoring function. Moreover, immunity is provided against variation in fibre tip-to-target distance, surface topography effects and drift in laser intensity in overall detection efficiency.

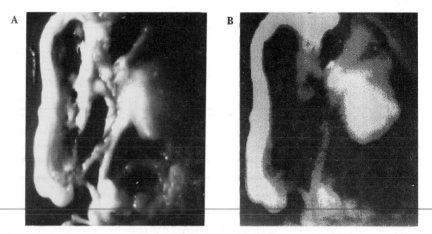

Fig. 12.5 In vitro photodiagnostic imaging of a rat duodenopancreatic bloc bearing a tumour after systemic injection of pheophorbide A. **A** Videoimage of duodenum (on the left) and tumour (on the right). **B** Contrast of fluorescence was maximum in the duodenum and in the tumour.

Wavelengths of the excitation lasers used in fluorescence imaging system range in the ultraviolet. Fluorescence is collected by a charge coupled device (CCD) camera and transmitted to a computer. Mathematical calculation increases the contrast between normal tissue and cancerous cells and produces a false colours fluorescence image on a video screen (Andersson Engels et al 1991).

KEY POINTS FOR CLINICAL PRACTICE

- Biological effects of a laser beam depend on its wavelength (tissue depth penetration) and its output (kinetic energy).
- Biological activity of light is due to the absorption phenomenon by natural chromophores like water, haemoglobin, melanin, etc.
- CO_2 and Nd-YAG lasers are used as thermal scalpels.
- Laser will probably find a specific field of application in telesurgery because of light transmission through flexible quartz fibres.
- Photodynamic therapy and imaging are two interesting applications of non-thermal lasers based on the selective retention of photosensitizers by malignant tissues and abnormal stroma. Absorption of light by the photosensitizer produces either free cytotoxic radicals (tumour destruction) or fluorescence (tumour detection).
- After debulking surgery, photodynamic therapy may be useful in destroying residual micrometastases dispersed in cellular fat or lymph nodes.
- Tissue laser-induced fluorescence is collected by a CCD camera and transmitted to a computer. A mathematical calculation increases the contrast between normal tissue and malignant cells and produces a false colours fluorescence image on a video screen.

REFERENCES

Amato I 1993 Hope for a magic bullet that moves at the speed of light. Science 262: 32–33
Andersson PS, Montan S, Svanberg S 1987a Multispectral system for medical fluorescence imaging. IEEE J Quantum Electron 23: 1798–1805
Andersson PS, Montan S, Persson T et al 1987b Fluorescence endoscopy instrumentation for improved tissue characterization. Med Phys 14: 633–636
Andersson-Engels S, Johansson J, Svanberg K et al 1991 Fluorescence imaging and point measurements of tissue: applications to the demarcation of malignant tumours and atherosclerotic lesions from normal tissue. Photochem Photobiol 53: 807–814
Aronoff BL 1981 The carbon dioxide laser in head and neck surgery. In: Goldman L (ed) The biomedical laser. Springer-Verlag, New York, p. 240–245
Balchum OJ, Doiron DR 1985 Photoradiation therapy of endobronchial lung cancer: large obstructing tumors, nonobstructing tumors, and early stage bronchial cancer lesions. Clin Chest Med 6: 255–275
Balchum OJ, Profio AE, Razum N 1987 Ratioing fluorometer probe for localizing carcinoma in situ in bronchi of the lung. Photochem Photobiol 46: 887
Barr H, Krasner N, Raouf A et al 1990 Prospective randomised trial of laser therapy only and laser therapy followed by endoscopic intubation for the palliation of malignant dysphagia. Gut 31: 252–258
Baumgartner R, Fisslinger H, Jocham D et al 1987 A fluorescence imaging device for

endoscopic detection of early stage cancer — instrumental and experimental studies. Photochem Photobiol 46: 759

Bouquet de la Jolinière J, Dubuisson JB, Tessier B 1989 Fibre CO_2 et infertilité. 2nd Congrès Mondial d'Endoscopie Gynécologique. Clermont-Ferrand Personal communication

Bruhat MA, Mage G 1979 Use of the CO_2 laser in neosalpingostomy. In: Kaplan J (ed) Proceedings of the 3rd international congress for laser surgery. Tel Aviv, Jerusalem. Academic Press, New York, p 271

Brunetaud JM, Maunoury V, Cochelard D et al 1990 Lasers in rectosigmoid tumours. Lasers Med Sci 5: 22

Chang BW, Pollock ME, Eugene J et al 1987 The potential for common duct injury during laser cholelitholysis. Lasers Surg Med 7: 88–92

Dayton MT, Decker DL, McClane R et al 1988 Copper vapor laser fragmentation of gallstones: In vitro measurements of wall heat transmission. J Surg Res 45: 90

Dixon JA 1988 Current laser applications in general surgery. Ann Surg 207: 355

Dixon JA, Berenson MM, McCloskey DW 1979 Neodymium YAG laser treatment of experimental canine gastric bleeding. Gastroenterol 77: 647–651

Dixon JA, Miller F, McCloskey D 1980 Laser partial splenectomy. Surg Res 10: 116

Donna GD 1981 Total pancreatectomy with the carbon dioxyde laser. In: Atsumi K, Nimsakul N (eds), Laser Tokyo 81. Inter-Group, Tokyo, p 43

Einstein A 1917 Zur Quantentheorie des Strahlung. Phys Z 19: 121–128

Evrard S, Aprahamian M, Marescaux J 1993 Intraabdominal photodynamic therapy: from theory to feasibility. Br J Surg 80: 298–303

Fleischer DE, Sivak MV 1984 Recurrent gastric adenocarcinoma treated by endoscopic Nd-YAG laser therapy. Gastroenterology 87: 815–820

Fleischer DE, Sivak MV 1985 Endoscopic Nd:YAG laser therapy as palliation for esophagogastric cancer. Gastroenterology 89: 827–831

Foote CS 1982 Light, oxygen and toxicity. In: Author AP (ed) Pathology of oxygen. Academic Press, New York, p 21–44

Fujimaki M, Nakayama K 1986 Endoscopic laser treatment of superficial esophageal cancer: Semin Surg Oncol 2: 248–256

Fuller T 1983 Fundamentals of lasers in surgery and medicine. In: Dixon JA (ed) Surgical application of lasers. Year Book, Chicago, pp 11–27

Gibson S, Hilf R 1983 Photosensitization of mitochondrial cytochrome C oxidase by hematoporphyrin derivative and related prophyrins in vitro and in vivo. Cancer Res 43: 4191–4197

Gitomer SJ, Jones RD 1987 Modeling laser ablation and fragmentation of renal and biliary stones. In: Conference on lasers and electro-optics. Society of Lasers and Electro-Optics, Baltimore

Grossweiner LI, Hill JH, Lobraico RV 1987 Photodynamic therapy of head and neck squamous cell carcinoma: optical dosimetry and clinical trial. Photochem Photobiol 46: 911–918

Herrera-Ornelas L, Petrelli NJ, Mittelman A et al 1986 Photodynamic therapy in patients with colorectal cancer. Cancer 57: 677–684

Hira N, Moore KC 1987 The use of the Nd-YAG contact laser in abdominal surgery. Lasers Surg Med 7: 86

Hunter JG 1991 Laser or electrocautery for laparoscopic cholecystectomy. Am J Surg 161: 345–349

Hunter JG, Becker JM, Dixon JA 1984 Lesser curvature laser myotomy. Lasers Surg Med 8: 362–363

Jin ML, Yang BQ, Zhang W, Ren P 1989 Photodynamic therapy for the treatment of advanced gastrointestinal tumours. Lasers Med Sci 4: 183–186

Joffe SN, Sankar MY, Salzer B 1985 Preliminary clinical application of the contact surgical rod and endoscopic microprobes with the Nd-YAG laser. Lasers Surg Med 5: 188

Kapadia CR, Cutruzzola FW, O'Brien KM et al 1990 Laser induced fluorescence spectroscopy of human colonic mucosa. Detection of adenomatous transformation Gastroenterology 99: 150–157.

Katkhouda N, Fabiani P, Benizri E et al 1992 Laser resection of a liver hydatid cyst under videolaparoscopy. Br J Surg 79: 560–561

Linsker R, Srinivasan R, Wynne JJ, Alonso DR 1984 Farultraviolet ablation of atherosclerotic lesions. Laser Surg Med 4: 201–206

Loizou LA, Grigg D, Boulos PB et al 1990 Endoscopic Nd-YAG laser treatment of rectosigmoid cancer. Gut 31: 812–816

McCaughan JS, Guy JT, Hicks W et al 1989a Photodynamic therapy for cutaneous and subcutaneous malignant neoplasms. Arch Surg 124: 211–216

McCaughan JS, Nims TA, Guy JT et al 1989b Photodynamic therapy for esophageal tumors. Arch Surg 124: 74–80

McCaughan JS, Mertens BF, Cho C et al 1991 Photodynamic therapy to treat tumors of the extrahepatic biliary ducts. Arch Surg 126: 111–113

Manni J 1992 Surgical diode laser. J Clin Laser Med Surg 10: 377–380

Marcus SL 1990 Photodynamic therapy of human cancer: clinical status, potential, and needs. In: Future directions and applications in photodynamic therapy. SPIE Institute Series vol IS6: 5–56

Murray A, Mitchell DC, Wood RFM 1992 Lasers in surgery. Br J Surg 79: 21–26

Nambisan RN, Karakousis CP, Holyoke ED et al 1988, Intraoperative photodynamic therapy for retroperitoneal sarcomas. Cancer 61: 1248–1252

Parrish JA, Wilson BC 1991 Current and future trends in laser medicine. Photochem Photobiol 53: 731–738

Patrice T, Foultier MT, Adam F et al 1989 Traitement palliatif par photochimiothérapie de 54 cancers digestifs. Essai clinique de phase 1. Ann Chir 43: 433–437

Reddick EJ, Olsen DO 1990 Outpatient laparoscopic laser cholecystectomy. Am J Surg 160: 485–489

Schroder T, Sankar MY, Brackett AKM 1987 Major liver resection using contact Nd-YAG laser. Lasers Surg Med 7: 89

Shapshay SM, Simpson GT 1983 Lasers in bronchology. Otolaryngol Clin North Am 16: 879–886

Shumaker BP, Hetzel FW 1987 Clinical laser photodynamic therapy in the treatment of bladder carcinoma. Photochem Photobiol 46: 899–901

Sindelar WF, DeLaney TF et al 1991 Technique of photodynamic therapy for disseminated intraperitoneal malignant neoplasms. Arch Surg 126: 318–324

Skobelkin OK, Breckow EI, Smoljiniov MB 1987 Resection of hollow abdominal organs with lasers. Lasers Surg Med 7: 101

Star WM, Marijnissen HPA, van den Berg Blok AE 1986 Destruction of rat mammary tumor and normal tissue microcirculation by hematoporphyrin derivative photoradiation observed in vivo in sandwich observation chambers. Cancer Res 46: 2532–2540

Svaasand LO, Doiron DR 1983 Thermal distribution during photoradiation therapy. In: Kessel D, Dougherty TJ (eds) Porphyrin photosensitization, Plenum Press, New York, p 77–90

Tranberg KG, Ricotti P, Brackett KA 1986 Liver resection – a comparison using the Nd-YAG laser, ultrasonic dissector or conventional blunt dissection. Am J Surg 151: 368–374

Valenzeno DP 1987 Photomodification of biological membranes with emphasis on singlet oxygen mechanisms. Photochem Photobiol 46: 147–160

Voyles CR, Meena AL, Petro AB et al 1990 Electrocautery is superior to laser for laparoscopic cholecystectomy. Am J Surg 160: 457

White BJ, Adkins WY 1986 The use of the carbon dioxide laser in head and neck lymphangiomas. Lasers Surg Med 6: 293–296

13

Innovations in paediatric surgery

R. Wheeler

Paediatric surgery may be considered one of the last bastions of general surgery, where subspecialization by anatomical region or system is least prevalent, age being the sole line of demarcation. This should be qualified by the recognition of paediatric urology as a growing and discrete entity: whether this will encompass all paediatric uropathy and hypospadias or simply complex malformations whose reconstruction would require tertiary level referral remains an issue for debate.

The first report of the National Confidential Enquiry into Perioperative Deaths (1989) highlighted the importance of specifically trained surgeons and anaesthetists caring for small children, and with the rising tide of litigation this advice seems likely to harden into a directive.

As a discipline covering all fields of general surgery, the evolution of paediatric surgery obviously reflects the developments in adult practice. However, there are different constraints as is demonstrated with laparoscopy which has more limited applications. Anatomical size has permitted developments in surgical approaches that would not be appropriate in adults, such as approaching the pylorus via the umbilicus. In topics dictated by age, such as the advent and consequences of antenatal diagnosis and the prospect of a single stage operation for Hirschsprung's disease in infancy, the advances remain exclusive to paediatric surgery.

VASCULAR ACCESS

Long-term vascular access of over 3–4 weeks' duration in children has undergone major changes. The population requiring this has increased, partly because of oncology protocols of intensive and prolonged chemotherapy, blood administration, parenteral nutrition and blood sampling. There is also now a population of patients with short bowel syndrome surviving and requiring parenteral nutrition. The development of central venous catheters suitable for children has encouraged this proliferation. The conventional material of silicone rubber had the disadvantage of a high ratio of wall thickness/lumen diameter, necessitated by the relatively poor tensile strength of the rubber. The poor flow rate of cerebral venous catheters that had a small enough external diameter to be inserted into an infant was thus a limiting factor. Although improvements in the silicone lead to long-term total parenteral nutrition being practicable in infancy, the penetration of the silicone molecule by lipids led to inevitable fragmentation and fracture of the catheter. The resultant multiple venous access procedures under general anaesthesia could lead to the destruction of all conventional sites of venous access, i.e. internal jugular, subclavian, saphenofemoral junction and azygous veins.

The development of new materials such as polyurethane have led to marked improvement in some of these areas. With a higher tensile strength, polyurethane catheters have thin walls and thus achieve improved flow rates with much smaller external diameters. There is no lipid penetration into the polyurethane ultrastructure and fracture has not occurred despite prolonged in vivo usage (Wheeler & Griffiths 1992). The configuration of some of these central venous catheters (Cuff Cath, Ohmeda, UK) permits a retrograde tunnelling technique which ensures immediate and permanent fixation (Wheeler et al 1991) (Fig. 13.1). This has reduced the rate of displacement, previously a major problem in the paediatric population, to zero.

The concept of completely implantable venous access reservoirs (Pegelow et al 1986) has been facilitated by the development of low profile devices

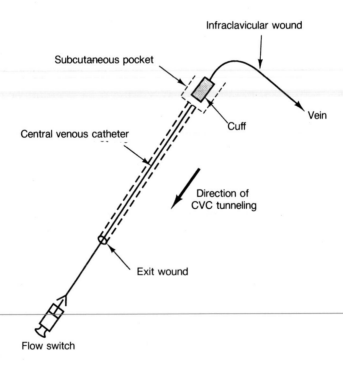

Fig. 13.1 The retrograde tunneling technique. (Reproduced with permission from Wheeler et al 1991.)

suitable for small children such as Vascuport (Ohmeda, UK). These have a clear advantage in that accidental (or wilful!) removal by the child is prevented and infection may be reduced. Swimming is also easier with a subcutaneous reservoir, although waterproof dressings allow submersion in children with more conventional catheters. However, there have been some complications of prolonged usage in children. They are sometimes reluctant to have the port accessed, despite the use of topical local anaesthetic creams, and cannulae have been developed to give overnight access to the port because of occasional problems with skin necrosis if the reservoir is used too frequently. Blood transfusion has been implicated in reservoir blockage.

The totally implantable reservoir undoubtedly has a vital role to play in the field of long-term venous access in children, but should not be considered as universally appropriate and venous access may have to be modified according to individual therapeutic requirements.

Further development in extrusion techniques has allowed the introduction of 'short long lines' — silicone catheters (Epicutaneo-cava Katheter, Vygon, Germany) 0.6 mm external diameter, 0.3 mm internal diameter, which thread via a peripherally punctured basilic or saphenous vein up to the right atrium. Although prone to blockage and thus only suitable for continuous infusion techniques, these catheters are ideal for the neonate or infant requiring medium term (e.g. up to 21 days) intravenous infusion (Stringer et al 1992). They have the advantage of requiring only local anaesthesia for insertion, which can be performed whilst a neonate is still in its incubator, thus avoiding the heat loss and disturbance that may be involved with open procedures in theatre. There is evidence that percutaneous central venous line insertion in neonates is associated with fewer complications than with those inserted surgically (Puntis et al 1987). There are further advantages: peripheral cannulation is not associated with the potentially serious mechanical complications of internal jugular or subclavian venous access, the percutaneous lines are cheaper and do not leave thoracic scars (Stringer et al 1992). Elective replacement of 27G polyurethane central venous catheters after a maximum 13 days led to a reported zero rate of line sepsis complicating a series of high-risk neonates weighing less than 1200 g (Nakamura et al 1990). The principle of central venous catheter exchange may thus be combined with peripheral percutaneous central venous cannulation to minimize sepsis if the need for prolonged parenteral access is anticipated.

MALONE STOMA AND ANTEGRADE CONTINENCE ENEMAS

In the same way that the Mitrofanoff catheterizable channel gave access to the bladder (Mitrofanoff 1980), and thus potential for urinary continence, the Malone stoma has prepared the way for a new approach to encopresis, leading to renewed pleas for appendiceal conservation in selected patients (Wheeler & Malone 1991), (Fig. 13.2). In children and adolescents with faecal incontinence associated with anorectal anomalies or neuropathic bowel, the success

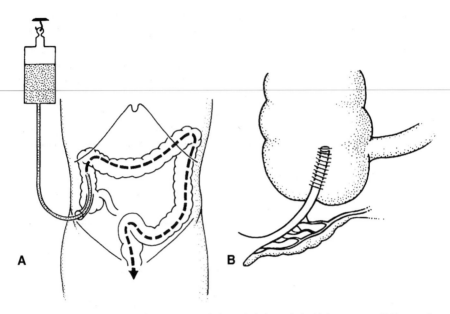

Fig. 13.2 A   Antegrade continence enema being administered via Malone stoma. **B** Reversed appendix re-implanted into caecum to form Malone stoma. (Reproduced with permission from Lancet 1990: 336.)

rate in terms of faecal continence has been devastatingly poor (Malone et al 1994). Therapies ranging from suppositories and enemas to washouts and manual evacuations may be inadequate to control the problem, making the individual absolutely reliant on assistance (particularly if the patient is paraplegic); the use of pads or nappies becomes mandatory.

The Malone stoma (Malone et al 1990) is a continent appendicocaecostomy. The original description was of a reversed appendix, reimplanted into the caecum with a submucosal tunnel to prevent reflux. The base of the appendix was led through the anterior abdominal wall. This has been modified by some authors (Squire et al 1993) to an orthotopic technique; the appendicular attachment to the caecum is left intact, but the caecum imbricated around the appendix base and the appendix tip merely exteriorized. In the absence of the appendix, a conduit may be fashioned from a tubulerized flap of caecal wall (Kiely et al 1994). Late complications of stomal stenosis may respond to dilatation, but some need formal surgical revision (Squire et al 1993). The stoma is usually sited in the right iliac fossa such that it can be readily accessible to the patient and is catheterized with an 8–12F Jacques® catheter. The patient sits on the lavatory throughout this procedure and can rapidly be taught how to administer the ACE (antegrade colonic enema), thus conferring both cleanliness and independence. The washouts, taking approximately 5 min to administer, are commenced with 60 ml of phosphate enema diluted with 60 mls of saline; this is followed with 100–200 ml of saline. There is considerable variation in the total volumes required once the children are practised with the ACE technique, varying from 0 to 1000 ml (Squire et al 1993). A full phosphate enema is sometimes necessary, but because of the risks of phosphate toxicity (McCabe et al 1991) no further phosphate should be administered if the enema is not evacuated. In this situation, an ACE with arachis oil has been shown to be effective. The washout process is usually complete within 30 min; 25% of patients will leak small quantities of enema fluid. Most patients perform their ACE before going to bed and, if necessary, wear an absorbent pad after the ACE to solve this problem. The procedure is repeated every 2 or 3 days. In the interim the patient has an empty colorectum and is clean. It has become clear that very careful patient selection is required and that to an extent the child needs time to earn the Malone stoma for their motivation to be sufficient to comply with the routine necessary for regular ACE washouts. There also remains a question over the group of children with primary constipation, who at least in the early stages fared less well with the antegrade washouts.

The results in the incontinent anorectal and neuropathic groups (Squire et al 1993) have been little short of spectacular and the subjective changes in the children's behaviour, demeanour and quality of life as reported by parents are very encouraging. The children rapidly achieve dependable cleanliness within 6 weeks of starting ACE washouts.

SINGLE STAGE SURGERY FOR HIRSCHSPRUNG'S DISEASE

Conventional treatment of Hirschsprung's disease involved infant resuscitation, tissue diagnosis and then defunctioning colostomy. The faecal diversion reduced the incidence of enterocolitis, recognized as a potentially fatal complication of Hirschsprung's disease. Definitive surgery to excise the aganglionic segment and transition zone was then performed towards the end of the first year of life. Some discussion continues as to whether the definitive surgery should be covered by a stoma, which is closed as a third stage (Philippart 1993), or whether the pull-through should incorporate stoma closure.

What is more controversial is the necessity of the preliminary stoma. In infants too ill to undergo colostomy, rectal washouts proved effective as a temporizing measure (Shim & Swenson 1966). Provided abdominal decompression was achieved effectively by rectal irrigation, colostomy was avoided; definitive surgery was performed early and the results were favorable (So et al 1980). The underlying concern over enterocolitis has encouraged earlier surgery in the non-stoma group, leading to the observation that the operation may be technically easier in early infancy (Ghinelli & Del Rossi 1993). In a series of 32 patients with Hirschsprung's disease, 81% underwent surgery within the first 3 months of life without colostomy (Carcassone et al 1989); infants with long segment Hirschsprung's disease decompress inadequately with washouts and are unsuitable for one stage management. It is usually unclear at presentation whether an infant will respond to rectal washouts, but the first 24 h can be usefully employed in attempting this management. Providing washouts obtain a satisfactory response, parents can be taught how to perform them and the infant is sent home with close follow-up. Washouts are not enemas. Washouts involve irrigation which is repeated two or three times daily through a wide-bore rectal tube with side holes. Normal saline is used to avoid electrolyte disturbances and irrigation continues until the abdomen is decompressed with minimal particulate matter in the effluent. Strenuous parental instruction is given on the signs of enterocolitis: progressive abdominal distension, unresponsive to the washouts, foul diarrhoea, bile-stained vomiting and rapid clinical deterioration. This disease occurs most commonly (although not exclusively) before the curative surgery has been performed. Because of the potentially catastrophic nature of Hirschsprung's enterocolitis (Philippart 1993) the parents clearly require careful selection in terms of both their temperament and the local availability of informed medical support. The infant will then undergo definitive surgery in the second or third month of life and will have avoided two additional operations. However, this should be tempered by reports of some large series suggesting a significantly increased complication rate when reconstruction is performed before 4 months of age (Sherman et al 1989).

LAPAROSCOPIC SURGERY AND COSMESIS

Paediatric laparoscopy was first described more than two decades ago (Gans & Berci 1971) and has a well-established role in the pursuit of the imperfectly descended testis, providing the most rapid and accurate means of localizing the impalpable gonad. The therapeutic options once the testis has been visualized include laparoscopic first stage orchidopexy by placing a clip on the testicular vessels or orchidectomy as appropriate (Elder 1993).

Paediatric surgeons have been relatively slow to react to the burgeoning development of minimally invasive surgery seen in adult practice, initially because the indications for cholecystectomy are relatively infrequent in childhood, whereas general surgeons have relied heavily on this procedure for the development of surgery through a laparoscope. As spectators at the development of laparoscopic surgery in adults, it was evident that, despite apparent advantages, the new procedures had to meet two criteria before they could be deemed superior to conventional surgery: the complication rate must be no worse and recurrence rates following repair or reconstructive procedures must be at the same level as in conventional operation.

Cholecystectomy modified or smaller patients (Holcomb 1993) is one of the applications of laparoscopic surgery with potential for wide acceptance by paediatric surgeons. Cholelithiasis (Rescorla & Grosfeld 1992), either due to haemolytic disease or related to ileal resection, cystic fibrosis or total parenteral nutrition, provides the usual indication for cholecystectomy. In a small series (Sigman et al 1991) only two patients were less than 10 years of age; the remainder were of small adult body mass and this really represents the lower end of the normal laparoscopic population rather than a procedure developed for the paediatric group.

Two of the obvious advantages of laparoscopy in adult practice — the pressing need to reduce both the hospital stay and the period of convalescence — are harder to justify in childhood. There are sporadic reports of other laparoscopic procedures in children including fundoplication, pyloromyotomy, appendicectomy and oophoropexy. Nissen's fundoplication has been successfully performed laparoscopically in a small series of children between ages of 3 months and 11 years (Lobe et al 1993).

The avoidance of a laparotomy incision in mentally retarded children who are resistant to physiotherapy may reduce the risk of postoperative chest complications. If the operation proves easier laparoscopically it could be justified in young children with a narrow subcostal angle in whom access to the oesophagogastric junction is difficult.

Gastrostomy is another potential indication; although minimally invasive endoscopic/percutaneous techniques are widely used for gastrostomy placement in children (Gauderer et al 1980), the procedure may be complicated by visceral impalement. Direct laparoscopic vision may make the procedure safer, particularly in the retarded kyphoscoliotic child with a previously fundoplicated stomach lying above the costal margin. The technique has the additional advantage that endoscopy is not an essential part of the procedure (Stringel et al 1993).

In America, laparoscopic appendicectomy has been performed in children in much greater numbers, e.g. a series of 465 in 1991 (Valla et al 1991), but this has not had such a dramatic impact in the UK. Advocates cite the ability to view the entire peritoneum for diagnosis and superior lavage compared with the open procedure as advantages of this technique (Naffis 1993).

Ramstedt's pyloromyotomy has been performed laparoscopically (Alain et al 1991). The open procedure would routinely involve a single 3 cm scar, 20 min anaesthesia and 24–36 h postoperative hospital course. The consequences of the laparoscopic approach (Tan & Najmaldin 1993) are three port scars totalling in excess of 3 cm and a similar postoperative course. The operation time is reported as 50 mins. There are insufficient data to comment fairly on the comparative complications.

Oophoropexy may be performed laparoscopically. This involves suturing the ovaries to the lateral abdominal wall to avoid subsequent damage from irradiation planned for pelvic malignancy (Tan et al 1993). Laparotomy in childhood malignancy which involves the use of chemotherapy carries morbidity from wound infection, dehiscence and hernia formation. The laparoscopic technique obviates these, and increases the accuracy of radiation needle placement if required.

Inguinal herniorraphy is another growing application for the laparoscope in adult surgery; there has been speculation that this might be appropriate for paediatric practice (Scharli 1993). The rapidity of herniotomy in a child, the fact that it is almost universally a day case procedure performed through a single 1–2 cm incision and that convalescence time is so short as to have no significant bearing on the child or its mother (albeit that she may be working), means that open inguinal herniotomy in childhood is here to stay.

The search for the less noticeable scar continues. Pyloromyotomy leaves a 2–3 cm scar, conventionally either in a skin crease in the right upper quadrant or in the upper midline. In an attempt to improve on this a circumumbilical skin incision combined with a midline approach has been proposed (Tan & Bianchi 1986) and has been adopted by some surgeons. There is no doubt that the scar is invisible to the cursory glance at the 6-month stage, but there is evidence of increased wound sepsis and concern that the pylorus is subjected to more traction injury than when using the conventional approach (Huddart et al 1993).

URINARY TRACT RECONSTRUCTION

Augmentation of the urinary bladder to increase volume in children with a neuropathic bladder, bladder exstrophy and posterior urethral valves is well established, but problems of metabolic derangement, excessive mucus production, recurrent urinary tract infections, spontaneous rupture and late neoplasia have led to the pursuit of alternatives to ileum and colon (Lorenz & Dewan 1993). The pedicled gastric graft, using the greater curve of the stomach based on the left or right gastroepiploic artery, is employed as a gastrocystoplasty. Bladder augmentation as a preliminary to renal transplantation is a modification to accepted adult practice (Burns et al 1992); unlike older patients, the contracted unused bladder of a child with end-stage renal failure does not distend following the inflow of dilute urine post-transplantation and remains a harmful high-pressure container. In a series of eight cases (Dykes & Ransley 1992) the graft performed satisfactorily, the authors observing that the size of the gastric patch was critical in determining the acid secretion and that immunosuppression related to subsequent renal transplantation may increase acid output. This has proved useful in children with chronic renal failure in whom aciduria is an advantage (Vaughan & Tiffany 1988). However, stone formation, the effect of acid output on metabolism and the risk of metaplasia in both the incorporated gastric mucosa and the native urothelium have given concern (Lorenz & Dewan 1993) and urethritis has proved sufficiently troublesome to limit its use to those who void via a Mitrofanoff stoma (Ransley 1994).

Autoaugmentation preserves the bladder mucosal continuity; a patch of bladder muscle is excised and the subdetrusor plane then mobilized until a wide-mouthed mucosal diverticulum is created. The bladder volume is thus increased, but scarring leads to shrinkage of the bulge. Small thick-walled bladders do not tend to give a favourable result and both vesicoureteric reflux and perforation are reported, although good results have been reported in paediatric series (Gordon et al 1991).

Autoaugmentation and gastrocystoplasty may be combined. To protect the urothelial diverticulum created by autoaugmentation from fibrosis and ultimate shrinkage, a pedicled graft of the gastric greater curve, from which the mucosa has been removed, maybe utilized to provide a seromuscular patch applied directly on to the diverticulum. The seromuscular layer rapidly interlaces with the detrusor and a bladder of improved capacity and compliance results (Dewan & Lorenz 1994). The medium- and long-term efficacy of this procedure remains speculative.

The recent advent of ureterocystoplasty (Churchill et al 1992), where a dilated ureter may be used as the augmenting tissue and its native kidney diverted via transureteroureterostomy, has the advantages of a stable urothelium and good compliance, although long-term results are awaited. If successful, this approach could lead to the preservation of an endstage kidney for the augmentation potential of its dilated upper tracts at a later date (Ransley 1994).

ANTENATAL DIAGNOSIS

The advent of prenatal diagnosis has had a profound effect on paediatric surgery. First, there is a discernible reduction in neonatal referrals, which may be partly attributable to termination of fetuses with antenatally diagnosed congenital heart disease, a population with a high incidence of associated congential malformations falling within the remit of general surgery. There is also an unknown number with an antenatal diagnosis of uropathy, abdominal wall defect, neural tube defect, gastrointestinal anomalies and specific conditions such as sacrococcygeal teratoma whose parents elect for termination of pregnancy (Needell 1994).

Secondly, the management of babies with a prenatally diagnosed 'surgical' condition who survive to delivery has changed radically in some cases. During 5 years in Glasgow 52 babies were diagnosed with anomalies falling within the remit of general surgery; 23 abdominal wall defects, 18 urinary tract malformations and eight with intestinal atresias or volvulus (Hutson et al 1985). Of this group, 35 were liveborn, 17 were terminated or stillborn and overall, 21 survived.

Defects of the anterior abdominal wall are important to identify antenatally because of both prognosis and planning. The diagnosis of exomphalos major (with a membranous sac covering the herniated viscera) confers a 30–70% risk of associated potentially lethal or lethal abnormality — either chromosomal such as trisomy 13 and 18 or multiple visceral and limb abnormalities (Lee & Blake 1977). It has not been established that the introduction of prenatal diagnosis of exomphalos improves overall survival (Suita et al 1992), the unavoidable factor limiting survival being the associated abnormality. The diagnosis of exomphalos major should prompt a detailed ultrasonographic examination for further anomalies and termination of the pregnancy may be offered.

The main differential diagnosis is of gastroschisis, where loops of bowel are observed to be outside the predicted abdominal contour, lying in the amniotic fluid. This is not associated with chromosomal abnormality and carries a <10% chance of associated malformation; termination of pregnancy would not normally be contemplated in this surgically correctable anomaly. The presence of gastroschisis may affect planning. The congenital equivalent of a burst abdomen, this is a surgical emergency and delay in closure is associated with increased rates of morbidity and mortality. Additionally, prolonged exposure of the gut leads to matting which may be responsible for an associated delay in the infant tolerating enteral nutrition (Sapin et al 1993). Thus, on the basis of gastroschisis, delivery might be planned within easy access of a neonatal surgical centre. There is no evidence that vaginal delivery is beneficial (Hasan & Hermansen 1986) but, following a spate of late gestational deaths, it has been suggested that the baby is delivered at 38 weeks; this is still debated (Roberts & Burge 1990).

Antenatal diagnosis of sacrococcygeal teratoma should influence obstetric care. Fetal hydrops may result from the high output cardiac failure as a consequence of the substantial arterio-venous fistula within the tumour (Langer et al 1989). Dystocia and fetal death during delivery, or due to haemorrhage from the ruptured tumour after delivery, is well documented leading to the suggestion that caesarian section should be mandatory in this situation (Flake et al 1986).

Antenatal diagnosis has also presented the opportunity of prenatal intervention. In utero surgery has been performed on fetuses with congenital diaphragmatic hernia (Harrison et al 1981) with varying degrees of success. The treatment of other pathologies such as fetal chylothorax and cystic adenomatoid malformation of the lung, which cause pulmonary hypoplasia and may present at birth with acute respiratory failure, has been attempted (Harrison & Adzick 1993).

In utero decompression of hydronephrosis as a closed technique (Schapps et al 1993) is practised and has been treated by vesicostomy as an open fetal procedure (Harrison & Adzick 1993). If gestation is allowed to continue in a fetus with bilateral high-grade urinary obstruction, renal dysplasia incompatible with life may result. Pulmonary hypoplasia may be caused by the resultant oligohydramnios. Thus, life-threatening respiratory and renal disease may be averted if the obstruction is relieved early enough in gestation. Prospective controlled data do not exist to allow comment on this hypothesis.

Antenatal diagnosis has also presented the opportunity to describe the natural history of hydronephrosis and it is becoming clear that many antenatally identified hydronephroses will eventually resolve into normal kidneys. It is estimated that 80% of infants with antenatally diagnosed hydronephrosis have neither signs nor symptoms at birth (Thomas & Gordon 1989). Of 142 hydronephrotic kidneys identified prenatally, 100 functioned well at assessment at 3 months with only 23 of this group requiring later pyeloplasty because of deterioration of function (Ransley et al 1990). The significance of hydronephrosis at the postnatal scan can only be assessed when considered in conjunction with data on differential function and there seems to be no indication for immediate pyeloplasty if the initial function is good. In a group of 85 children with idiopathic hydronephrosis and good function managed conservatively from the postnatal period, none deteriorated (O'Flynn et al 1993). It is unsurprising that empirical antenatal intervention into 'pathology' whose natural history has still to be defined remains highly controversial.

To describe intrauterine surgery as a recent advance is contentious. The ability to operate on the unborn child exists. Whether it has any relevance in the foreseeable future remains to be seen.

KEY POINTS FOR CLINICAL PRACTICE

- As subspecialization within general surgery continues, it is appropriate that the referral of infants and toddlers to established paediatric surgical centres increases. This philosophy is reinforced by the report of the National Confidential Enquiry into Perioperative Deaths.
- Central venous access in children has been facilitated by new materials such as polyurethane. The use of percutaneously introduced 'short long lines' has made the delivery of medium-term total parenteral nutrition or antibiotic therapy much easier in infants and neonates. The opportunity for elective catheter replacement may lead to a reduction in the rate of infection.
- Antegrade colonic enemas administered via an appendicocaecostomy have radically altered the lives of children with intractable faecal incontinence related to anorectal malformations and neuropathic bowel. Reliable cleanliness is maintained with two or three washouts a week; phosphate toxicity remains a potential problem.
- The recognition that carefully selected neonates with Hirschsprung's disease may be successfully managed with rectal washouts as a temporizing manoeuvre has reduced the need for immediate colostomy. This has resulted in single stage curative surgery becoming feasible and has lead to definitive surgery earlier in infancy. Enthusiasm for this development must be tempered with the dangers of enterocolitis before surgery.
- The value of laparoscopy in diagnosis is undisputed. Laparoscopic surgery is currently restricted to fields of major surgery where the open access is limited, such as at the gastro-oesphageal junction in kyphoscoliotic children.
- Transumbilical pyloromyotomy represents a new approach to minimize scarring without changing the underlying operating technique.
- The undoubted early success of bladder augmentation with bowel has been tempered with problems of metabolic derangement, excessive mucus production, neoplasia and rupture. Attempts to increase the urothelial surface area by diverticulum creation were complicated by shrinkage and

the application of a gastric seromuscular graft may alleviate this. Ureterocystoplasty may offer a long-term solution.

• Antenatal diagnosis gives the opportunity for prognosis, perinatal planning and raises the issue of either open or closed techniques of interventional in utero surgery. As the natural history of the various antenatally identified conditions is defined, the role of intervention becomes increasingly uncertain in the absence of prospective controlled data.

REFERENCES

Alain JL Grosseau D, Terrier G 1991 Extramucosal pyloromyotomy by laparoscopy. J Padiatr Surg 26: 1191–1192
Burns MW, Watkins SL, Mitchell ME et al 1992 Treatment of bladder dysfunction in children with end-stage renal disease. J Pediatr Surg 27: 170–174
Carcassone M, Guys JM, Morrison-Lacombe G 1989 Management of Hirschsprung's disease: curative surgery before three months of age. J Pediatr Surg 24: 1032–1034
Churchill BM, Aliabadi H, Landau EH et al 1992 Bladder reconstruction using ureteral augmentation constructed from megaureter. Am Acad Pediatr: October
Dewan PA, Loenz C 1994 Autoaugmentation gastrocystoplasty: the initial clinical experience. Br J Urol (in press)
Dykes EH, Ransley PG 1992 Gastrocystoplasty in children. Br J Urol 69: 91–95
Elder JS 1993 Laparoscopy for the non palpable testis. Semin Pediatr Surg 2: 168–173
Flake AW, Harrison MR, Adzick NS et al 1986 Fetal sacrococcygeal teratoma. J Pediatr Surg 21: 563–566
Gans SL, Berci G 1971 Advances in endoscopy of infants and children. J. Pediatr Surg 6: 199–234
Gauderer MWL, Ponsky JL, Inzant RJ 1980 Gastrostomy without laparotomy: A percutaneous endoscopic technique. J. Pediatr Surg 26: 1145–1147
Ghinelli C, Del Rossi C 1993 Treatment of Hirschsprung's disease without colostomy. Pediatr Surg Int 8: 27–30
Gordon E, Malone PS, Duffy PG et al 1991 The place of autocystoplasty in the management of the neuropathic bladder. Br J Urol 68: 644
Harrison MR, Adzick NS 1993 In utero interventions. In: Ashcraft KW, Holder TM (eds) Pediatric surgery, 2nd edn. WB Saunders, Philadelphia, p 1103–1013
Harrison MR, Globus MS, Filley RA 1981 Management of the fetus with a correctable congenital defect. JAMA 246: 774–777
Hasan S, Hermansen MC 1986 The prenatal diagnosis of ventral abdominal wall defects. Am J Obstet Gynecol 155: 842–845
Holcomb GW 1993 Laparoscopic cholecystectomy. Semin Pediatr Surg 2: 159–167
Huddart SN, Bianchi A, Kumar V et al 1993 Ramstedt's pyloromyotomy: circumumbilical versus transverse approach. Pediatr Surg Int 8: 395–396
Hutson JM, McNay MB, MacKenzie JR et al 1985 Antenatal diagnosis of surgical disorders by ultrasonography. Lancet 1: 621–623
Kiely EM, Ade-Ajayi N, Wheeler RA 1994 When there is no appendix: a modification of the Malone stoma. Br J Surg (in press)
Langer JC, Harrison MR, Schmidt KG et al 1989 Fetal hydrops and demise from sacrococcygeal teratoma. Rationale for fetal surgery. Am J Obstet Gynecol 160: 1145–1150
Lee TG, Blake S 1977 Prenatal fetal abnormality. Radiology 124: 475–478
Lobe TE, Schropp KP, Lunsford K 1993 Laparoscopic Nissen fundoplication in childhood. J Pediatr Surg 28: 358–361
Lorenz C, Dewan PA 1993 The evolution of autoaugmentation gastrocystoplasty. Pediatr Surg Int 8: 491–495
McCabe M, Sibert JR, Routledge PA 1991 Phosphate enemas in childhood: cause for concern. Br Med J 302: 1074
Malone PS, Ransley PG, Kiely E M 1990 Preliminary report: the antegrade continence enema. Lancet 336: 1217–1218

Malone PS, Wheeler RA, Williams JE 1994 Continence in patients with spina bifida: long term results. Arch Dis Child 70: 107–110

Mitrofanoff P 1980 Cystomie continente trans-appendiculare dans le traitment des vessies neurologiques. Chir Pediatr 21: 297–305

Naffis D 1993 Laparoscopic appendectomy in children. Semin Pediatr Surg 2: 174–177

Nakamura KT, Sato Y, Erenberg A 1990 Evaluation of a percutaneously placed 27G central venous catheter in neonates weighing <1200 g. JPEN 14: 295–299

National Confidential Enquiry into Perioperative Deaths (NCEPOD) 1989 Report of the National Confidential Enquiry into Perioperative Deaths. Royal College of Surgeons, London

Needell JC 1994 Wessex Regional Genetics Service Personal communication.

O'Flynn KJ, Gough DCS, Gupta S et al 993 Prediction of recovery in antenatally diagnosed hydronephrosis. Br J Urol 71: 478–480

Pegelow CH, Narvael M, Toledano SR et al 1986 Experience with a totally implantable venous device in children. Am J Dis Child 140: 69–71

Philippart AT 1993 Hirschsprung's disease In: Ashcraft KW, Holder TM (eds) Pediatric surgery, 2nd edn. WB Saunders, Philadelphia, p 358–371

Puntis JWL, Ball PA, Booth IW 1987 Percutaneous central venous feeding lines in infants: do they perform as well as surgically positioned catheters? Z Kinderchir 42: 354–357

Ransley PG 1994 Personal communication

Ransley PG, Dhillon HK, Gordon I et al 1990 The postnatal management of hydronephrosis diagnosed by prenatal ultrasonography. J Urol 144: 584–587

Rescorla FJ, Grosfeld JL 1992 Cholecystitis and cholelithiasis in children. Semin Pediatr Surg 1: 98–106

Roberts JP, Burge MD 1990 Antenatal diagnosis of abdominal wall defects: a missed opportunity? Arch Dis Child 65: 687–689

Sapin E, Lewin F, Baron JM et al 1993 Prenatal diagnosis and management of gastroschisis. Pediatr Surg Int 8: 31–33

Schapps JP, Thomisin H, Lambotta R 1983 Intrauterine unilateral nephrostomy. Am J Obstet Gynecol 146: 105–106

Scharli AF 1993 Laparoscopic surgery. Pediatr Surg Int 8: 375

Sherman JO, Snyder ME, Weitzman JJ et al 1989 A 40 year multinational retrospective study of 880 Swenson procedures. J Pediatr Surg 24: 833

Shim WKT, Swenson O 1966 Treatment of congenital megacolon in 50 infants. Pediatrics 38: 185–193

Sigman HH, Laberge JM, Croitoru D et al 1991 Laparoscopic cholecystectomy: a treatment option for gallbladder disease in children. J Pediatr Surg 26: 1181–1183

Squire R, Kiely EM, Carr B et al 1993 The clinical application of the Malone antegrade colonic enema. J Pediatr Surg 28: 1012–1015

So HB, Schwartz DL, Becker J et al 1980 Endorectal pullthrough without preliminary colostomy in neonates with Hirschsprung's disease. J Pediatr Surg 15: 470–471

Stringel G, Robinson E, Maisel S 1993 Laparoscopic gastrostomy. Pediatr Surg Int 8: 382–384

Stringer MD, Brerecton RJ, Wright VM 1992 Performance of percutaneous silastic central venous feeding catheters in surgical neonates. Pediatr Surg Int 7: 79–81

Suita S, Sakaguichi T, Nakano H et al 1992 Significance of antenatal diagnosis of omphalocoele. Pediatr Surg Int 7: 37–40

Tan KC, Bianchi A 1986 Circumumbilical incision for pyloromyotomy. Br J Surg 73: 399

Tan HL, Najmaldin AS 1993 Laparoscopic pyloromyotomy for infantile hypertrophic pyloric stenosis. Pediatr Surg Int 8: 376–378

Tan HL, Scorpio RJ, Hutson JM et al 1993 Laparoscopic ovariopexy for paediatric pelvic malignancy. Pediatr Surg Int 8: 379–381

Thomas DFM, Gordon AC 1989 Management of prenatally diagnosed uropathy. Arch Dis Child 64: 58–63

Valla JS, Limmone B, Valla V 1991 Laparoscopic appendectomy in children. Report of 465 cases. Surg Laparosc Endosc 1: 166–172

Vaughan ED, Tiffany P 1988 The use of gastrocystoplasty. Dialysis Pediatr Urol 11: 6

Wheeler RA, Griffiths DM 1992 Cuff Cath: an initial experience of cuffed polyurethane central venous catheters in children. JPEN 16: 384–385

Wheeler RA, Malone PS 1991 The use of the appendix in reconstructive surgery: a case against incidental appendicectomy. A review. Br J Surg 78: 1283–1285
Wheeler RA, Griffiths DM, Burge DM 1991 The retrograde tunnel: a new method of long term paediatric CVC fixation. JPEN 15: 114–115

14

Recent advances in general surgery

I. Taylor

This review will concentrate on important publications which have appeared over the last year and which might eventually influence surgical practice. Of necessity it is selective and by no means intended to be comprehensive. The subspeciality topics chosen are emergency surgery, upper gastrointestinal surgery, pancreatico biliary, liver, lower gastrointestinal surgery and breast.

Reviews of vascular surgery and paediatric surgery appear in Chs 8 and 13 respectively.

EMERGENCY SURGERY

Appendix

There has been a resurgence of interest in acute appendicitis stimulated predominantly by laparoscopy. It has been suggested that laparoscopy prior to emergency surgery may significantly reduce management errors and enhance surgical practice. A review by Patterson-Brown (1993) provides firm evidence for this approach, particularly in acute appendicitis. The normal appendix can be visualized at laparoscopy in at least three-quarters of patients, a figure that with experience approaches 100%. Scott et al (1993) reported results in 67 laparoscopies performed over an 18-month period in which the diagnosis was altered in 19% of cases and management in 13% of cases.

Diagnostic laparoscopy is of benefit in excluding other acute situations, for example perforated duodenal ulcer and acute diverticulitis. In each case management strategies can be decided by laparoscopic appearances.

Laparoscopic appendicectomy has been assessed as a therapeutic manoeuvre in several studies. Techniques vary depending upon preference for delivering the appendix to the abdominal wall surface (Byrne et al 1992) or for one in which an endoloop ligature is passed around the appendix and secured at its base (Tate et al 1993). In experienced hands laparoscopic appendicectomy is successful in 90% of patients with conversion to open operation usually due to marked inflammatory adhesions around the appendix. In prospective randomized trials, however, laparoscopic appendicectomy has not convincingly demonstrated benefit over an open approach. There is a similar incidence of wound complications and wound pain after leaving hospital. Operating time, however, is significantly longer in laparoscopic compared to open appendicectomy (Tate et al 1993, McAnena et al 1992).

The timing of surgery for supposed appendicitis is important. Two studies have suggested that the decision to operate for suspected acute appendicitis should not be made hastily in the small hours of the morning. Although early appendicectomy remains the treatment of choice it can be safely postponed overnight without increasing morbidity and mortality (McLean et al 1993, Surana et al 1993).

Finally, a review of carcinoid tumours of the appendix has provided a logical management strategy (Roggo et al 1993). Tumours of less than 1 cm are adequately managed by appendicectomy, whereas right hemicolectomy is recommended for tumours larger than 2 cm.

Management of septic shock

There appears to be biological variation in the development of sepsis after surgery or trauma, particularly if this is major. Some patients remain at high risk of morbidity and mortality after postoperative or post-traumatic sepsis and antibiotic prophylaxis has not made major improvement in the prognosis for these patients. Multisystem organ failure causes 80% of late deaths after trauma. The heterogeneity of leucocyte reaction is a biological variability and this is thought to play an important part in determining the development of postoperative sepsis (Guillou 1993). Important aspects in the management of septic shock include early recognition and supportive measures enhanced by intensive care units. The role of specific antagonists or antibodies to inflammatory mediators released at the end organ is still controversial. These drugs are no substitute for the important basic resuscitative measures (Edwards 1993).

Small bowel obstruction

The majority of patients with small bowel obstruction have postoperative adhesion formation as a major aetiological factor. Menzies (1993) has reviewed in depth the treatment of adhesion formation as it relates to small bowel obstruction. It is possible that troublesome adhesive problems may be reduced by peritoneal lavage with plasminogen activators following surgery. Adhesions following laparotomy for appendicectomy or tubo-ovarian surgery are more likely to result in obstruction which does not resolve with non-operative management. In one series bowel resection was required more frequently in this group and it was considered that conservative management was not worthwhile in patients with obstruction following earlier appendicectomy or tubo-ovarian surgery (Meagher et al 1993).

UPPER GASTROINTESTINAL SURGERY

Oesophagus

Long-term results of Nissen fundoplication for reflux oesophagitis have been reported (Luostarinen 1993). Provided that an adequate fundic wrap has been performed the results are satisfactory and cure of oesophagitis has been achieved in the majority of cases. Of 24 patients with a defective wrap 14 had continuing oesophagitis.

A report has confirmed the hypothesis that complications in Barrett's columnar lined oesophagus develop in association with increased exposure to an alkaline environment which appears to be secondary to duodenogastric reflux; 24-h ambulatory gastric pH monitoring in conjunction with oesophageal pH monitoring can identify patients at risk (Attwood et al 1993).

The management of oesophageal carcinoma continues to be both problematic and depressing. Accordingly non-surgical treatment to deal with dysphagia is generating much interest (Griffin & Robertson 1993). Laser recanalization in association with radiotherapy is being assessed in a prospective randomized trial. Other techniques requiring assessment are brachyherapy and other means of intubation.

One trial has indicated the possible benefit of multimodality therapy for operable oesophageal carcinoma. In a randomized trial patients received either preoperative chemotherapy and surgery, surgery alone, preoperative radiotherapy and surgery, and a combination of chemotherapy, radiotherapy and surgery (Nygaard et al 1993). The results indicate that preoperative radiotherapy has a beneficial effect on survival whereas the chemotherapy regimen does not influence survival.

Gastroduodenal

Gastric infection with *Helicobactes pylori* seems to be a risk factor for gastric carcinoma. A multicentre epidemiological study has investigated this relationship further. An approximately sixfold increased risk of gastric cancer has been demonstrated in populations with 100% *H. pylori* infection compared to populations with no infection (The Eurogast Study Group 1993). In addition, certain features of primary low-grade B-cell gastric lymphoma of mucosa-associated lymphoid tissue suggest that the tumour might be antigen responsive. Withersppon et al (1993) suggest that eradication of *H. pylori* might inhibit the tumour. They were able to eradicate *H. pylori* in five of six patients and repeat biopsy showed no evidence of lymphoma.

A review of molecular aspects of gastric carcinoma suggests that new therapeutic targets and hopefully more effective treatments with fewer side-effects are feasible (Wright & Williams 1993). In addition, it is likely also that a better understanding of cell kinetics and proliferation in both normal gastric mucosa (Patel et al 1993b) and in early gastric carcinoma (Brito et al 1993) might improve our understanding. Aneuploidy is recognized in 39% of gastric carcinomas but is more frequent in submucosal than in mucosal tumours. It is likely that these studies will eventually provide information of prognostic significance.

CD44 is a cell surface molecule which is attracting interest because of its association with metastasis. Mayer et al (1993) have observed an association between CD44 expression and distal metastases at the time of diagnosis. It appears to be associated with an increased incidence of both tumour recurrence and mortality.

Preoperative staging for gastric cancer using different imaging modalities has proved disappointing. In a prospective study of 180 consecutive patients treated by total gastrectomy and previously evaluated with computed tomography (CT), endogastric ultrasonography and intraoperative surgical assessment, CT was found to be of little value and endoscopic ultrasonography most sensitive. In particular CT has a tendency to understage nodal involvement of gastric carcinomas.

As a result of the Japanese experience, there have been increasing attempts to diagnose and treat early gastric cancer. Moreaux & Bougaran (1993) have presented a 25-year experience of early gastric cancer (101 patients). They recommend subtotal gastrectomy except for proximal lesions, and the prognosis is significantly better for cancers confined to mucosa; 5- and 10-year actuarial survival rates were 88% and 65% respectively. Sue-Ling et al (1993) have similarly reviewed a large prospective series of patients with gastric carcinoma. They report a significant increase in potentially curative resections from 35% in the first 5-year period to 53% in the last 5-year period. The incidence of early gastric cancer was between 1% and 15%. There was a 98% 5-year survival in patients with early gastric cancer.

Guadagni et al (1993) reported the post-operative course of 159 patients with early gastric carcinoma followed for a median of 7 years. An overall 10-year survival rate of 77% was achieved with significant improvement in those cancers confined to the mucosa. Finally a Norwegian multicentre study has reviewed the results of curative surgery in 532 patients (Haugstvedt et al 1993). Once again the stage of the disease was the single most important factor in determining survival and patients with early stage I disease had 5-year survivals in excess of 70%. All of these studies have demonstrated the importance of adequate surgical clearance for early gastric carcinoma.

There is no doubt that duodenal polyposis associated with familial adenomatous polyposis (FAP) will become an increasing problem. A report of 12 patients from two institutions has noted a high incidence of recurrence following local excisions and regard this as an unsatisfactory treatment option. However, the ideal management for patients with FAP and severe duodenal polyposis remains uncertain (Penna et al 1993).

Peptic ulceration

Eradication of *H. pylori* significantly decreases basal acid secretion in duodenal ulcer patients and heals the ulcer (Moss & Calman 1993). Labenz et al (1993) have demonstrated that 2 weeks of treatment with omeprazole plus amoxycillin is as good as triple therapy plus ranitidine in eradicating *H. pylori* and in addition seems to offer better safety, pain relief and ulcer healing. They recommend amoxycillin plus omeprazole as the treatment of choice for eradicating *H. pylori* in duodenal ulcer patients. However, Armstrong et al (1993) in a large German study of 1923 patients with endoscopically proven recurrent duodenal ulcers have shown that delay in healing is associated with multiple factors (smoking, frequent prior recurrence, heavy physical workload and psychological stress) and that the effects of these are cumulative. For patients with two or more easily identifiable risk factors, more than 2 weeks of treatment with an H2 receptor antagonist is required to achieve healing.

The most effective endoscopic injection therapy to prevent rebleeding in peptic ulcers is still problematic. Rutgeerts et al (1993) have included 75 patients in a randomized controlled trial to compare the efficacy of injection with epinephrine followed by polidocanol, injection of absolute alcohol and sham injection. They have demonstrated that absolute alcohol was superior to epinephrine and polidocanol which in fact was not significantly better than sham therapy.

Laparoscopic techniques in the treatment of peptic ulceration have been suggested. There has been a dramatic reduction in the practice of peptic ulcer surgery in the last 15 years but perhaps an increased interest in laparoscopic lesser curve seromyotomy with posterior truncal vagotomy will alter the balance. There is no doubt, however, that properly conducted trials will be necessary to confirm this (Taylor et al 1993). In the meantime innovative technical challenges are being presented by the laparoscope.

BILIARY SURGERY

Laparoscopic cholecystectomy is now the standard treatment for patients with gallbladder stones. The development and techniques involved have been described in a number of publications (Russell 1993, Macintyre & Wilson 1993). Patients can expect to be in hospital for 1–2 days and return to work within 2 weeks. In large series the results are good and indicate that any increased incidence of bile duct injury should decrease with proper training and experience. In most respects the long-term results of laparoscopic cholecystectomy are similar to those following open cholecystectomy. Qureshi et al (1993) have demonstrated a similar incidence of postcholecystectomy symptoms with the two procedures, although in a further study (Van der Velpen et al 1993) patient appreciation of a satisfactory cosmetic result was better following laparoscopic cholecystectomy. Despite the persistence of de novo occurrence of symptoms, 95% of patients considered that they had obtained overall symptomatic improvement by surgical treatment regardless of the access used.

Ventilatory and blood gas changes do occur and in one study during laparoscopic cholecystectomy a substantial but variable increase in minute ventilation was required to compensate for the carbon dioxide absorption from the peritoneum (McMahon et al 1993b). In a randomized trial the metabolic responses were compared in laparoscopic cholecystectomy and minilaparotomy cholecystectomy. There were similar changes in the two procedures. Thus despite less postoperative pain and more rapid recovery the metabolic responses following laparoscopic cholecystectomy are similar to those following open surgery.

There is increasing evidence that laparoscopic cholecystectomy can be offered as a day case in selected patients (Stephenson et al 1993) and innovative techniques for pain relief are likely to increase this. For example, Chundrigar et al (1993) in a randomized trial have demonstrated that less postoperative pain was recorded when bupivacaine was given intraperitoneally.

The indications for operative cholangiography in laparoscopic surgery are still being defined. Soper & Dunnegan (1993) have demonstrated that, in patients without indications for cholangiography, the performance of static cholangiograms markedly increased the operative time and cost of laparoscopic cholecystectomy. In very few cases was management changed and it is thought that laparoscopic cholecystectomy can be performed safely in the absence of cholangiography with little risk of injury to the major ductal system or retained calculi. This view is shared by others and a selective policy is now generally advised (Keane et al 1993). Sharma et al (1993) in a further randomized trial of operative cholangiography in open cholecystectomy have arrived at similar conclusions. The presence of common bile duct stones can be recognized preoperatively by ultrasonography and liver function tests in over 85% of patients. There is increasing evidence that common bile duct stones can be treated in the vast majority of patients by endoscopic surgery. ERCP and endoscopic sphincterotomy are successful in many, but laparoscopic approaches can also be used (Martin et al 1993). MacMathuna et al (1993) have advocated endoscopic balloon sphincteroplasty as a safe alternative to papillotomy for removal of bile duct stones. The procedure is said to be easy to learn and requires less operator skill than endoscopic papillotomy.

In critically ill patients with severe acute cholecystitis, a useful technique is ultrasound-guided puncture and aspiration of the gallbladder. One study has suggested that this is both safe and effective (Verbanck et al 1993). Finally it should not be forgotten that elective open cholecystectomy is also both safe and effective. Clavien et al (1993) in a series of 1252 elective open cholecystectomy reported no deaths and a low incidence of serious complications.

PANCREAS

Pancreatitis

Acute pancreatitis continues to be a most troublesome condition with significant morbidity. The timing of intervention is crucial and the decision can be extremely difficult. Dynamic CT is an accurate method for determining the extent of necrosis in acute pancreatitis but patient selection and timing for this investigation is still not certain. Lucarotti et al (1993) reported a study in 120 patients with acute pancreatitis in which dynamic CT was performed if a number of criteria were identified; these included a biochemically severe attack, a high C-reactive protein and failure of clinical resolution within 7 days. They concluded that not all patients require CT for prognostic purposes and that this investigation should be limited to this selected group of patients. Johnson (1993) has reviewed the indications for timing and intervention. Patients with gallstones should be offered endoscopic sphincterotomy within 48 h; when complications develop early necrosectomy is indicated only if conservative measures fail. Fan et al (1993) do not advise endoscopic retrograde cholangio pancreatography (ERCP) in all patients with acute pancreatitis especially in areas where the prevalence of biliary pancreatitis is lower than alcoholic pancreatitis. Patients with non-biliary pancreatitis do not benefit from the added morbidity of ERCP.

Neoptolemos (1993) has reviewed the role of endoscopic sphincterotomy in acute gallstone pancreatitis. His indications are patients with severe gallstone pancreatitis, patients with mild pancreatitis who have failed to improve, patients who require surgery for local pancreatic complications such as necrosis, and as an alternative to cholecystectomy in the prevention of further attacks of pancreatitis in frail elderly patients.

A recent review (McKay et al 1993) adds further evidence to the view that somatostatin and its analogues are not sufficiently effective in treatment or prophylaxis against acute pancreatitis to recommend their use in routine clinical practice.

A thoughtful review has indicated a logical strategy for dealing with pancreatic pseudocysts (Grace & Williamson 1993). Whether these should be dealt with percutaneously, endoscopically or surgically depends on several factors including size and appearance on CT.

Cancer

Little progress is being made in enhancing the overall prognosis following surgery for pancreatic carcinoma. Bakkevold & Kambestad (1993) have reported morbidity and mortality from a large prospective multicentre study involving 442 patients with adenocarcinoma of the pancreas and 30 with carcinoma of the papilla of Vater. Morbidity rates of 43% were noted with a mortality of 11% after radical surgery and 14% after palliative surgery. Preoperative biliary drainage had no impact on the risks and can usefully be abandoned.

Non-surgical palliation is now preferred to surgery for most patients with destructive jaundice. Anderson et al (1993) have supported previous conclusions with regard to relief to metastatic biliary obstruction by stent placement. Worthwhile palliation was achieved by endoscopic stent placement and half the patients in their study had a suggestion of prolonged symptom-free survival.

Sadly a prospective randomized trial of tamoxifen in patients with irresectable pancreatic adenocarcinoma failed to demonstrate any significant difference between the groups in terms of survival and quality of life assessement (Taylor et al 1993).

LIVER

Tumours

Benign tumours of the liver are common but rarely cause problems. When cavernous haemangiomas become larger than 4 cm in diameter they are regarded as 'giant' and can be troublesome. Baer et al (1993a) have described a technique of enucleation of haemangiomas with a low blood loss. Occasionally benign tumours are mistaken for malignant lesions. A recent report of a little known tumour (inflammatory pseudotumour of the liver) indicates that this lesion can be treated conservatively and resolves spontaneously (Karatsis et al 1993).

Primary malignant tumours of the liver provide the surgeon with a number of challenges. Small localized lesions are best treated by resection but in patients with hepatocellular carcinoma and cirrhosis other options should be considered, including transplantation (McMaster et al 1993). Nagasue et at (1993a) have reported the results of 229 patients with primary hepatocellular carcinoma treated by radical resection over an 11-year period. The 30-day operative mortality was 7% and 5- and 10-year survival rates were 26.4% and 19.4% respectively. Age, liver cirrhosis, tumour size and postoperative chemotherapy were significant prognostic factors. This same group (Nagasue et al 1993b) have demonstrated that the treatment policy for hepatocellular carcinoma in patients over the age of 70 years is identical to that in younger patients. Reports have also appeared from specialized centres in which resection for recurrent hepatocellular carcinoma have been undertaken (Jeng et al 1992). The data suggest that the cumulative survival is significantly better in patients who undergo recurrent resection compared to patients treated conservatively. In addition the results appear better than that obtained following chemoembolization in patients with cirrhosis.

Hilar cholangiocarcinoma is also a difficult tumour to treat adequately. With improvements in imaging and technical refinement a more aggressive resection approach has been advocated. Baer et al (1993b) have reported the results of a resectional policy with curative intent in 29 patients. Mean actuarial survival of 32 months was reported with a low postoperative mortality and morbidity.

Metastases

Duplex colour Doppler sonography has been demonstrated to be of value in recognizing early occult liver metastases and this may have therapeutic implications (Leen et al 1993). The quantitative assessment of involvement of the liver with tumour is difficult. Purkis & Williams (1993) have utilized a technique of planimetry of CT images to assess this more accurately.

Liver resection is now established as a major treatment for patients with localized metastases from colorectal cancer (Scheele 1993, Barr et al 1993). The indications for resection vary in different studies as indeed does the timing following primary colorectal resection. Most individuals feel that a period of 6 weeks to 3 months is satisfactory. There is no doubt that the results of hepatic resection in experienced centres are good. For example, Habib et al (1993) have reported results in 60 consecutive elective hepatic resections within two operative deaths and a mean operative blood transfusion of 900 ml.

Following liver resection for metastases, approximately half the patients who develop recurrence do so within the liver. The remainder develop metastases in other sites such as lung and abdominal cavity (Sugihara et al 1993). Two papers have advocated selective repeat liver resection for patients with recurrent colorectal metastases. Vaillant et al (1993) report 60 patients in whom 18 underwent repeat liver resection; four of these patients were free of disease 26–93 months after resection and three others were alive with recurrence. Similar results from Gouillat et al (1993) have re-emphasized the possible role for this technique in selected patients. Other treatments which should be considered include cryotherapy and regional cytotoxic perfusion (Morris et al 1993) and superselective intra-arterial chemotherapy with mitomycin C (Makela et al 1993).

Oesophageal varices

Injection sclerotherapy still remains an important aspect of treatment for patients with portal hypertension. A review of indications and complications, however, suggests that surgery still has a role to play (Heaton & Howard 1993). This is particularly so in patients with uncontrolled bleeding and oesophageal ulceration. An extensive survey of sclerotherapy from Japan has demonstrated that this is the leading method of treatment and less than 16% of patients required surgical procedures (Idezuke et al 1992). Two other techniques for treatment of bleeding oesophageal varices have been compared with injection sclerotherapy. In a randomized trial of 100 patients, bleeding was equally controlled by emergency sclerotherapy (in 90%) and by octreotide infusion (in 84%) (Sung et al 1993). Gimson et al (1993) have compared variceal banding ligation with injection sclerotherapy for bleeding varices. Both treatments were highly effective in controlling active haemorrhage (91% and 92% respectively). Complication rates were similar in the two groups. It is suggested that variceal banding ligation is safe and effective and obliterates varices more quickly with a lower rebleeding rate than injection sclerotherapy.

Trauma

The management of traumatic liver injuries continues to be a major problem with a high mortality. However, two reviews suggest that emphasis would be placed on non-resectional treatment. Schweizer et al (1993) in a review of 175 patients demonstrated a 40% rate of non-operative treatment with an overall mortality rate of 12%. Few deaths in patients with multiple injuries resulted specifically from liver trauma. Similarly, John et al (1992) reported a 10-year experience of liver trauma in 73 patients. They advocate the use of suture for simple injuries and a resectional approach with packing for more complex injuries. There is no doubt that careful clinical assessment and radiological monitoring can reduce the number of unnecessary laparotomies.

COLORECTAL SURGERY

Cancer

The outcome for patients with colorectal carcinoma has improved in recent years. A study from Aberdeen comparing patients treated in 1968–1969 with those treated in 1980–1982 has indicated tht there is now a lower operative mortality even in the elderly. Palliative resection can now be offered to over 80% of patients. However, some 40% of patients are not curable when they present (Gordon et al 1993). Undoubtedly patients presenting as an emergency are in poorer physical condition than those presenting electively. The operative mortality for emergency patients is significantly higher than for elective patients (Kingston et al 1993). In addition the 5-year survival is poorer in patients presenting as an emergency. Delay in diagnosis is still a problem and the most common error appears to be a failure to investigate iron deficiency anaemia. In one study of 152 consecutive patients with carcinoma of the right colon 40% suffered delays in treatment of more than 12 weeks with a mean delay of 8 weeks (Goodman & Irvin 1993).

Early diagnosis of colorectal cancer and prediction of patients at risk are clearly important. Colonoscopic follow-up after resection for colorectal cancer is probably of benefit in younger patients who are at risk of continuing polyp formation and therefore at high risk of developing metachronous carcinoma (Barlow & Thompson 1993). Other studies have indicated that frequent surveillance is not justified in the early postoperative years but colonoscopy should be confined to a single procedure to exclude synchronous lesions (Patchett et al 1993). Hall et al (1993) have studied the efficacy of faecal occult blood detection with colonoscopy in the detection of metachronous tumours. The results suggest that haemoccult alone is not sufficient to recognize metachronous lesions in the absence of colonoscopic surveillance.

Faecal occult blood screening has also been used also to recognize patients at high risk of colorectal neoplasia. The sensitivity for cancer was 68% and specificity 96% with a positive predictive value of neoplasia of 29% in high-risk patients. As expected this is higher than the detection rate in an unselected population (Caffarey et al 1993).

There is increasing interest in the possibility that a better understanding of genetics would enable more sensitive screening for familial colorectal cancer to take place. Several studies have investigated and reviewed this aspect (Thomas 1993, Scott et al 1993, Mulcahey & O'Donoghue 1993, Scott & Quirke 1993). Another possible method of preventing colorectal cancer which has been investigated and promulgated in the last year is a single flexible colonoscopy at the age of 50–60 years with appropriate colonoscopic surveillance for the 3–5% of patients found to have high-risk adenomas. It is suggested that a randomized trial to evaluate single flexible sigmoidoscopy should be initiated (Atkin et al 1993).

There is increasing interest on whether aspirin can in fact prevent colorectal cancer by its effect on polyps (Paganini-Hill 1993). A case-controlled study of subjects participating in a faecal occult blood screening programme for colorectal cancer has been reviewed to determine the relationship between the use of aspirin and non-steroidal anti-inflammatory drugs (NSAIDs) and the presence of asymptomatic colorectal adenomas. The estimated relative risk was 0.49 (95% confidence interval 0.3–0.8). These findings support the hypothesis that aspirin and NSAIDs may protect against the development of colorectral neoplasia (Logan et al 1993). Other studies investigating the cell kinetics of patients with adenomatous polyps have indicated that prolonged supplementation with vitamin C may also reduce the incidence of adenomatous polyps and further studies on this are indicated (Cahill et al 1993). Finally, an interesting association has been recognized between the increased risk of colorectal cancer and congenital anomalies of the urinary tract. A family history of congenital anomalies of the urinary tract may be a useful marker in screening (Atwell et al 1993).

There have been interesting developments in surgical technique for colorectal cancer. Chief amongst these has been the increasing interest in laparoscopic surgery. Two reviews have indicated that the evidence supporting this form of surgery is weak at present and that the technique should really be regarded as experimental when used for malignant conditions (O'Rourke & Heald 1993, Taylor 1993). The operation is technically feasible and may be associated with an increased return to mobility. However, postoperative stay and complications are not significantly reduced and the long-term effects and prognosis are still to be assessed. Tate et al (1993b) have reported a prospective comparison of laparoscopically assisted and conventional anterior resection. Postoperative analgesic requirement was less and there was a suggestion of reduced length of hospital stay although this did not reach statistical significance. Histopathological examination of the resection specimens showed similar lymph node harvest for the two procedures.

However, the possibility of local recurrence due to spillage of malignant cells is still a source of concern. Studies of the presence of malignant cells in the mesenteric blood and peritoneal cavity following this procedure should be performed. Leather et al (1993) have demonstrated immuno-cytochemical techniques for the detection and enumeration of circulating tumour cells.

It is possible that laparoscopically assisted reversal of Hartmann's procedure will prove valuable (Gorey et al 1993). Phillips et al (1993) have described 51 colonic resection procedures in which 14% were converted. A whole range of pathological conditions were included. Operative time averaged 2.3 h with a mean of 4.6 days' hospitalization. Few other groups have achieved such satisfactory results.

There have been other technical innovations. Total mesorectal excision for rectal carcinoma now appears to be the standard procedure with very low local recurrence rates. MacFarlane et al (1993) report an actuarial local recurrence rate of 4% after curative anterior resection at 5 years, with an overall recurrence rate of 18%. These data are exceptional and should be regarded as the 'gold standard'. Other studies have suggested that more conservative treatment, such as radical local excision for rectal carcinoma, should be considered. Lock et al (1993) regard this as suitable for low-grade tumours but not for average-grade tumours. Rouanet et al (1993) combined local excision with radiotherapy and have achieved good control in selected patients. They advocate small minimally infiltrating and well-differentiated adenocarcinomas for this treatment. Endoscopic transanal resection is also becoming popular in selected patients with adenomas or indeed those with locally advanced malignancy requiring palliation. It is regarded as both quick and safe with a low complication rate (Wetherall et al 1993).

A large series from Japan has reported a 5-year survival of 79.8% with an operative mortality of approximately 1.5% for low anterior resection (Konn et al 1993). Other technical aspects of note are that the double-stapled anastomosis for low anterior resection is now accepted as a safe technique with an acceptable local recurrence rate (Redmond et al 1993). Following total rectal excision a coloanal anastomosis can be performed and a colonic reservoir may improve function (Leo et al 1993).

Finally, Sagar et al (1993) in a prospective randomized trial have suggested that suction drainage following colorectal resection is probably unnecessary. Palliation of advanced colorectal carcinoma using endoscopic laser treatment is becoming increasingly popular and the results are satisfactory, particularly when combined with radiotherapy (Mesko et al 1993, Sargeant et al 1993).

The role of preoperative radiotherapy in patients with resectable rectal carcinoma is still controversial. A Swedish trial on 1168 patients (Swedish Rectal Cancer Trial 1993) has suggested that this form of treatment can be given in high doses without major acute effects. No difference in the incidence of complications or anastomotic dehiscence was reported. It is likely that endorectal ultrasonography will be used increasingly as a technique for evaluating patients both before and after radiotherapy treatment.

Inflammatory disease

Restorative proctocolectomy is becoming increasingly popular in the management of ulcerative colitis and the results are improving with experience. However, there are problems associated with bowel function and aspects of quality of life (Carty et al 1993).

Acute pouchitis is a common complication and resembles acute ulcerative colitis. The cause of this is not entirely clear but one study has indicated that, unlike ulcerative colitis, it is not associated with the carriage of adhesive *Escherichia coli* (Lobo et al 1993).

In Crohn's disease, perianal fistulae are an extremely difficult problem to deal with. A recent classification by Hughes has been utilized by a number of groups to predict the outcome of anal perineal fistulae (Francois et al 1993). Patients presenting with a specific fistula fared much worse than those with non-specific fistulae. They required repeated surgery and frequently suffered from impaired continence. The role of elemental diet in Crohn's disease has been investigated extensively. It is thought to be effective in producing remission but most patients relapse soon after resumption of a normal diet. One trial has investigated the efficiency of dietary modification and oral corticosteroids in maintaining remission achieved with elemental diet. This involved a multicentre trial of 136 patients with active Crohn's disease. Clinical improvement occurred in the diet group and this was associated with significant changes in plasma albumin and erythrocyte sedimentation rate. Undoubtedly diet provides an additional therapeutic strategy in active Crohn's disease (O'Riordan et al 1993).

Although ischaemic colitis is a rare condition, it provides major problems for both surgeons and physicians. The majority of patients with ischaemic colitis respond favourably to conservative treatment such as bed rest and antibiotics. However, a number of patients require early surgical intervention often without the benefit of preoperative diagnosis. In these patients treatment involves resection of all ischaemic colon (Robert et al 1993).

Because of a number of similar epidemiological characteristics between colon cancer and diverticulosis it has been hypothesized that patients with diverticular disease are at increased risk of developing colon cancer. However, this does not appear to be the case and in one cohort study no cause or relationship was found between diverticular disease and cancer of the left colon (Stefansson et al 1993). In recent years there has been an increasing emphasis on radiological investigations in acute diverticulitis not only in diagnosis (ultrasonography and CT) but also in following the progression or resolution of suppuration and in particular in guiding percutaneous aspiration where appropriate. A recent review has demonstrated the value of both ultrasonography and CT in this regard (McKee et al 1993).

BREAST CANCER

Screening

National breast cancer screening in the UK is now well established and the results from 1991–1992 have been published (Chamberlain et al 1993). The overall acceptance rate was 71.3% and the breast cancer detection rate was 6.2 cancers per 1000 women screened; 95% of programmes achieved a recall rate of less than 10%. These results can be regarded as extremely satisfactory.

An overview of the Swedish screening trials has shown no evidence of detrimental effects in terms of breast cancer mortality. The largest reduction in breast cancer mortality was observed amongst women aged 50–69 years (29%). Amongst women aged 40–49 years there was no significant reduction in mortality. This and other evidence suggests that no benefit has been demonstrated for screening women under the age of 50 years and there are indeed potentially harmful effects (Jatoi & Baum 1993).

With increasing experience new techniques for removal of mammographically detected breast lesions are being reported. The importance of specimen-oriented radiography (Dixon et al 1993) and careful histopathological examination of excision margins is being increasingly emphasized (Mueller et al 1993, Holme et al 1993). Undoubtedly screening detects tumours at an earlier biological stage. Crisp et al (1993) have reported results from one centre which confirm that a higher proportion of tumours with a more favourable histological grade and type are recognized with expected survival advantage.

Treatment

The management of early breast cancer is still highly controversial (Rubens 1993). The most effective method of dealing with the axilla is a constant source of discussion. Optimal treatment should combine accurate determination of node status and avoidance of unnecessary morbidity. Ranaboldo et al (1993) have reported that 31% of women with screen-detected cancer have lymph node involvement. Of these 33% have an 'impalpable' tumour. Similar data have been obtained by Walls et al (1993). Of 180 screen-detected cancers which were invasive, 40 had associated lymph node metastases. However, patients with tumours less than 1 cm in diameter or those with grade 1 tumours of less than 3 cm in diameter could probably be spared axillary surgery with an expected reduction in morbidity and operating time. There is no doubt that with lymph node immunohistochemistry the incidence of involvement in apparently node-negative breast cancers is increased. In one study patients with occult metastases diagnosed in this way had a shorter time to disease recurrence but not death (Hainsworth et al 1993).

In early breast cancer the most effective surgical procedure is still controversial with recent emphasis on conservation therapy. Staunton et al (1993), however, have reviewed a prospective study of 193 patients treated by

Patey mastectomy. The results are remarkably good with a 10-year survival of 79% for stage I and 64% for stage II. This treatment should still be considered for patients with T1 and T2 tumours who prefer mastectomy to breast conservation. For patients with ductal carcinoma in situ, wide excision is generally regarded as the treatment of choice. In a recent randomized prospective trial of 818 women with ductal carcinoma in situ treated by wide excision with or without radiotherapy, the 5-year event-free survival was 84.4% versus 73.8%. The improvement was due to a reduction in the occurrence of a second ipsilateral breast cancer (Fisher et al 1993). Similar data advocating conservative surgery with radiotherapy in patients with small breast cancers (less than 2.5 cm diameter) have demonstrated a significantly reduced local recurrence rate with radiotherapy (0.3% versus 8.8%). Radiotherapy appears to have an important role in reducing the risk of local recurrence both in ductal carcinoma in situ and in small early breast cancers (Veronesi et al 1993).

Adjuvant therapy is now regarded as an important modality for early breast cancer. However, the exact place of oophorectomy in premenopausal women is still subject to debate. The Scottish Cancer Trials Breast Group (1993) have published the results of ovarian ablation versus CMF (cyclophosphamide–methotrexate–5-fluorouracil) chemotherapy in premenopausal women with stage II breast carcinoma. After a maximum follow-up of 12 years patient outcome analysed in terms of oestrogen receptor (ER) concentration showed that patients with high ER concentrations had a better response to oophorectomy than patients with a low ER concentration within the primary tumour.

The role of primary tamoxifen therapy in older women with breast cancer has generated much interest. It may well be that those women with ER-positive tumours, as detected by immunocytochemical methods, respond better than those without a high ER content (Low et al 1992). This was also suggested in a study by Gaskell et al (1993) in which the survival of patients with and without ER activity was statistically significant.

Two other important management aspects require comment. Subcutaneous mastectomy and axillary dissection combined with immediate reconstruction have been advocated in many reports. Local recurrence rates do not appear to be excessive and local control is achieved. Prophylactic radiotherapy can be avoided in the majority of patients (Palmer et al 1992, Patel et al 1993b).

It is still unclear as to whether the timing of surgery for breast cancer in relation to the menstrual cycle is associated with survival differences. Studies appear to be split and the most recent one (Nathan et al 1993) suggests no adverse relationship.

Finally, a number of papers have identified more prognostic markers for breast cancer. These correlations include: p53 mutations and histopathological changes (Dunn et al 1993); expression of proliferating cell nuclear antigen association with a poor histological grade and increased cell proliferation rate (Betta et al 1993); c-erb B-2 proto-oncogene expression and nuclear DNA content in node-positive patients (Schimmelpenning et al 1992); plasma prolactin level and poor prognosis in patients with advanced disease (Bhatavdekar et al 1993). In addition there is increasing evidence that genetic risk prediction by genetic linkage analysis may enable high-risk screening clinic resources to be concentrated on women who are most likely to benefit (Porter et al 1993).

REFERENCES

Anderson ID, Manson JM, Martin DF et al 1993 Relief of metastatic biliary obstruction by stent placement: is it worthwhile? Surg Oncol 2: 113–117

Armstrong D, Arnold R, Classen M et al and the RUDER Study Group 1993 Prospective multicentre study of risk factors associated with delayed healing of recurrent duodenal ulcers (RUDER). Gut 34: 1319–1326

Atkin WS, Cuzick J, Northover JMA et al 1993 Prevention of colorectal cancer by once-only sigmoidoscopy. Lancet 341: 736–740

Attwood SEA, Ball CS, Barlow AP et al 1993 Role of intragastric and intraoesophageal alkalinisation in the genesis of complications in barret's columnar lined lower oesophagus. Gut 34: 11–15

Atwell JD, Taylor I, Cruddas M 1993 Increased risk of colorectal cancer associated with congenital anomalies of the urinary tract. Br J Surg 80: 785–787

Baer HU, Dennison SR, Mouton W et al 1993a Enucleation of giant hemangiomas of the liver. Ann Surg 216: 673–676

Baer HU, Stain SC, Dennison AR et al 1993b Improvements in survival by aggressive resections of hilar cholangiocarcinoma.

Bakkevold KE, Kambestad B 1993 Morbidity and mortality after radical and palliative pancreative cancer surgery. Ann Surg 217: 356–368

Barlow AP, Thompson MH 1993 Colonoscopic follow-up after resection for colorectal cancer: a selective policy. Br J Surg 80: 781–784

Barr LC, Skene AI, Meiron Thomas J 1992 Metastasectomy. Br J Surg 79: 1268–1274

Betta PG, Bottero G, Pavesi M et al 1993 Cell proliferation in breast carcinoma assessed by a PCNA grading system and its relation to other prognostic variables. Surg Oncol 2: 59–63

Bhatavdekar JM, Patel DD, Sherbet GV 1993 Prognostic significance of plasma prolactin in breast cancer: comparison with the expression of c erb B-2 oncoprotein. Eur J Surg Oncol 19: 409–413

Brito MJ, Filipe MI, Williams GT et al 1993 DNA ploidy in early gastric carcinoma: a flow cytometric study of 100 european cases. Gut 34: 230–234

Byrne DS, Bell G, Morrice JJ et al 1992 Technique for laparoscopic appendicetomy. Br J Surg 79: 574–575

Caffarey SM, Broughton CIM, Marks CG 1993 Faecal occult blood screening for colorectal neoplasia in a targeted high-risk population. Br J Surg 80: 1399–1400

Cahil RJ, O'Sullivan KR, Mathias PM et al 1993 Effects of vitamin antioxidant supplementation on cell kinetics of patients with adenomatous polyps. Gut 34: 963–967

Carty NJ, Corder A, Johnson CD 1993 Restorative proctocolectomy is a major advance in the management of ulcerative colitis. Ann R Coll Surg Engl 75: 275–280

Chamberlain J, Moss SM, Kirkpatrick AE et al 1993. National Health Service breast screening programme results for 1991–92. Br Med J 307: 353–356

Chundrigar T, Hedges AR, Morris R et al 1993 Intraperitoneal bupivacaine for effective pain relief after laparoscopic cholecystectomy. Ann R Coll Surg Engl 75: 437–439

Clavien P et al 1993 Recent results of elective open cholecystectomy in a North American and a European Centre. Ann Surg 216: 618–626

Crisp WJ, Higgs MJ, Cowan WK et al 1993 Screening for breast cancer detects tumours at an earlier biological stage. Br J Surg 80: 863–865

Dixon JM, Ravid Sekar O, Walsh J et al 1993 Specimen-orientated radiography helps define excision margins of malignant lesions detected by breast screening. Br J Surg 80: 1001–1002

Dunn JM, Hastrich DJ, Newcomb P et al 1993 Correlation between p53 mutations and antibody staining in breast carcinoma. Br J Surg 80: 1410–1412

Edwards JD 1993 Management of septic shock. Br Med J 306: 1661–1664

Fan ST, Lai ECS, Mock FPT et al 1993 Early treatment of acute biliary pancreatitis by endoscopic papillotomy. N Engl J Med 328: 228–232

Fisher B, Costantino J, Redmond C et al 1993 Lumpectomy compared with lumpectomy and radioation therapy for the treatment of intraductal breast cancer. N Engl J Med 328: 1581–1586

Francois Y, Vignal J, Descos L 1993 Outcome of perianal fistulae in Crohn's disease – value of Hughes' pathogenic classification. Int J Colorectal Dis 8: 39–41

Gaffarey SM, Broughton CIM, Marks CG 1993 Faecal occult blood screening for colorectal neoplasia in a targeted high-risk population. Br J Surg 80: 1399–1400

Gaskell DJ, Hawkins RA, de Carteret S et al 1993 Indications for primary tamoxifen therapy in elderly women with breast cancer. Br J Surg 79: 1317–1320

Gimson AES, Ramage JK, Panos MZ et al 1993 Randomised trial of variceal banding ligation versus injection sclerotherapy for bleeding oesophageal varices. Lancet 342: 391–394

Gouillant C, Ducerf C, Partensky et al 1993 Repeated hepatic resections for colorectal metastasess. Eur J Surg Oncol 19: 443–447

Goodman D, Irvin TT 1993 Delay in the diagnosis and prognosis of carcinoma of the right colon. Br J Surg 80: 1327–1329

Gordon NLM, Dawson AA, Bennett B et al 1993 Outcome in colorectal adenocarcinoma: two seven-year studies of a population. Br Med J 307: 707–710

Gorey TF, O'Connell, Waldron D 1993 Laparoscopically assisted reversal of Hartmann's procedure. Br J Surg 80: 109

Grace PA, Williamson RCN 1993 Moderan management of pancreatic pseudocysts. Br J Surg 80: 573–581

Griffin SM, Robertson CS 1993 Non-surgical treatment of cancer of the oesophagus. Br J Surg 80: 412–413

Guadagni S, Reed PI, Johnston BJ et al 1993 Early gastric cancer: follow-up after gastrectomy in 159 patients. Br J Surg 80: 325–328

Guillou PJ 1993 Biological variation in the development of sepsis after surgery or trauma. Lancet 342: 217–220

Habib NA, Kok MK, Zografos G et al 1993 Elective hepatic resection for benign and malignant liver disease: early results. Br J Surg 80: 1039–1041

Hainsworth PJ, Tjandra JJ, Stillwell RG 1993 Detection and significance of occult metastases in node-negative breast cancer. Br J Surg 80: 459–463

Hall C, Griffin J, Dykes PW et al 1993 Haemoccult does not reduce the need for colonoscopy in surveillance after curative resection for colorectal cancer. Gut 34: 227–229

Haugstvedt TK, Viste A, Eide G 1993 Norwegian multicentre study of survival and prognostic factors in patients undergoing curative resection for gastric carcinoma. Br J Surg 80: 475–478

Heaton ND, Howard ER 1993 Complications and limitations of injection sclerotherapy in portal hypertension. Gut 34: 7–10

Holme TC, Reis MM, Thompson A et al 1993 Is mammographic microcalcification of biological significance? Eur J Surg Oncol 19: 250–253

Idezuke Y and the Japanese Research Society for Portal Hypertension and Japanese Research Society for Sclerotherapy of Esophageal Varices, 1992 Present status of sclerotherapy and surgical treatment of oesophageal varices in Japan. World J Surg 16: 1193–1201

Jatoi I, Baum M 1993 American and European recommendations for screening mammography in younger women: a cultural divide? Br Med J 307: 1481–1483

Jeng K, Yang F, Chiang H et al 1992 Repeat operation for nodular recurrent hepatocellular carcinoma within the cirrhotic liver remnant: a comparison with transcatheter arterial chemoembolization. World J Surg 16: 1188–1192

John TG, Greig JD, Johnstone AJ et al 1992 Liver trauma: a 10-year experience. Br J Surg 79: 1352–1356

Johnson CD 1993 Timing of intervention in acute pancreatitis. Postgrad Med J 69: 509–515

Karatsis P, Wyman A, Sweetland HM et al 1993 Inflammatory pseudotumour of the liver. Eur J Surg Oncol 20: 384–387

Keane FBV, Tanner WA, Gillen P 1993 Operative cholangiography and laparoscopic bile duct exploration. Br J Surg 80: 957–958

Kingston RD, Walsh SH, Jeacock J 1993 Physical status is the principal determinant of outcome after emergency admission of patients with colorectal cancer. Ann R Coll Surg 75: 335–338

Konn M, Morita T, Engl Hada R et al 1993 Survival and recurrence after low anterior resection and abdominoperineal resection for rectal cancer: the results of a long term study with a review of the literature. Jpn J Surg 23: 21–30

Labenz J, Gyenes E, Ruhl GH et al 1993 Amoxicillin plus omeprazole versus triple therapy for eradication of *Helicobacter pylori* in duodenal ulcer disease: a prospective, randomized and controlled study. Gut 34: 1167–1170

Leather AJM, Gallegos NC, Kocjan et al 1993 Detection and enumeration of circulating tumour cells in colorectal cancer. Br J Surg 80: 777–780

Leen E, Goldberg JA, Robertson J et al 1993 Early detection of occult colorectal hepatic metastases using duplex colour Doppler sonography. Br J Surg 80: 1249–1251

Leo E, Belli F, Baldini MT et al 1993 Total rectal resection, colo-endoanal anastomosis and colic reservoir for cancer of the lower third of the rectum. Eur J Surg Oncol 19: 283–293

Lobo AJ, Sagar PM, Rothwell J et al 1993 Carriage of adhesive *Escherichia coli* after restorative proctocolectomy and pouch anal anastomosis: relation with functional outcome and inflammation. Gut 34: 1379–1383

Lock MR, Ritchie JK, Hawley PR 1993 Reappraisal of radical local excision for carcinoma of the rectum. Br J Surg 80: 928–929

Logan RFA, Little J, Hawtin PG et al 1993 Effect of aspirin and non-steroidal anti-inflammatory drugs on colorectal adenomas: case-control study of subjects participating in the Nottingham faecal occult blood screening programme. Br Med J 307: 285–289

Low SC, Dixon AR, Bell J et al 1992 Tumour oestrogen receptor content allows selection of elderly patients with breast cancer for conservative tamoxifen treatment. Br J Surg 79: 1314–1316

Lucarotti ME, Virjee J, Alderson D 1993 Patient selection and timing of dynamic computed tomography in acute pancreatitis. Br J Surg 80: 1393–1395

Luostarinen M 1993 Nissen fundoplication for reflux oesophagitis. Ann Surg 217: 329–337

McAnena OJ, Austin O, O'Connel PR et al 1992 Laparoscopic versus open appendicectomy: a propsective evaluation. Br J Surg 79: 818–820

MacFarlane JK, Ryall RDH, Heald RJ, 1993 Mesorectal excision for rectal cancer. Lancet 341: 457–460

Macintyre IM, Wilson RG 1993 Laparoscopic cholecystectomy. Br J Surg 80: 552–559

McKay CJ, Imrie CW, Baxter JN 1993 Somatostatin and somatostatin analgoues – are they indicated in the management of acute pancreatitis: Gut 34: 1622–1626

McKee RF, Deignan RW, Krukowski ZH 1993 Radiological investigation in acute diverticulitis. Br J Surg 80: 560–565

McLean AD, Stonebridge PA, Bradbury AW et al 1993 Time of presentation, time of operation and unnecessary appendicectomy. Br Med J 306: 307

McMahon AJ, Baxter JN, Kenny G, et al 1993a Ventilatory and blood gas changes during laparoscopic and open cholecystectomy. Br J Surg 80: 1252–1254

McMahon AJ, O'Dwyer PJ, Cruikshank AM et al 1993b Comparison of metabolic responses to laparoscopic and minlaparotomy cholecystectomy. Br J Surg 80: 1255–1258

McMaster P, Mirza D, Harrison JD 1993 Surgical options for primary hepatocellular carcinoma. Br J Surg 80: 1365–1367

MacMathuna P, White P, Clark E et al 1993 Endoscopic sphicteroplasty — a novel and safe alternative to papillotomy in the management of bile duct stones. Gut 35: 127–129

Makela J, Tikkakoski T, Leionen A et al 1993 Superselective intra-arterial chemotherapy with mitomycin C in hepatic neoplasms. Eur J Surg Oncol 19: 348–354

Martin IG, Curley P, McMahon MJ 1993 Minimally invasive treatment for common bile duct stones. Br J Surg 80: 103–106

Mayer B, Jauch KW, Gunthert U et al 1993 De-novo expression of CD44 and survival in gastric cancer. Lancet 342: 1019–1022

Meagher AP, Moller C, Hoffmann DC 1993 Non-operative treatment of small bowel obstruction following appendicectomy or operation on the ovary or tube. Br J Surg 80: 1310–1311

Menzies D 1993 Post-operative adhesions: their treatment and relevance in clinical practice. Ann R Coll Surg Engl 75: 147–153

Mesko TW, Petrelli NJ, Rodriguiez-Bigas M et al 1993 Endoscopic laser treatment for palliation of colorectal adenocarcinoma. Surg Oncol 2: 25–30

Moreaux J, Bougaran J 1993 Early gastric cancer. Ann Surg 217: 347–355

Morris DL, Horton MDA'C, Dilley AV et al 1993 Treatment of hepatic metastases by cryotherapy and regional cytotoxic perfusion. Gut 34: 1156–1157

Moss SF, Calman J 1993 Acid, ulcers and *H. pylori*. Lancet 342: 384–385

Mueller X, Amery A, Lallemand RC 1993 Biopsy of mammographically-detected breast lesions in a district hospital. Eur J Surg Oncol 19: 415–419

Mulcahey HE, O'Donoghue DP 1993 Molecular biology. Setting the stage in colorectal cancer? Gut 34: 1476–1477

Nagasue N, Chang Y, Takemoto Y 1993a Liver resection in the aged (seventy years or older) with hepatocellular carcinoma. Surgery 113: 148–154

Nagasue N, Kohno H, Chang Y et al 1993b Liver resection for hepatocellular carcinoma. Ann Surg 217: 375–384

Nathan B, Bates T, Anbazhagen R et al 1993 Timing of surgery for breast cancer in relation to the menstrual cycle and survival of premenopausal women. Br J Surg 80: 43

Neoptolemos JP 1993 Endoscopic sphincterotomy in acute gallstone pancreatitis. Br J Surg 80: 547–549

Nygaard K, Hagen S, Nansen HS et al 1993 Pre-operative radiotherapy prolongs survival in operable oesophageal carcinoma: a randomized multi-centre study of pre-operative radiotherapy and chemotherapy. The Second Scandinavian Trial in Esophageal Cancer. World J Surg 16: 1104–1110

Nystrom L, Rutqvist LE, Wall S et al 1993 Breast cancer screening with mammography: overview of Swedish randomised trials. Lancet 341: 973–978

Riordan AM, Hunder JO, Cowan RE et al 1993 Treatment of active Crohn's disease by exclusion diet: East Anglian Multicentre Controlled Trial. Lancet 342: 1131–1134

O'Rourke NA, Heald RJ 1993 Laparoscopic surgery for colorectal cancer. Br J Surg 80: 1229–1230

Paganini-Hill A 1993 Aspirin and colorectal cancer. Br Med J 307: 278–279

Palmer BV, Mannur KR, Ross WB 1992 Subcutaneous mastectomy with immediate reconstruction as treatment for early breast cancer. Br J Surg 79: 1309–1311

Patchett SE, Mulcahy HE, O'Donoghue DP 1993 Colonoscopic surveillance after curative resection for colorectal cancer. Br J Surg 80: 1330–1332

Patel RT, Webster DJT, Mansel RE et al 1993a Is immediate postmastectomy reconstruction safe in the long-term? Eur J Surg Oncol 19: 372–375

Patel S, Rew DA, Taylor I et al 1993b Study of the proliferation in human gastric mucosa after in vivo bromodeoxyuridine labelling. Gut 34: 893–896

Patterson-Brown S 1993 Emergency laparoscopic surgery. Br J Surg 80: 279–263

Penna C, Phillips RKS, Tiret E et al 1993 Surgical polypectomy of duodenal adenomas in familial adenomatous polyposi: experience of two European centres. Br J Surg 80: 1027–1029

Phillips EH, Franklin M, Carroll BJ 1993 Laparoscopic colectomy. Ann Surg 216: 703–707

Porter DE, Steel CM, Cohen BB et al 1993 Genetic linkage analysis applied to unaffected women from families with breast cancer can discriminate high from low risk individuals. Br J Surg 80: 1381–1385

Purkiss SF, Williams NS 1993 Growth rate and percentage hepatic replacement of colorectal liver metastases. Br J Surg 80: 1036–1038

Qureshi MA, Brindley NM, Osborne DH et al 1993 Post-cholecystectomy symptoms after laparoscopic cholecystectomy. Ann R Coll Surg Engl 75: 349–353

Ranaboldo CJ, Mitchell A, Royle GT et al 1993 Axillary nodal status in women with screen-detected breast cancer. Eur J Surg Oncol 19: 130–133

Redmond HP, Austin OMB, Clery AP et al 1993 Safety of double-stapled anastomosis in low anterior resection. Br J Surg 80: 924–927

Riordan AM, Hunter JO, Cowan RE et al 1993 Treatment of active Crohn's disease by exclusion diet: East Anglian Multicentre Controlled Trial. Lancet 342: 1131–1134

Robert JH, Mentha G, Rohner A 1993 Ischaemic colitis: two distinct patterns of severity. Gut 34: 4–6

Roggo A, Wood WC, Ottinger LW 1993 Carcinoid tumours of the appendix. Ann Surg 217: 385–390

Rouanet P, Saint Auber B, Fabre JM et al 1993 Conservative treatment for low rectal carcinoma by local excision with or without radiotherapy. Br J Surg 80: 1452–1456

Rubens RD 1993 Management of early breast cancer. Br Med J 304: 1361–1364

Russell RCG 1993 General surgery: biliary surgery. Br Med J 307: 1266–1269

Rutgeerts P, Gevers AM, Hiele M et al 1993 Endoscopic injection therapy to prevent rebleeding from peptic ulcers with a protruding vessel: a controlled comparative trial. Gut 34: 348–350

Sagar PM, Couse N, Kerin M et al 1993 Randomized trial of drainage of colorectal anastomosis. Br J Surg 80: 769–771

Sargeant IR, Tobias JS, Blackman G et al 1993 Radiation enhancement of laser palliation for advanced rectal and rectosigmoid cancer: a pilot study. Gut 34: 958–962

Scheele J 1993 Hepatectomy for liver metastases. Br J Surg 80: 274–276

Schimmelpenning H, Eriksson ET, Falkmer UG et al 1992 Prognostic significance of immunohistochemical C-erbB-2 proto-oncogene expression and nuclear DNA content in human breast cancer. Eur J Surg Oncol 18: 530–537

Schweizer W, Tanner S, Baer HU et al 1993 Management of traumatic liver injuries. Br J Surg 80: 86–88

Scott N, Quirke P 1993 Molecular biology of colorectal neoplasia. Gut 34: 289–292

Scott HI, Rosin RD 1993 The influence of diagnostic and therapeutic laparoscopy on patients presenting with an acute abdomen. J R Soc Med 86: 699–701

Scott N, Bell SM, Sagar P et al 1993 p53 expression and K-ras mutation in colorectal adenomas. Gut 34: 621–624

Scottish Cancer Trials Breast Group and ICRF Breast Unit, Guy's Hospital 1993 Adjuvant ovarian ablation versus CMF chemotherapy in premenopausal women with pathological stage II breast carcinoma: the Scottish trial. Lancet 341: 1293–1298

Sharma AK, Cherry R, Fielding JWL 1993 A randomised trial of selective or routine on-table cholangiography. Ann R Col Surg Eng 75: 245–248

Soper NJ, Dunnegan DL 1993 Routine versus selective intro-operative cholangiography during laparoscopic cholecystectomy. World J Surg 16: 1133–1140

Staunton MD, Melville DM, Monterrosa A et al 1993 A 25 year prospective study of modified radical mastectomy (Patey) in 193 patients. J R Soc Med 86: 381–384

Stefansson T, Ekbom A, Sparen P et al 1993 Increased risk of left sided colon cancer in patients with diverticular disease. Gut 34: 499–502

Stephenson BM, Callander C, Sage M et al 1993 Feasibility of 'day case' laparoscopic cholecystectomy. Ann R Coll Surg Engl 75: 249–251

Sue-Ling HM, Johnston D, Martin IG et al 1993 Gastric cancer: a curable disease in Britain. Br Med J 307: 591–596

Sugihara K, Hojo K, Moriya Y 1993 Pattern of recurrence after hepatic resection for colorectal metastases. Br J Surg 80: 1032–1035

Sung JJY, Chung SCS, Lai CW et al 1993 Ocreotide infusion or emergency sclerotherapy for variceal haemorrhage. Lancet 342: 637–641

Surana R, Quinn F, Puri P 1993 Is it necessary to perform appendicectomy in the middle of the night in children? Br Med J 306: 1168

Swedish Rectal Cancer Trial 1993 Initial report from a Swedish multicentre study examining the role of preoperative irradiation in the treatment of patients with resectable rectal carcinoma. Br J Surg 80: 1333–1336

Tate JJT, Dawson JW, Chung SCS et al 1993a Laparoscopic versus open appendicectomy: prospective randomised trial. Lancet 342: 633–637

Tate JJT, Kwok S, Dawson JW et al 1993b. Prospective comparison of laparoscopic and conventional anterior resection. Br J Surg 80: 1396–1398

Taylor I 1993 Keyhole colon surgery. Cancer Topics 9: 37–38

Taylor OM, Benson EA, McMahon MJ and the Yorkshire Gastrointestinal Group 1993 Clinical trial of tamoxifen in patients with irresectable pancreatic adenocarcinoma. Br J Surg 80: 384–386

The Eurogast Study Group 1993 An international association between Helicobacter pylori infection and gastric cancer. Lancet 341: 1359–1362

Thomas HJW 1993 Familial colorectal cancer. Br Med J 307: 277–278

Vallant J-C, Balladur P, Nordlinger B et al 1993 Repeat liver resection of recurrent colorectal metastases. Br J Surg 80: 340–344

Van der Velpen GC, Smith SM, Cuschieri A 1993 Outcome after cholecystectomy for symptomatic gall stone disease and effect of surgical access: laparoscopic v open approach. Gut 34: 1448–1451

Verbanck JJ, Demol JW, Ghillebert GL et al 1993 Ultrasound-guided puncture of the gallbladder for acute cholecystitis. Lancet 341: 1132–1133

Veronesi U, Luini A, Del Vecchio M et al 1993 Radiotherapy after breast-preserving surgery in women with localised cancer of the breast. N Engl J Med 328: 1587–1591

Walls J, Boggis CRM, Wilson M 1993 Treatment of the axilla in patients with screen-detected breast cancer. Br J Surg 80: 436–438

Wetherall AP, Williams NMA, Kelly MJ 1993 Endoscopic transanal resection in the management of patients with sessile rectal adenomas, anastomotic stricture and rectal cancer. Br J Surg 80: 788–793

Witherspoon AC, Doglioni C, Diss TC et al 1993 Regression of primary low-grade B-cell gastric lymphoma of mucosa-associated lymphoid tissue type after eradication of *Helicobacter pylori*. Lancet 342: 575–577

Wright PA, Williams GT 1993 Molecular biology and gastric carcinoma. Gut 34: 145–147

Zielgler K, Sanft T, Zimmer et al 1993 Comparison of computed tomography, endosonography, and intraoperative assessment in TN staging of gastric carcinoma. Gut 34: 604–610

RECENT ADVANCES IN SURGERY

Provisional Contents of Number 19
Edited by: C. D. Johnson, I. Taylor

Index